'This is an important and timely book. Wind power is an essential element of our response to climate change. This book shows that the spread of the technology has been slowed by misinformation, misunderstanding and barefaced lies. Everyone concerned about the need to slow climate change should read this book and use it to counter the dishonest campaign against renewable energy.'

—Emeritus Professor Ian Lowe AO FTSE, president of the Australian Conservation Foundation 2004–14

'The book is a fantastic achievement. Its great strength is in pulling together multiple strands of work on the same issue, providing a robust, in-depth and fascinating account of how "wind turbine syndrome" has come into existence and, hopefully, how it can fade into the background.'

—Dr James Rubin, Psychological Medicine, Kings College London

'Simon Chapman has become a touchstone for everything the extreme right hates: arguments grounded in fact, a passion for a healthier planet, and sometimes just a dose of plain common sense. His writing is erudition and conviction combined. Read on!'

—The Hon. Peter Garrett AM, lead singer of Midnight Oil and former federal minister for the environment

'Are windfarms a threat to human health? Public health expert Simon Chapman and health psychology PhD Fiona Crichton blow away the bad science, rumours and misinformation in an illuminating, fascinating and entertaining look at the makings of a health scare. "Tilting at windmills" is an analogy for the activities of those who passionately believe that windfarms are a threat to human health. This book shows that these fears are not backed by persuasive evidence, and that not all the critics have the grace and dignity of the original windmill-tilter, Don Quixote.'
—Professor Sir Simon Wessely, Regius Professor of Psychiatry, IOPPN, KCL, President Royal Society of Medicine, Past President Royal College of Psychiatrists

‘Our policies on issues such as climate change and health should be based on science, not emotion, distortion and invention. This lively and thorough account of the wind turbines story in Australia should be required reading for all those interested not only in climate change, but also the way public policy can and should be shaped.’

—Professor Fiona Stanley AC FAA FASSA, Australian of the Year 2003

‘Simon Chapman has a finely tuned bullshit detector and a thick hide. He was the first public health expert to see confected windfarm health reports for what they were – a powerful and almost plausible tool for scuttling wind development. With his tireless research, keen eye for “killer facts” and media savvy, nobody has done more than Simon Chapman, globally, to exile the windfarm health scare back to the fringes from which it emerged.’

—Simon Holmes à Court, community renewable energy pioneer and Senior Advisor to the Energy Transition Hub at the University of Melbourne

Wind turbine syndrome

PUBLIC AND SOCIAL POLICY SERIES

Marian Baird and Gaby Ramia, Series Editors

The Public and Social Policy series publishes books that pose challenging questions about policy from national, comparative and international perspectives. The series explores policy design, implementation and evaluation; the politics of policy making; and analyses of particular areas of public and social policy.

Markets, rights and power in Australian social policy
Gabrielle Meagher and Susan Goodwin (eds)

Risking together: how finance is dominating everyday life in Australia
Dick Bryan and Mike Rafferty

Wind turbine syndrome: a communicated disease
Simon Chapman and Fiona Crichton

Wind turbine syndrome

A communicated disease

Simon Chapman and Fiona Crichton

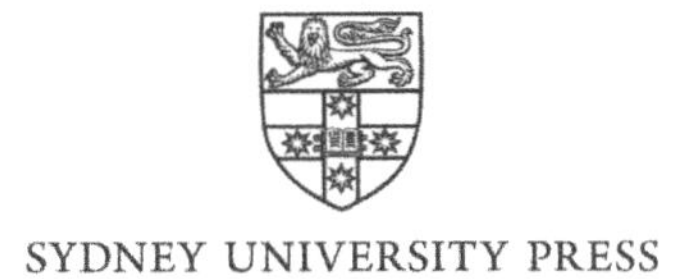

SYDNEY UNIVERSITY PRESS

First published by Sydney University Press

Sydney University Press
Fisher Library F03
University of Sydney NSW 2006
AUSTRALIA
sup.info@sydney.edu.au
sydney.edu.au/sup

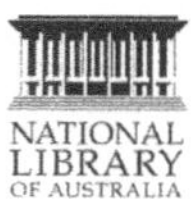

A catalogue record for this book is available from the National Library of Australia

ISBN 9781743324967 paperback
ISBN 9781743324974 ebook

Cover image credit iStock/Eddisonphotos by Getty Images.
Cover design by Miguel Yamin.

Contents

List of figures	ix
Editorial note	xi
Acknowledgements	xiii
Introduction	xv
1 The history and growth of windfarms, and early objections	1
2 The advent of noise and health complaints	33
3 Core problems with health claims about windfarms	67
4 The best evidence opponents have to offer	103
5 The psychogenics of wind turbine complaints	139
6 Opponents of windfarms in Australia	179
7 How the anti-wind lobby reacts when challenged	225
8 Strategies for reducing anxiety and complaints	259
Appendix: 247 symptoms, diseases and aberrant behaviours attributed to wind turbine exposure	279
Works cited	285
Further reading	319
Index	323

List of figures

Figure i.1 The progression of nervousness. xix

Figure 1.1 James Blyth's first electricity generating windmill. 3

Figure 1.2 *Rodney and Otamatea Times* (New Zealand), 14 August 1912. 3

Figure 1.3 The windmill at Westerfield, photographed in 1925. 6

Figure 1.4 Dunlite windmill in Toowoomba, Queensland, Australia. Photograph by John Nielsen. 8

Figure 1.5 Southern Cross windmills in Australia. 9

Figure 1.6 Windfarm projects under construction in Australia, 2017. 10

Figure 1.7 My most retweeted tweet. 14

Figure 1.8 Water-bombing aircraft at Waterloo windfarm in South Australia. 30

Figure 2.1a Google Trend worldwide data 'wind turbine syndrome', 8 March 2017. 40

Figure 2.1b Google Trend Australian data for 'wind turbine syndrome', 8 March 2017. 41

Figure 2.2 Spectrum of sound by frequency (Hz to kHz). 51

Figure 2.3 Hearing thresholds for a young adult. 51

Figure 3.1 The village of Avignonet-Lauragais in the commune of Haute-Garonne in south-western France. 73

Figure 3.2 Wind turbines surrounding suburban Copenhagen, Denmark. 74

Figure 3.3 A micro-turbine in Jubilee Park in the inner Sydney surburb of Glebe, New South Wales. 80

Figure 3.4 David Mortimer as pictured in the *King Island Courier* in April 2013. 87

Figure 4.1 Extract from a Korean fan manual warning people not to sleep with the fan running, for fear of 'fan death'. 134

Figure 5.1 Subject being contemporaneously exposed to infrasound and audible windfarm sound in the Acoustic Research Centre listening room. 159

Figure 5.2 Subject undergoing hearing screening test in the listening room with view into the sound control room. 160

Figure 5.3 Changes from baseline in symptom number, symptom intensity, and mood scores. 164

Figure 6.1 A desultory anti-windfarm rally organised by Stop These Things, Canberra, 18 June 2013. 184

Editorial note

Simon Chapman began writing this book in 2016. After some 65,000 words had been written, he invited Fiona Crichton to join him in writing what remained to be done. Fiona's 2016 PhD thesis, completed at the University of Auckland, explored psychogenic aspects of complaints about windfarm noise, so her involvement in the book was invaluable, particularly in Chapter 5.

Where the first person (I, me, my) is used in the book, it refers to Simon. The rest of the book reflects our combined efforts.

Acknowledgements

The following people have been invaluable to us both in developing our understanding and awareness of the science, psychology and politics of wind energy and in providing support to us in many ways as the book was written: Mike Barnard, David Clarke, Christophe Delaire, Simon Holmes à Court, Marita Hefler, Ketan Joshi, Geoff Leventhall, Chris Ollson, Keith Petrie and James Rubin.

This is Simon's fifth book with Sydney University Press since 2010. Like this book, three of these were published in both paperback and as open-access ebooks. Together these three books have been downloaded some 90,000 times.

Knowing how strong the readership numbers, retweets and Facebook shares have been for our 17 columns for *The Conversation*[1] on windfarm issues (272,313 readers, 2678 tweets and 24,801 Facebook shares), we are hoping this book will eclipse all of those combined, such is the global concern for the importance of renewable energy. We are extremely grateful to Sydney University Press for their wonderful support in allowing the ebook to be freely accessible to all. Agata Mrva-Montoya has edited each of these five books. Her patience, good humour and unfailing eye for detail have been constant. Denise O'Dea's copy editing of this book was way beyond first-class. Every page, and quite nearly every paragraph, was improved by her professionalism. We can't thank them both enough.

1 Unlike many other media outlets, *The Conversation* provides its authors with data on article accesses, updated every 15 minutes.

Introduction

> 'To tilt at windmills' is a venerable English idiom meaning to pursue an unrealistic, impractical, or impossible goal, or to battle imaginary enemies. In current usage, 'tilting at windmills' carries connotations of engaging in a noble but unrealistic (usually wildly unrealistic) effort, an endeavour which may garner the admiration of onlookers but which usually strikes other people as delusional.—*The Word Detective*[1]

The introduction of new technology has a long history of being accompanied by beliefs that take root among small proportions of the population who believe that rapidly proliferating inventions are silently eroding people's health. Railway travel and electric light were early villains to those who saw such developments as Mephistophelian artifice that could bring only harm to communities and society. At the advent of electric light in the late 19th century, the belief was common that the night was divinely ordained to be dark. For some, artificially lighting up the darkness was a profanity that was likely to reap hubris.

Historian Linda Simon in her book *Dark light: electricity and anxiety from the telegraph to the X-ray*, notes that although the discovery of electricity generated excitement and electrical companies worked hard to build the market for electrical power:

1 See http://www.word-detective.com/2009/03/tilting-at-windmills/.

> more than thirty years after Thomas Edison invented the incandescent bulb in 1879 and soon afterwards installed a lighting system in a business section of lower Manhattan, barely 10 per cent of American homes were wired. Even after the First World War that percentage rose only to 20 per cent.[2]

One reason for this was that community concerns about the safety of electricity were widespread. The electrical companies ran advertising as late as 1923 assuring the public that 'electric light is safe'. Simon notes that 'Newspapers frequently reported electrical fires and accidental electrocutions, and magazines offered long lists of cautions for those who dared to install electricity'.[3] Some worried about going blind from reading by electric light. On 10 May 1889, *Science* noted:

> A new disease, called photo-electric opthalmia, is described as due to the continual action of the electric light on the eyes. The patient is awakened in the night by severe pain around the eye, accompanied by an excessive secretion of tears.[4]

On 24 September in the same year, the *British Medical Journal* carried a report that the newly popular telephone could cause 'telephone tinnitus', claiming that victims 'suffered from nervous excitability, with buzzing noises in the ear, giddiness, and neuralgic pains'. The article contextualised the perils of these new contraptions:

> As civilization advances, new diseases are not only discovered, but are actually produced by the novel agencies which are brought to bear on man's body and mind … almost every addition which science makes to the convenience of the majority seems to bring with it some new forms of suffering to the few. Railway travelling has its *amari aliquid* in the shape of slight but possibly not unimportant jolting of the nervous centres; the electric light has already created a special form of opthalmia; and now we have the telephone indicted as a cause of ear troubles, which react on the spirits, and indirectly on general health.

---

2 Simon 2005, 4.
3 Simon 2005, 91.
4 Simon 2005, 367.

> M Gellé has observed, not in women only, but in strong-minded and able-bodied men, symptoms of what we may call 'aural overpressure' caused by the condition of almost constant strain of the auditory apparatus, in which persons who use the telephone much have to spend a considerable portion of each working day. In some cases, also, the ear seemed to be irritated, by the constantly recurring sharp tinkle of the bell, or by the nearness of the sounds conveyed through the tube, into a state of over sensitiveness which made it intolerant of sound, as the eye, when inflamed or irritable, becomes unable to bear the light.[5]

George Miller Beard was a prominent US neurologist who from around 1869 began promoting the diagnosis of 'neurasthenia' in his prolific clinical writings and books. His central thesis was that modern living and the pace of life among the well-to-do was causing a proliferation in a range of progressive symptoms shown in Figure i.1.

In what today reads like the quintessence of sexist ideology permeating clinical guidelines, the recommended treatment for women suffering from neurasthenia was the rest cure. This consisted of: 'Undisturbed seclusion from children, family members, and friends combined with … uplifting literature and light exercise.' Women were thought to be:

> particularly sensitive to the draining effects of strenuous mental effort, the dangers from which the Rest Cure protected them. Those with the worst cases were prescribed complete bed rest for six to eight weeks in dim rooms with only soothing activities, sometimes excluding books or substantive conversations.[6]

Men, being made of sterner stuff, were prescribed 'vigorous, even strenuous exercise in natural areas away from the pernicious influences of modern life.' They were ordered to travel to remote areas, such as the cattle ranches of the American west or the European Alps.

Among the causes of all this nervousness, Beard included several new-fangled inventions: 'wireless telegraphy, science, steam power, newspapers and the education of women; in other words modern civilization.'

---

5 Anon. 1889.

6 Claude Moore Health Sciences Library 2007.

In the years since, power lines, televisions, electric blankets, hair dryers and washing machines, microwave ovens, computer screens, mobile phones and transmission towers, and, most recently, wi-fi, smart electricity meters, LED light bulbs and even solar electricity roofing panels are examples of new technologies where claims of potential calamitous consequences – typically 'cancer', but sometimes problems of biblical plague proportions – have been megaphoned by activist groups opposed to them.[7] Typically, these waves of anxiety arise in a very small proportion of the population, are promoted by electrophobic groups (these days online), attract an initial burst of media coverage and then dissipate as the technology in question proliferates and becomes commonplace and valued, making the alarmist claims harder to sustain when the threatened disease increases fail to materialise.

My family had the first television set in our small street in Bathurst, New South Wales in the early 1960s. CBN Channel 8 began broadcasting from the town of Orange on 17 March 1962. The kids from the street would gather in our living room after school to watch programs like *The Mickey Mouse Club*, but some were anxious that their parents would find out, as they had been told not to watch television because of the danger of 'rays' being emitted.

Today, someone expressing constant anxiety about the dangers of radiation exposure from watching television would be seen as decidedly technophobic, or plain wacky.

When mobile telephones were introduced into Australia in the 1980s, there was considerable popular anxiety about transmission towers causing unspecified disease in those who were exposed. In 1995, Tony Abbott, who would go on to disparage wind energy as Australian prime minister, publicly stoked local anxiety about a mobile base station in the northern beaches area of Sydney, where he was the federal MP for Warringah. A collection of Sydney television news clips from 1995 gives the flavour.[8] I wrote about this in the *Sydney Morning Herald*

---

7 See: powerlines (Safespace n.d.); televisions (EM Watch n.d.a), electric blankets (Mercola 2009), hair dryers, washing machines (Carpenter 2012), microwave ovens (Wayne and Newell n.d.), computer screens (EM Watch n.d.b), mobile phones (EMR Australia 2015) and transmission towers (Chapman and Wutzke 1997), and, most recently, wi-fi (Group 2015), smart electricity meters (EMR Australia n.d.), LED light bulbs (Mercola 2016), and solar electricity roofing panels (Chapman 2015a).

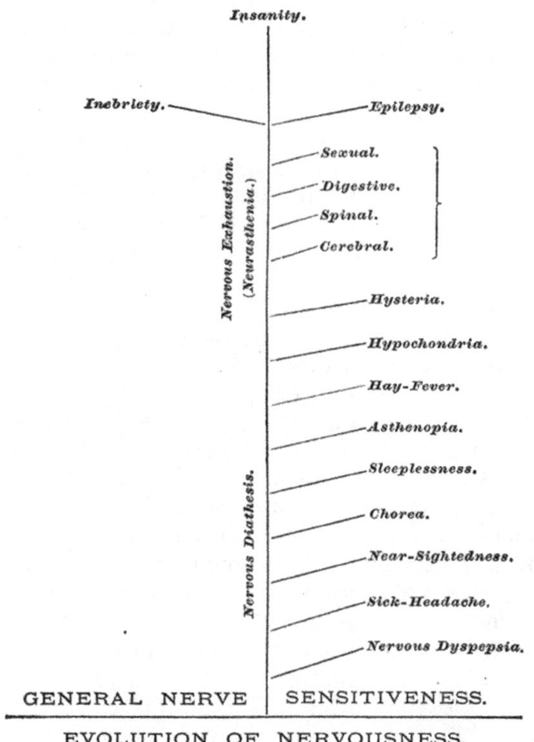

Figure i.1 The progression of nervousness. Source: George M. Beard (1880), *American nervousness: with its causes and consequences* (Claude Moore Health Sciences Library 2007).

in March 1997, noting the utter irrationality of the Lane Cove local council's regulations regarding where transmission towers could be placed in relation to different types of buildings and facilities.

8 Chapman 2014a.

> Local councils in Sydney have struggled to respond to growing resident action about the placement of mobile phone towers across their municipalities. Recently I received a letter from one informing me about decisions regarding minimum distances towers can be located from people.
>
> Note here that it is 'distances' not 'distance'. If you live in the council district, the council will not allow a tower within 300 metres of your house. But if you work in the area, the towers can come as close as specified in any deal struck between your employer or a landowner and a phone company. They can plonk one right outside your office or factory window, in your car park, wherever.
>
> The council wrote that it had taken 'potential health impact' into account in fashioning its resolutions. From this, we can draw one of two conclusions: that the council believes people at work are somehow more robust than people in houses to resisting the alleged health effects of radio frequency radiation (RFR) emitting from the towers; or that it finds this a preposterous idea and instead believes that workers are less uptight about exposure than residents and won't mind a tower or two. What the thousands who work and live in the area are supposed to make of this is anyone's guess.
>
> But wait, there is more. If you are in a school, any sort of child-care facility, a hospital or, most intriguingly, 'any recreational facility', you won't find a tower within 450 metres of you. Observe that yet further layers have now been added to this emerging hierarchical model of radiation susceptibility.
>
> Someone playing golf, bowls or having a picnic apparently cannot resist RFR like a worker can. Along with infants, children, the sick and the elderly, those taking recreation get to enjoy an extra 150 metres buffer zone. Or at least while the kids are at day care or school. When they go home in the afternoon, the council thinks it's OK to locate the towers up to 150 metres closer. Given that children spend more time at home than in school, the two different minimum distances cannot reflect any rational concern to minimum exposure.[9]

This sort of utterly capricious and bizarre approach to distance zoning was repeated years later in policies on the minimum distance that wind turbines could be placed from residences (see Chapter 3).

9 Chapman 1997.

Today, more than 30 years since the introduction of mobile phones into Australia, we still see very occasional instances of concern, as in the case of the distressed woman seen in a 2013 news report wearing a cloth head cover, convinced that it will somehow protect her from the feared radio frequency radiation being emitted from mobile phone transmission towers.[10] Such expressions of anxiety are now extremely uncommon. Near universal use of cell phones and the accompanying widespread rollout of transmission towers, together with no evidence of any rise in the national incidence of brain cancer (the condition most frequently nominated by alarmists as likely to arise from exposure to mobile phones),[11] make the claims sound incredible.

Early close personal encounters

I first saw windfarms while living in Lyon, France in 2006 during a research sabbatical. On various trips I saw occasional clusters of them and thought they looked quite majestic: they seemed emblematic of an exciting future in which the world would start moving to renewable energy. Like many, I saw them as being all about the non-polluting harvesting of an endless, free resource. Here was this century's natural progression of previous centuries' use of wind to sail ships and turn windmills, but to a degree that offered part of the solution to the growing problem of global warming from carbon dioxide and other greenhouse gas emissions: a problem that 97 percent of the world's climate scientists agree is real, increasingly caused by humans, and likely to be catastrophic if not rapidly abated.[12] As has often been remarked, if 97 percent of the world's leading relevant specialist doctors told you that you needed a lifesaving operation and 3 percent said that you need not worry, a decision to trust the 3 percent would almost certainly be 'brave' or utterly unwise. Moving to replace polluting energy sources with renewable energy, including that generated by windfarms, is at the very front line of solutions that offer some hope of averting or reducing the size of that catastrophe. Yet a small but determined number of people are determined to wreck that hope.

---

10 See https://www.youtube.com/watch?v=t5LZMFZF4F4.

11 Chapman, Azizi et al. 2016

12 NASA 2013.

Three Australian Senate inquiries

Political opponents of windfarms in Australia caused there to be three Senate inquiries into windfarms in the five years between 2011 and 2015. There have also been two state government inquiries, in South Australia and New South Wales, both in 2012. The 2015 Senate inquiry saw the main political opponents of windfarms dominate the Senate committee, with just one member, Senator Anne Urquhart, Labor Senator for Tasmania, taking a contrary position.[13]

The majority report that was published is an utter travesty of impartial inquiry. It was the report of a committee set up and populated by four sworn enemies of windfarms, exercising their power within a parliament led by a prime minister (Tony Abbott) who infamously declared that climate change was 'crap' and who in 2015 recalled that the only wind turbine he had ever been close to (on Rottnest Island) was 'ugly and noisy'.[14] 'Local authorities said this was the first complaint they had ever heard,' he observed.[15] Abbott found no difficulty in throwing a juicy bone to four salivating members of the Senate crossbench (John Madigan, Bob Day, David Leyonhjelm and Nick Xenophon) and encouraging them to unleash their contempt for windfarms and give a major stage to a wide range of impassioned, unswerving opponents. Abbott would have hoped that by indulging their fantasies, he would ingratiate himself to them and *quid pro quo* secure their vital votes on government legislation. At various places throughout the book we look at what this oddball committee had to say about the evidence relevant to health issues that it received. The main outcome of the committee's report was the establishment of a National Wind Farm Commissioner charged with investigating complaints about windfarms. In March 2017, the much anticipated first report was released by the commissioner, Andrew Dyer. We will consider this report and its findings in Chapter 6.

When I saw windfarms occasionally in France in 2006 I gave them little thought. It certainly never occurred to me that I was looking at agents that might cause health problems. I was unaware that at that time in Australia, there were already some 22 windfarms operating. I'd never seen any at home nor even read of their existence. In the

13 Commonwealth of Australia 2015e.

14 O'Brien 2010.

15 Cox and Arup 2015.

European autumn of 2008, I holidayed in the Minervois district of Languedoc in southern France and this time I saw many clusters of them. They were unavoidable on any trip in any direction in that part of France. I drove up very near several of these and became fascinated. At that time, I'd still never encountered any suggestion that they might be somehow toxic to those living near them. Villages and farm houses were all around them.

I first encountered this claim in February 2010 when I heard a radio report about some distressed residents living near the newly opened windfarm near the central Victorian hamlet of Waubra, near Ballarat. At the time I was writing regularly for the online news source *Crikey* and its health-focused cousin, *Croakey*.[16]

I decided to write a piece triggered by the news report. I asked whether the health claims being made were:

> calculated displays from a few people seeking to cash in on hopes of land sales or compensation? Do they reflect genuine health effects actually caused by the noise from the wind farm? Or are they equally genuine health effects caused by residents' anxiety about the towers?[17]

In Chapter 7, I describe the reaction caused by this first dip of my toe into the shark-infested waters of windfarm opposition and my subsequent five years of public engagement with this issue.

In May 2014 (just an hour after reading online that the then Australian treasurer, Joe Hockey, had described windfarms as 'utterly offensive'),[18] my wife and I were driving through the Andalusian plains of southern Spain past hundreds of wind turbines quietly turning on ridges, often near towns. Spain is one of many European nations that has taken wind energy very seriously, with 23.1 gigawatts (GW) of installed capacity, the fifth most in any nation. Australia has just 4.237 GW, putting us in 17th position (see Table i.1).

Seeing windfarms and solar energy expanding, I felt hopeful that my children and grandchildren will grow up in a world in which clean energy will complement, then match, and eventually replace polluting

16 Sweet, Chapman et al. 2009.

17 Chapman 2010.

18 Bourke 2014.

Country	Gigawatts installed	Country	Gigawatts installed
1 China	168.732	11 Sweden	6.520
2 USA	82.184	12 Turkey	6.081
3 Germany	50.018	13 Poland	5.782
4 India	26.700	14 Portugal	5.316
5 Spain	23.074	15 Denmark	5.298
6 UK	14.543	16 Netherlands	4.328
7 France	12.066	17 Australia	4.327
8 Canada	11.900	18 Mexico	3.527
9 Brazil	10.740	19 Japan	3.234
10 Italy	9.257	20 Romania	3.026

Table i.1 Top 20 nations by installed wind power capacity (Global Wind Energy Council 2017).

fuels, at prices commensurate with the fact that the fuel it uses is free and boundless. What's not to like?

In 2015, I drove with my wife down to Waubra, to get up close to some of the 128 turbines on Australia's most publicised windfarm. In 2010 Waubra had been chosen by a small group of anti-windfarm activists in naming their Waubra Foundation, an organisation subsequently stripped of its Australian Charities and Not-for-Profits Commission 'health promotion' status in 2014.[19] In 2013, it ignored a petition signed by more than 300 Waubra residents asking the Waubra Foundation to stop running down the town's name for its self-absorbed cause.[20] I wanted to see for myself what the fuss in Waubra was about. For several hours we drove around the local roads, stopping the car a dozen or so times near different turbine clusters. It was a warm, sunny day, with a mild yet obvious wind blowing. All the turbines were turning, powering what one turbine-hosting farmer told us later was enough for 110,000 homes, just from this one windfarm.

19 Conroy 2014.
20 McGrath 2013.

Inside the car with the windows up, we could hear nothing. Outside the car, the overwhelming sound was that of the wind blowing in our ears. Beneath that sound was the barely audible sound of the gently turning blades. To even call it a 'whooshing' sound would be very misleading. That's a word I would use to describe convoys of large trucks driving past you at speed as you stood on the side of a road. It was more like the sound of a slightly amplified whisper in the distance. In Chapter 3, we provide a sample of some of the more colourful turns of phrase that windfarm opponents use to describe this slight sound.

My wife, who had not been near an Australian windfarm before but had often heard me talk about the Waubra objectors, was incredulous. The first time we stopped the car, turned off the motor and stepped outside, she opened with a forceful 'You *must* by joking!', followed by 'This is just *nothing* compared to what hundreds of millions live with every day in the world's cities.'

Indeed. And in fact people like us. I live in Sydney's inner western suburb. Depending on the wind direction, we, along with hundreds of thousands of others living under Sydney's three flight paths, get these planes sometimes as frequently as every two minutes, from the moment the second hand sweeps past 6am until a last boomer takes off at about 10.40pm each night. The planes are often 300 to 400 metres above our roof.

The planes always stop conversation outdoors and sometimes rattle our double-glazed soundproofed windows. On days with low cloud, the noise is very much louder, with echoes of trapped noise flashing back and forth as the planes pass overhead. We've lived under the main flight path for 26 years, raised three children and two grandchildren here, and had countless dinner parties and conversations. The noise that surrounds every city resident is incomparably louder and more constant than that experienced by people living near windfarms. And as we shall see in Chapter 2, city residents are also bathed in infrasound, the sub-audible component of total wind turbine sound that is the focus of much of their opponents' anger and anxiety.

At Waubra we visited a turbine host who had seven or so towers on his sheep farm. We made our way to the nearest turbine, about 500 metres from his house. Hundreds of sheep grazed contentedly in the shade of the tower, many of them having sought it out to rest. My collection of 247 symptoms and diseases said to be caused by windfarms (see Appendix 1) contains several entries about sheep, but apparently no one had told these sheep that they should feel disturbed.

Our host chuckled about the local objectors: 'I think for most of them, being complainers has become part of their identity. They get to see their name in the newspaper. They get to travel around the place telling their story.'

Understanding public health anxieties

Our interest as authors in this issue has been in no small part an extension of a longstanding interest we've both had in the ways in which putative risks to health are understood and communicated within communities and in the news media. Risk-communication researchers have long identified elements of risk perception which are likely to amplify community anxiety and outrage about alleged environmental hazards. In 1997, I co-authored a paper on this as it applied to community concerns about mobile telephone towers.[21] When a hazard is believed to arise from exposure to a natural source or agent, anxiety is low compared to when the source or agent is thought to be industrial or artificial. We rarely hear of communities living in windy locations describing symptoms caused by the sound of wind itself, despite wind having frequencies in the audible and sub-audible ranges (see Chapter 2). But with windfarms the sound is perceived as being somehow artificial in origin, and so of greater concern. Hazards that are imposed on people, as opposed to voluntary exposures, also increase outrage. People who ski voluntarily and enthusiastically expose themselves to a high risk of serious injury without complaint. But there are legions of examples of extremely low-level risks 'imposed' on communities causing mild panics. In Chapter 5, we provide a chart looking at factors known to be relevant to panic and outrage about often low-risk agents, illustrating the case of wind turbines.

Similarly, the 'new' can provoke anxiety. Mobile phone towers went through a phase of alarming some citizens who had for many years blithely walked without a care in the world past suburban electricity substations and TV and radio towers. Today communities are used to the sight of mobile phone transmission base stations and the outrage sometimes seen in the past is now rare.

21 Chapman and Wutzke 1997.

In public health, when the goal is to have people change their behaviour in some way, there are two broad risk communication goals. If people are unaware of or indifferent to a serious risk, the task is to find ways of making them more aware and sufficiently concerned to take action, whether this be to avoid exposure to an agent, to stop or reduce doing something like smoking, eating a poor diet or drinking and driving, or to start or increase a behaviour like immunisation, physical activity or safe sex.

But there are also many issues where people's behaviours reflect sometimes wildly exaggerated concerns about things that in fact pose negligible risk. Such health anxieties can cause large numbers of people to worry needlessly about extremely low-probability risks, seeking medical advice and testing and self-medicating unnecessarily. Some get clinically anxious and consumed by their fears. (Worse, some may misattribute illness to the wrong cause, and thereby deprive themselves of readily available and effective treatments.)

People's lives can be significantly adversely impacted when they become preoccupied by erroneous beliefs. In extreme cases they can develop excessive anxiety or debilitating phobias about extremely low risks such as air travel, household 'germs', 'chemicals', or radio signals. When such personal irrationalities are championed by those in power, like politicians and sections of the news media, it is not just the irrational whose lives can be affected. If those opposed to wind energy were to succeed in greatly inhibiting the rollout of windfarms in Australia and the handful of other nations where windfarm opposition has occurred, the speed with which we can combat climate change could be greatly compromised. Successful opposition to windfarms globally could have extremely serious consequences for life on earth.

Outline of this book

In the first chapter, we sketch the history of the development of wind turbines, from the iconic windmills most readily identified with the Netherlands, to early small-scale prototypes of electricity-generating windmills that began to be designed late in the 19th century, through to today's global explosion in the harvesting of wind as renewable energy and the exciting recent developments in battery storage that are rapidly expanding as we write.

We then review the various objections initially made by those opposed to windfarms. These included concerns about aesthetics, and the economic and local environmental impacts of windfarms, their alleged negative impact on land values, and their supposed propensity to decimate bird and bat populations. It was only later that objectors decided to turbo-charge the idea that living (or even spending short amounts of time) near wind turbines could endanger human health. Non-health concerns are still voiced today, although health issues are probably those most often advanced by objectors in the handful of nations where anti-windfarm groups are active.

The book's central focus is on claims that wind turbines are the *direct* cause of illness in some of those exposed to them, and in Chapter 2 we explore the emergence of this proposition. The notion began to attract minor attention from around 2002, when claims made in unpublished 'research' by a British doctor were covered by a few news outlets and began to be circulated among objectors.[22] The 2009 appearance of a self-published book, *Wind turbine syndrome*, by a US paediatrician, Nina Pierpont, acted like petrol thrown onto a fire of latent anxiety in a small number of communities where activists were doing their utmost to spread concern and to urge people to attribute common health problems to sub-audible sound emitted by the turbines.[23] The book put the alleged health issue on the global map, although as we shall see, concerns about windfarms and health are virtually unknown in most nations which have windfarms today. In Chapter 2 we also look forensically at a sister 'disease' to the non-disease of wind turbine syndrome: vibroacoustic disease (VAD). We show its origins as a concept developed by a heavily self-citing Portuguese research group.[24] On the basis of a case study about a single person presented at a conference, VAD was suddenly also deemed by this research group to be caused by wind turbines. VAD remains largely unrecognised by others. While there are occasionally claims made about the audible sound of wind turbines turning, it is the sub-audible low frequency infrasound emitted (at entirely unspectacular levels) by wind turbines (and importantly for the argument we will develop in this book, also by wind itself) that has been the focus of most of the claims that wind turbines cause humans and animals to become ill.

22 Harry 2007.

23 Pierpont 2009.

24 Chapman and St George 2013.

So in Chapter 2 we critically examine the proposition that infrasound from wind turbines might be noxious while that emanating from a wide range of other natural and mechanical sources is, judging by the lack of claims about them, apparently harmless.

We then examine the seemingly unending number of symptoms and diseases that windfarm opponents have claimed afflict humans and animals exposed to turbines. I have been vigilantly collecting these claims since early in 2012, much to the amusing chagrin of windfarm opponents, who seem confused about whether they believe the many problems on the list are real, or privately understand that the publicity I have generated about the range of problems being advanced is harming their cause, simply because many of the claims are so ludicrous. Take the time to read through the list in Appendix 1 and decide for yourself.

In Chapters 3 and 4, we consider in detail the flaws inherent in claims made by windfarm opponents that exposure to wind turbines is a *direct* cause of health problems. In Chapter 3 we critically examine a series of 'gotcha' arguments repeatedly used by windfarm opponents, such as the claims that only those 'susceptible' suffer and that turbine hosts are contractually gagged to not complain. We consider the peculiar tendency for windfarm complaints to appear mostly in English-speaking nations and how the 'drug' of money seems to be a wonderful antidote against complaining. We finish Chapter 3 with a close examination of claims that in Australia 'over 40' families have had to abandon their homes because of wind turbine noise. My attempts to chase down the evidence behind this factoid saw efforts mounted to try and stop me doing so. We describe those efforts in Chapter 7.

In Chapter 4 we look at studies that have been repeatedly exalted by opponents as allegedly constituting serious evidence that wind turbines cause direct harms to humans and animals. These arguments and papers appear to be the best shots that windfarm opponents have been able to muster. Readers queasy about blood sport are warned that this section is not for the faint-hearted. Some of the studies we review here are appallingly inept and pointing out their many weaknesses may appear cruel.

By 2015, there had been 25 reviews published of the evidence that windfarms are a direct cause of health problems. In Chapter 4 we summarise the conclusions of these reviews, highlighting that published in 2015 by an expert committee of Australia's National Health and Medical Research Council.[25] We end Chapter 4 by summarising the findings of what is by any assessment the largest and most important study of whether wind turbines adversely affect health: the 2014 Health Canada Study.[26]

In Chapter 5 we turn to the main argument of this book: that 'wind turbine syndrome' and the various claims that go along with it are a casebook example of what we have called a *communicated* disease: a 'disease' that can be spread by people talking, reading, and writing about it. We will first explore the phenomenon of the nocebo effect, the inverse of the well-known placebo effect (*placebo* is Latin for 'I shall help'; *nocebo* means 'I shall harm'). Placebo effects occur when personal expectations that something will make a symptom improve or disappear lead to it doing just that, even when the agent involved is completely inert. Nocebos work in the opposite direction: being told that exposure to something is likely to have an adverse outcome will often produce such an outcome, even when the agent concerned is inert or non-existent.

We argue that concerns about wind turbines can foment anxiety in some people who have those concerns. Anxiety can produce real affective somatic symptoms, and some of those who loathe windfarms attribute their symptoms to direct impacts of the turbines, not to their anxiety about those alleged impacts. We look closely at several areas of evidence that make the case for direct effects impossible to sustain.

In Chapter 6, we will introduce readers to some of the main opponents of windfarms in Australia. We will look at the main organisations that have operated in Australia; an anonymous, frequently defamatory website that daily posts poisonous material about wind energy and anyone seen to be supporting it; acousticians who have worked with windfarm opponents; and the principal politicians who have lead the charge against windfarms in Australia.

A small number of anti-wind activists operating mainly in parts of Canada, the USA, the UK, Ireland, New Zealand and Australia have made wind turbine syndrome their *cause célèbre*. Without exception, they see themselves as contemporary Galileos, fearlessly holding aloft the truth in the face of doctrinaire, conspiratorial denial from the scientific establishment, which has now published 25 reviews of the evidence since 2003. These conclude there is very poor evidence for claims of direct health effects from wind turbines. The activists point knowingly to the historical denials of harm by the asbestos and tobacco

25 National Health and Medical Research Council 2015.
26 Health Canada 2014.

industries, convinced that the pernicious 'Big Wind' industry is reading from the very same playbook (see Chapter 3).

In a career in public health of some 40 years, I have rarely encountered the virulence and sheer nastiness that I have experienced since becoming involved in this issue. Chapter 7 describes the main attacks used by anti-windfarm interests that I have experienced since first writing about this issue in 2010. Sunlight makes a powerful antiseptic.

In the final chapter, we attempt to look at what governments, the wind industry and communities might do to reduce anxiety and opposition to wind turbines. Many nations have experienced few or no health claims about windfarms or indeed much anti-windfarm sentiment at all. There are lessons to be drawn from this.

We are both social scientists. In Chapter 6, we describe windfarm opponents' efforts to narrow the range of expertise deemed relevant to evidence and policy debate about alleged windfarm harms. Social scientists, unless their findings are considered useful to anti-wind agendas, have frequently been pilloried by opponents as unqualified to contribute. This is because the questions that social scientists bring to the debate are both obvious and unavoidable, and threaten efforts to frame the debate narrowly in terms of soundwaves striking human ears.

Social scientists working in health and medicine have long asked fundamental questions about patterns of illness that do not conform to the predictions of medical models. We ask questions about the social, cultural, economic and communicative environments that see often highly variable susceptibility in populations to putative risks.

Anyone who has been near a windfarm knows how quiet they are compared to the many noises that we are all surrounded by, particularly if we live in cities. If you have never visited a windfarm, we would strongly encourage you to do so. (Some windfarms allow the public, by special arrangement, to sleep out in very close proximity to turbines.) The difference between what you may have heard about the sound of wind turbines and what you will experience is a major 'penny drop' experience. We hope this book will provide a valuable truth serum for readers wanting background on how to interpret the manufactured controversy about wind turbines causing disease.

1 The history and growth of windfarms, and early objections

Wind has been used for millennia as an energy source to propel sailing boats, and to mill grain and pump water via windmills. Neolithic humans are thought to have used primitive sails to help move their watercraft, the ancient Egyptians had sailing boats in 3400 BC, and across the 5400 years since, most civilisations, including the Romans, Greeks, Phoenicians, and Vikings, saw major developments in the use of sail, with the largest happening in the 16th century. David Newton's 2015 book *Wind energy* provides a useful review of developments in wind power, from sails through to today's modern windfarms.[1]

The Persians appear to have been the first civilisation to develop windmills, using them to crush grain from 500 to 900 AD, with the English using them for the same purpose from 1100. There was a windmill in Arles, France, in 1105.[2] Today, windmills are emblematic of the Dutch, who used them to pump water from lowland areas from the 1300s. Dutch colonisers in New Amsterdam (now New York) erected windmills in the 1600s and by the 1800s their use had followed settlers and the railway as they moved westward. The world's first electricity-generating windmill was erected by Scottish engineer James Blyth in his garden at Marykirk, Kincardineshire in 1887; he used it to help power his house (see Figure 1.1). In 1895, he licensed the Glasgow engineering firm Mavor and Coulson to construct a larger improved version of his

1 Newton 2015.

2 Charlier and Justus 1993.

prototype.[3] In 1910, the *Daily Mail* newspaper in England explained the basics of wind-powered electricity generation to its readers:

> ELECTRICITY FROM WIND
>
> ECONOMICAL WAY OF OBTAINING POWER AND LIGHT
>
> Successful efforts are now being made to convert wind into electricity. Quite a large farm near Hamburg is being supplied with electrical energy generated by wind power, threshing machines, pumps, and various farm appliances being elecrically driven, while some hundreds of incandescent lamps are lighted in various sheds and houses on the farm. A large wind turbine is placed at the top of a tower, and as this is revolved by the wind it actuates a dynamo, which charges accumulators; consequently the electricity generated by a wind during the night can be stored up for the following day. An auxiliary oil engine has been installed for times when the wind fails.
>
> This is not the only wind plant for generating electricity. A firm of electrical engineers at Willesden Green have for some time had one running successfully. An ingenious arrangement is used by them to check the vagaries of the wind. When a strong wind is blowing the turbine naturally revolves quicker than in the case of a light breeze, hence the dynamo is driven quicker. The voltage or pressure of a dynamo rises in direct proportion to its speed, and a considerable rise might easily ruin the accumulators it was charging. This arrangement referred to automatically checks any change in voltage, so that a sudden change in the wind is instantly counterbalanced.
>
> Several country houses are being fitted with wind plants, as where fuel is difficult to obtain or abnormally dear the wind proves a useful substitute.

In 1888, Charles Brush built the first electricity-generating windmill in the USA in Cleveland, Ohio, with an output of just 12 kilowatts (kW).[4] It was abandoned in 1908. By the 1920s many farms across the great plains of the USA not connected to the electricity grid were being partly powered by electricity generated by windmills, built in a factory in Minneapolis that produced some 30,000 over the next

3 Aberdeenshire Council 2016.

4 A watt is a measure of the transfer of energy equivalent to 1 joule per second. A kilowatt (kW) is 1000 watts; a megawatt (MW) is a million watts; and a gigawatt (GW) is a thousand MW.

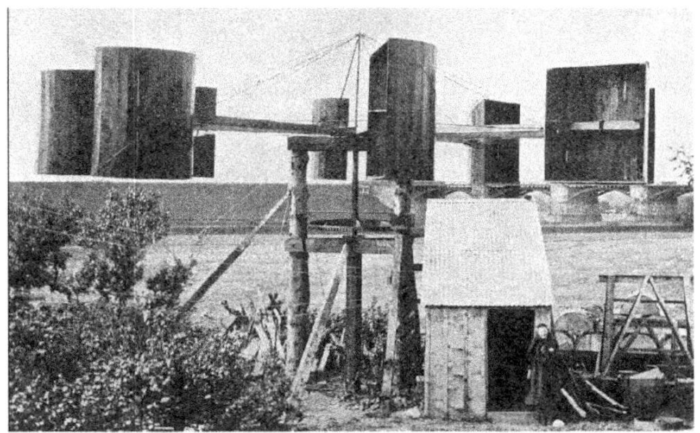

Figure 1.1 James Blyth's first electricity generating windmill. Source: Wikipedia.

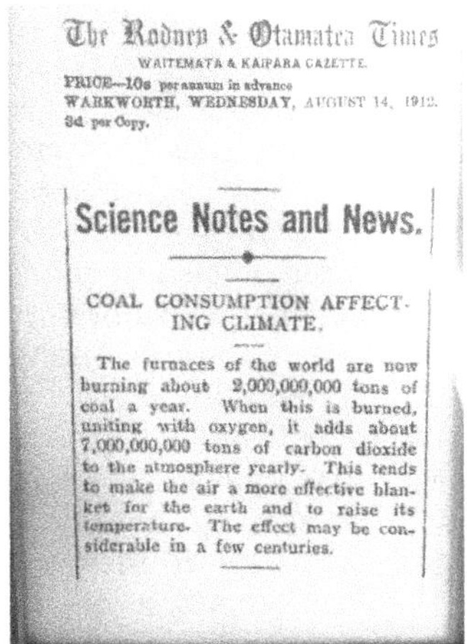

The Rodney & Otamatea Times

WAITEMATA & KAIPARA GAZETTE.

PRICE—10s per annum in advance
WARKWORTH, WEDNESDAY, AUGUST 14, 1912.
3d. per Copy.

Science Notes and News.

COAL CONSUMPTION AFFECTING CLIMATE.

The furnaces of the world are now burning about 2,000,000,000 tons of coal a year. When this is burned, uniting with oxygen, it adds about 7,000,000,000 tons of carbon dioxide to the atmosphere yearly. This tends to make the air a more effective blanket for the earth and to raise its temperature. The effect may be considerable in a few centuries.

Figure 1.2 *Rodney and Otamatea Times* (New Zealand), 14 August 1912.

30 years. These wind turbines were very small by today's standards, and it was not until 1941 that the world's first megawatt-sized turbine (1.25 MW) was connected to the local electricity grid and began operating in Castleton, Vermont. It operated for 1100 hours before suffering a mechanical failure caused by a wartime shortage of reinforcement material. Interest in wind energy went into the doldrums until the 1960s because of the widespread availability of cheap fossil fuels. In 1980 in the USA, electricity generated by coal- or oil-fired power stations cost around 5 cents per kilowatt hour, while that from wind was about 55 cents.[5] Wind energy, at the time, could not compete economically with fossil fuels, and there was only marginal awareness of the environmental consequences of burning fossil fuels. It was only in the 1980s that concern about climate change began to take root, although the problem had been identified much earlier. Figure 1.2 shows an interesting example of very early reporting about these problems.

As awareness of the possibility of 'peak oil' emerged in the 1950s interest in renewable energy rekindled.[6] This was boosted significantly following the 1973 Arab oil embargo, and by President Richard Nixon's Project Independence (announced in 1973), which was designed to make the USA less reliant on imported energy. However, renewable energy was given only some emphasis in a summary of the project, and wind energy was never mentioned. The large rise in oil prices from 1973 saw major attention focused on renewable energy, with the US government forming the United States Department of Energy in 1977 and the National Renewable Energy Laboratory (formerly the Solar Energy Research Institute) established in Boulder, Colorado. The US government began providing renewable energy tax credits in the 1980s to encourage investment in wind energy development.

In the mid 1970s Canada's Quebec Hydro constructed a number of 40 kW vertical-axis turbines, which became known as 'egg beaters'. The world's first windfarm (with 20 turbines) was constructed in New Hampshire, USA in 1980 and the first offshore farm commenced operation off the Danish coast in 1991. Canada's first windfarm began generating power at Crowley Ridge, Alberta in 1994.[7]

5 McVeigh, Burtraw, Darmstadter and Palmer 1999.
6 Hubbert 1956.
7 An illustrated timeline showing these early turbines can be found at http://www.cbc.ca/doczone/features/timeline1.

Denmark takes the lead

Danish polymath Poul La Cour – sometimes referred to as Denmark's Nikolai Tesla – contributed greatly to the development of wind technology. Well ahead of his time, in 1895 La Cour built a wind turbine system that separated hydrogen and oxygen from water and provided lighting for the Askov Folk High School. As happened elsewhere, the technology was sidelined for much of the 20th century.

As a small but windy nation with no petrochemical wealth, Denmark was hit particularly hard by the 1970s oil crisis. Proposals to address Denmark's energy dependency with nuclear energy were met with massive resistance and calls to harness renewable energy.

While energy experts at the time were debating whether large scale wind energy would ever be practical, an alternative school in Ullborg built a 1 MW turbine in 1975. Standing 50 metres high, the Tvindkraft turbine still operates today and is revered as an important industrial artefact.

The Global Wind Energy Council provides the most comprehensive overview of the global wind industry today. In 2015, the GWEC estimated there were some 314,000 turbines generating electricity in 80 nations.[8] In 2016, there were 486.79 GB of installed wind power throughout the world. This represented a 17 percent increase on the 2015 total and approximately a 20.4-fold increase in 16 years. Over 40 percent (42.8 percent) of global capacity added between 2015 and 2016 occurred in China.[9]

In 2016, China, with 169 GW of installed wind energy capacity, had more than double that of the USA, in second place with 82 GW. Australia ranked 17th, with 4.327 GW of installed capacity from wind power (see Table i.1). Denmark, with a land mass of 43,094 square kilometres smaller than Tasmania and a 2017 population of 5.7 million (less than a quarter of Australia's 24.6 million) had 5.2 GW of installed wind power capacity, 17 percent more than Australia.

8 Global Wind Energy Council 2016.
9 Global Wind Energy Council 2017.

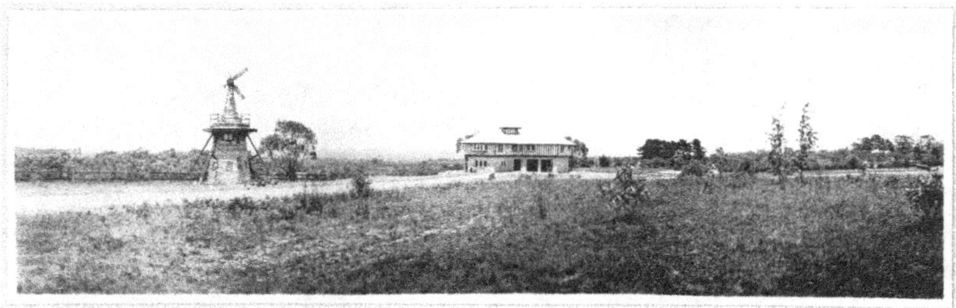

Figure 1.3 The windmill at Westerfield, photographed in 1925. Source: Melbourne University Archives.

Windfarms in Australia

It's quite likely that the first attempt to generate electricity from wind in Australia was with a Burne wind turbine (Figure 1.3) installed at Westerfield, the Mornington Peninsula farm of Russell and Mabel Grimwade, in the 1920s. The turbine was only sporadically useful.

Lloyd Dunn (1912–1978) founded the Dunlite Electrical Company in Adelaide in 1935 and manufactured a range of wind generators from 300 W to 5 kW, until 1975 (figure 1.4).[10] Many were manufactured, and the power generated was fed into lead acid batteries and used for homesteads, farm workshops, lighthouses and remote telecommunications repeater stations; the Dunlite company also had a thriving business exporting wind generators to North America. In the middle of the 20th century, seemingly almost every farm across Australia had either Southern Cross or Comet windmills (see Figure 1.5) drawing up bore water, helping immeasurably to develop the Australian rural landscape. The repetitive clanking sounds made by these windmills were part of the Australian rural soundscape for decades. Not too long ago, rural communities saw wind and the machinery to harvest it as essential to their livelihoods.

Australia's first modern, grid-connected wind turbines began operation in 1987 at Salmon Beach near Esperance in Western Australia. Six 60 kW turbines ran for 15 years, until they were decommissioned and dismantled in 2002, by which time the turbines

10 Pearen 2010.

were considered inefficient relative to newer, larger turbines. New turbines (now totalling nine) began operating from 1993, with a further six 600 kW turbines added at Nine Mile Beach in 2003.

Today, there are 80 operating windfarms across Australia. The smallest 'farm' is the single 60 kW Westwind turbine operating at Breamlea, near Geelong in Victoria,[11] which was erected shortly after the Salmon Beach turbines and celebrates its 30th birthday in 2017. At the time of writing, the largest windfarm in Australia is the 140-turbine Macarthur windfarm, located in south-western Victoria. Macarthur commenced operation in April 2013 and has a capacity of 420 MW. This will soon be eclipsed by the 530 MW windfarm at Stockyard Hill, 35 kilometres west of Ballarat. This is a project that the founder of the anti-windfarm Waubra Foundation, Peter Mitchell (see Chapter 6), tried unsuccessfully to have stopped several years ago. Some 35 projects are under construction or due to be completed in 2017 (Figure 1.6). These projects will deliver an unprecedented $7.4 billion in investment, produce more than 3300 MW of new renewable energy capacity, and create more than 4100 direct jobs.[12]

The total electricity-generating capacity of the Australian wind energy sector today stands at 4.3 GW.[13] Wind energy has made the greatest proportional contribution to local energy supplies in South Australia, with around 40 percent of the state's energy coming from wind in 2016,[14] although Victoria and New South Wales are fast catching up. The amount of wind energy produced in Australia is expected to double before 2021. Any data we might cite in this book will already be out of date when it is published, so fast is the pace of new windfarm developments.

---

11 Wong 2011.

12 A regularly updated, highly detailed timeline of the history of construction and operation of Australian windfarms is maintained by South Australian David Clarke at http://ramblingsdc.net/Australia/WindPower.html#chronology_of_wind_farm_construction.

13 Global Wind Energy Council 2017.

14 Parkinson 2016.

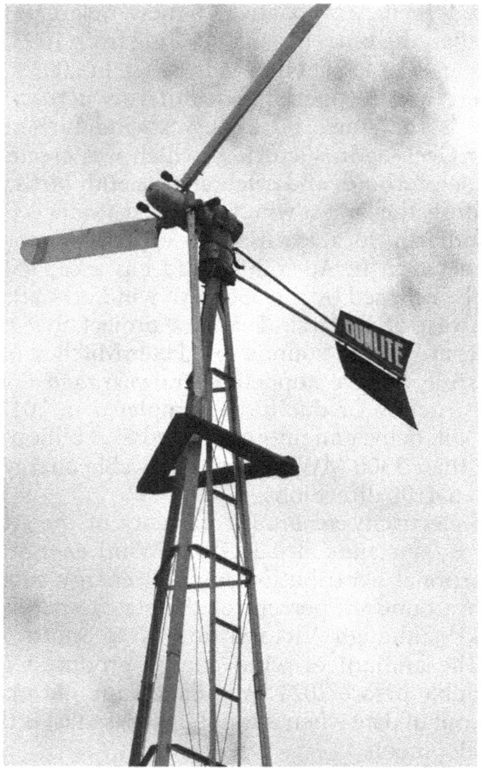

Figure 1.4 Dunlite windmill in Toowoomba, Queensland, Australia. Photograph by John Nielsen, http://bit.ly/2z6ZFW0.

Early objections in Australia

Complaints about windfarms in Australia appear to date from the early 2000s, when press reports mentioned occasional negative reactions in rural communities to the perceived intrusiveness of turbines in bucolic landscapes (one 2002 report described them as 'white behemoths',[15] and the Victorian premier Ted Baillieu spoke of 'towering triffids'[16]), allegations that threatened bird species were in danger of

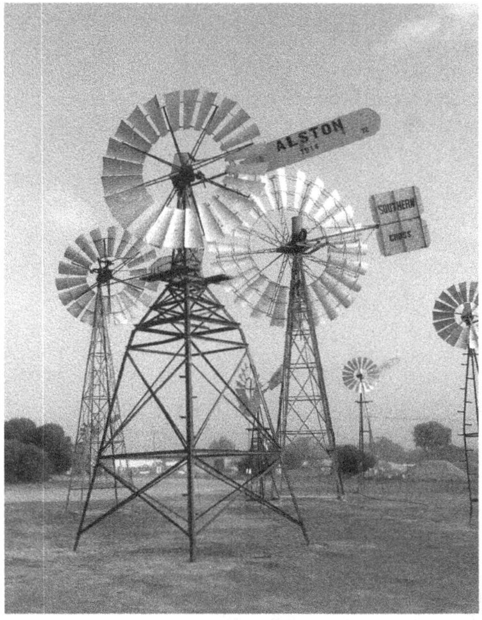

Figure 1.5 Southern Cross windmills in Australia. Source: Penong Windmill Museum. Photograph by Tony Hill.

being struck by turbine blades, the divisiveness engendered in communities by the perceived unfairness of some landowners being paid hosting fees of up to $21,000 per year per turbine while neighbours received none (see Chapter 3), and debates about the economics of green energy. Unapologetic NIMBYism ('I'm quite happy to admit that this is a not-in-my-backyard thing, because my backyard is very special') was also evident as far back as 2002.[17] Groups opposing windfarms ostensibly in order to preserve pristine bush and rural environments were active from these early years and included various

15 Fyfe 2002.
16 Fyfe 2004.
17 Fyfe 2002.

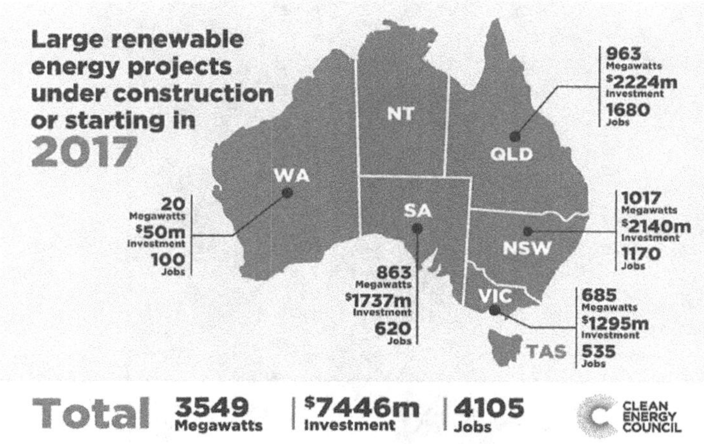

Figure 1.6 Windfarm projects under construction in Australia, 2017. Source: Clean Energy Council.

branches of the Australian Landscape Guardians (see Chapter 6). Interest groups with overt climate change denial agendas also actively opposed windfarm developments, particularly in Victoria. Chief among these was the Australian Environment Foundation,[18] registered in February 2005 out of the office of the Institute of Public Affairs and run for many years by Max Rheese, who later went on to advise Senator David Leyonhjelm, also a strong critic of windfarms.[19]

Six non-health arguments against windfarms

This book is about noise and health objections to windfarms. However, besides health arguments (see Chapters 3 and 4), those opposed to windfarms argue in six main, often intertwined domains: economic viablity; landscape aesthetics; devaluation of surrounding property;

18 See http://www.australianenvironment.org.

19 Parkinson 2014.

Economic unviability	Proximity to a gas pipeline
Electromagnetic interference	Light pollution
Absence of the neighbouring shire in proceedings	Confidentiality of lease arrangements
Distraction to passing drivers	Blade flicker effect on cattle
Hazard to overflying aircraft	Concerns for soil stability
Impact on social fabric	Lightning strikes
Groundwater contamination from underground power cables	Possibility of human remains buried in the vicinity
Interruption of spring water flows	Denial of natural justice
Leaching from concrete foundations	Violation of human rights
Blasting for foundations, causing vibration and other unknown impacts	Difficulties accessing the turbines if they caught on fire

Table 1.1 Objections made about the Hepburn Community Wind Project.

danger to birds and bats; danger to aircraft; and fire hazards. We will summarise and critically comment on each of these shortly.

Opponents also have a reserve arsenal of minor arguments which are often thrown in for good measure. Simon Holmes à Court, who chaired the Hepburn Community Wind Project in Victoria, provided a list of 22 objections used by the Daylesford and Districts Landscape Guardians (in addition to noise, health, blade flicker and visual amenity) in their unsuccessful appeal against Hepburn Wind's planning application (Table 1.1)

'Wind energy is unreliable and uneconomical'

The first major argument advanced by those opposed to windfarms is that electricity generated from wind is unreliable and uneconomical to produce because wind is intermittent and other forms of generation (especially coal, gas-fired and nuclear) are said to be far cheaper and more reliable. They argue that windfarms can only be erected and operate because they are vastly subsidised by governments duped by a global conspiracy of lies generated by climate change advocates and scientists, most of whom promote their arguments simply to keep their snouts comfortably in the trough of government-funded research grants.

China is far and away the world leader in both economic growth and the installation of new wind energy capacity – 23.4 GW added in 2016 alone (nearly 5.5 times in one year what Australia has installed in total). Try to imagine a conversation between China's energy minister and the then Abbott government's Business Advisory Council czars, Maurice Newman[20] and Dick Warburton, both of whom loathed wind energy.[21] These two would explain to the Chinese leaders that their economic understanding of wind energy, and their commitment to trying to greatly increase China's use of clean, renewable energy, were simply all wrong. While Newman and Warburton were publicly running down wind, in late 2015 global wind energy capacity (432 GW) surpassed that from nuclear generation (383 GW) for the first time.[22] By 2021 global wind energy is expected to almost double to 800 GW,[23] while the global nuclear power industry is in a state of torpor. In January 2017, Bloomberg reported that global investment in wind energy was $110.3 billion in 2016, down 11 percent compared with the previous year.[24] This was largely due to an 18 percent reduction by China. As Bloomberg noted, 'Because the vast majority of clean energy investment goes into financing assets in the world's most carbon-polluting nation, when China's market dips it moves the needle on global numbers.' The article continued:

> Offshore wind in particular saw a banner year in 2016. Capital spending commitments reached $29.9 billion in 2016, up 40 percent over the previous year. The availability of larger turbines and improved economics prompted greater investment from developers in Europe and China.
>
> Last year saw the approval of the largest-ever offshore wind project – Dong Energy's 1.2-gigawatt Hornsea array off the UK coast, with a price tag of $5.7 billion. An additional 14 parks greater than 100 megawatts also received the go-ahead last year, in British,

20 Newman 2012.
21 Ludlow 2015.
22 Anon. 2016.
23 Global Wind Energy Council 2017.
24 Pyper 2017.

> German, Belgian, Danish and Chinese waters. Going forward, new offshore wind markets are set to open in North America and Taiwan.

Then there's that other economic powerhouse, Germany, which led new wind energy capacity growth in Europe in 2016 with another 5.4 GW in newly installed capacity.[25] How is it that Newman's and Warburton's sources of information on wind energy being uneconomic seem to have passed by China's and Germany's most senior energy policy planners? And then there's multi-billionaire Warren Buffett, who in 2013 pumped US$1.9 billion into wind development in Iowa and by 2016, even more enthusiastic, was planning to construct the USA's largest windfarm of 2000 MW with a $3.6 billion investment.[26] Another windfarm critic, former Australian treasurer Joe Hockey, should have got on the phone and let Buffett know which side of the energy bread was really buttered. Farmers have always harvested the sun and the rain to feed humanity, and for a long time they relied upon the wind to pump water and mill grain. Farmers are now harvesting the wind as just another farm activity, with the welcome side effect of jamming an exponentially increasing brake on pollution and greenhouse gas production. Anyone with solar panels on their roof knows how they silently smash your power bill. Anyone who has grown their own fruit and vegetables 'gets' the natural wisdom of putting nature to work. It's not hard for ordinary people to understand that wind, as a free energy source available to any investor installing turbines, ought to be harvested wherever it can be.

So from what possible set of bizarre values could someone look at the application of the minds of some the world's best energy engineers to vastly improving the efficiency of modern wind turbines and call their work not just a bad idea, but 'utterly offensive', as Joe Hockey did in 2014? Community studies consistently show wide support for renewable energy, so Hockey's comment would have struck the great majority of the population as plain weird.

Would Hockey have preferred to drive past a vast, filthy, open-cut coal mine on his way to Parliament House in Canberra? We suspect not. On any long drive in Australia one sees quarries, highways, tall silos, towns, tunnels, bridges, massive power lines and their towers, radio towers, airports, rail lines, land clearance for cropping, and urban

---

25 Global Wind Energy Council 2017.
26 D'Angelo 2016.

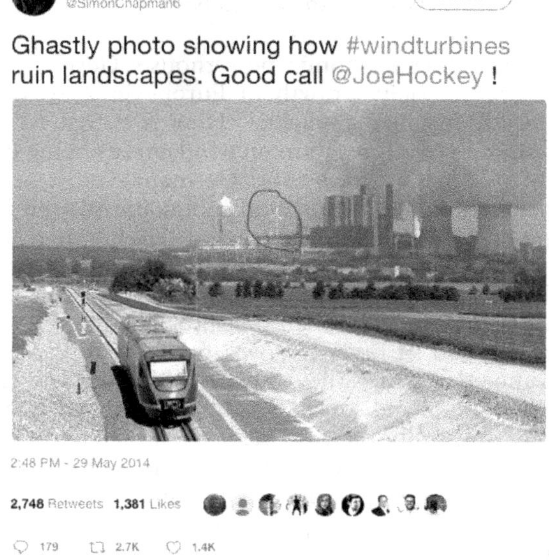

Figure 1.7 My most retweeted tweet.

development. Over the decades, bucolic sentimentalists have used language like Joe Hockey's to oppose all of these developments. Thankfully, few of them were in positions of power to ban them.

I tweeted the photo in Figure 1.7 on 30 May 2014 with the caption 'Ghastly photo showing how wind farms ruin landscapes'. It has so far received 2753 retweets and been favourited 1382 times. As of 22 September 2017 it had had 135,420 Twitter impressions and 10,572 engagements. My second-most retweeted tweet has received a distant 1598 retweets.

'Wind power is only viable if subsidised by the taxpayer'

Governments have long encouraged or discouraged the production and markets for various commodities by a range of taxes, subsidies and taxation policies. An example of this is tobacco tax, with Australian governments having set tobacco tax increases explicitly to reduce demand (which it does more than any other measure).[27] We pay less for low-alcohol beer than for brands with higher levels because low-strength beers are taxed at a lower rate. Various arrangements have long applied to fuels, and since 2000 the production of renewable energy in Australia has been effectively encouraged by arrangements set in place by the government's Renewable Energy Target (RET). Australia's *Renewable Energy (Electricity) Act 2000* provides a financial incentive to encourage the supply of electricity from renewable sources to reduce greenhouse gas emissions from the electricity sector. It operates for both large-scale and small-scale renewable projects. The Large-scale Renewable Energy Target Scheme requires Australia to generate progressively more renewable energy each year, towards a 2020 target of 33 terawatt hours (i.e. 33 million megawatt hours) above a 1997 baseline. This is enough energy to fully supply power to some five million houses. Wholesale purchasers of electricity (which then retail it to consumers) are obligated under the act to obtain and annually 'surrender' proportionately towards the generation of additional renewable electricity. They do this by purchasing large-scale generation certificates (LGCs). These are recorded in the online Renewable Energy Certificate (REC) Registry, having been registered there by renewable energy power stations like wind and solar energy farms and hydroelectricity power stations. One LGC is equivalent to one megawatt hour of eligible renewable electricity generated above the power station's baseline.

LGCs can be traded via electronic transfer between REC Registry account holders. Supply and demand determines the price of LGCs, with certificate prices not regulated by the Clean Energy Regulator. However, there is a price cap: if retailers don't surrender, they are fined $65 per LGC they fall short. For tax reasons – fines are not deductible expenses – it is expected that most retailers will pay up to a maximum $93 per LGC before choosing to take the penalty. While prices have come close to this, especially after the Abbott government's own-goal from restricting supply, the long-term average has been below half this price.

This complex alphabet soup of arrangements is explained in detail by the Clean Energy Regulator[28] but for our purposes here, the Australian government policy of providing what are in effect

27 Scollo and Winstanley 2017.
28 Clean Energy Regulator n.d.

incentive subsidies for the development of renewable energy has always caused a bizarre apoplexy among opponents of renewable energy. They argue that without such subsidies and concessions, renewable energy could not compete with fossil fuels. Windfarm opponents are unrelenting in their attacks on the financial support the wind industry receives from governments, but always silent on the massively greater supports received by the fossil fuel and mining industries. In the weeks before the 2016 Australian federal election a coalition of groups called on the government to cut the $7.7 billion in subsidies that were then being provided to fossil fuel industries. This sum included '$5.5 billion of non-agricultural fuel tax credits, $1.24 billion for concessional rates of fuel excise on aviation fuel and $650 million of tax deductions for exploration and prospecting by the mining industry', part of which would have gone to support coal, coal-seam gas and oil exploration.[29] The total subsidy received by the Australian wind sector to date has been calculated at approximately $2.7 billion in total over 16 years.[30]

Every coal-fired power station in Australia (and the pylons and wires to connect them to the population centres) was made possible by a government providing financing arrangements that modern developers can only dream of: government debt rates and guaranteed power purchase for the asset's entire life.

By contrast, nearly all wind and solar energy projects in the country have been built with private money. The RET has provided an essential subsidy to the renewable sector, but this is orders of magnitude smaller than the government support paid to the fossil fuel sector. It is important to note that the RET is effectively a self-destructing subsidy. Over time, as costs of energy from non-renewable generators rise (which they are) and renewable costs fall (as they are), the LGC price falls. The current RET ends in 2030, however generators in Latrobe Valley will still be paying little more than the current 25.2 cents per gigajoule for their coal in real terms – i.e. they are paying around three dollars to the state in real terms for the coal they burn to generate one megawatt hour, a unit they frequently sell for 20 to 30 times more, and, until policy settings change, paying nothing for the tens of millions of tons of carbon dioxide, nitrous oxides and heavy metals that each emits annually.

29 Karp 2016.
30 Holmes à Court 2017.

Transmission lines to fossil fuel power stations have all been built at government expense, as have transmission lines such as the 230 kilometres of lines from Port Augusta to the Olympic Dam copper, uranium and gold mine in South Australia. High voltage power lines cost around one million dollars per kilometre. No transmission lines have been built in Australia specifically for windfarms at taxpayer expense. The needed transmission lines from the windfarms to connect to the grid are built at the expense of the windfarm developers.

'Wind is intermittent, so wind power can never be a serious source of power'

Just as the sun does not shine at night, so does the wind not blow constantly. From this, critics of wind and solar energy argue that these renewable sources could never replace fuel sources that can generate power continually, like coal, gas, nuclear or hydro.

There are several obvious things wrong with this argument. First, it is true that in any nation the sun does not shine nor does the wind blow all the time. However, in a large nation like Australia where several states (Queensland, New South Wales, Victoria and South Australia) are connected with one another via the same electricity grid, the wind may not be blowing in some areas but blowing strongly in others. For example, if the wind is blowing hard in South Australia, the wind energy generated there can be exported into other eastern states if it is surplus to local consumption.

The aggregate wind energy in the electricity network is much less variable than that of a single turbine. While it is true that there are many times in a year when the aggregate energy output of all windfarms is relatively small, the grid is built to deal with this. Even the largest coal-fired power stations can and do go offline without warning, often during extreme events, as occurred when violent storms hit South Australia on 28 September 2016. Likewise, transmission lines can fail. Australian network operators always strive to have reserve power equal to the capacity of the largest generating unit in the system. At any time, a fleet of generators is ready to ramp up to replace a sudden loss of generation far larger than any windfarm in the country can generate. In reality, wind energy is very predictable – the Australian Wind Energy Forecasting System (AWEFS) is highly successful, providing accurate forecasts and ample time for the network operator and the market to adjust to variability. If there were to be a freak event that resulted in zero wind across the entire grid, there is surplus capacity across other operators. Every generator in the network effectively backs up every other generator. While it is undisputed that managing the grid becomes more complex as more and more variable generation is added to the network, the network operator AEMO has repeatedly confirmed that there is no reason to believe the challenge won't be met.

Those who initially advanced the argument that wind energy is unreliable made it in the era when developments in energy storage were in their infancy. This of course is rapidly changing. The dramatic advances in battery storage (and fast-decreasing costs) that we have seen in recent years, largely driven by the transport sector, are for the first time enabling business models for large-scale grid-connected battery farms. The high-profile offer to the South Australian government by Tesla's Elon Musk in May 2017 to install a 100 MW battery facility within 100 days and to forfeit all payment if the facility was not operating by that time perfectly illustrates how far battery storage has come.[31]

New-found enthusiasm for pumped hydro energy storage (PHES), whereby water is pumped uphill when energy is cheap (generally at night) and flows downhill through turbines at times of peak demand, has the potential to create a low-tech but powerful 'water battery'. Prime Minister Malcolm Turnbull said after the 2017 federal budget that the Commonwealth may consider buying out the New South Wales and Victorian governments' stakes in the Snowy Hydro Scheme, at a cost of $5.25 billion on top of a planned $2 billon upgrade.[32] Batteries and PHES will both give gas-powered generators a run for their money over the coming decades, especially as society moves, as it inevitably must, towards pricing emitters of carbon pollution.

'Wind turbines are ugly and ruin landscapes': aesthetic objections

Opponents often claim that wind turbines (or 'industrial wind turbines' – IWTs, as they like to call them), are ugly: that the towers are ghastly 'industrial' monstrosities imposed on pristine rural landscapes by large, often foreign-owned corporations, abetted by politicians and faceless bureaucrats who live far away from these eyesores in cities. They utterly devastate the bucolic aesthetic of the landscapes where

31 Parker 2017.

32 Potter and Ludlow 2017.

they are constructed, the argument runs. Case studies from Ireland and Scotland support the idea 'that aesthetic perceptions, both positive and negative, are the strongest single influence on individuals' attitudes towards wind power projects.'[33]

People are at perfect liberty to dislike the look of wind turbines and to feel that they should be located somewhere other than rural settings. All local governments have zoning regulations so that industries such as heavy manufacturing, or those thought likely to attract excessive traffic or undesirable patrons (as with brothel zoning regulations), are prevented from operating in inappropriate areas. But every person making this NIMBY ('not in my backyard') or BANANA ('build absolutely nothing anywhere near anyone') criticism about windfarms lives in the modern world, where homes and workplaces are powered by electricity. Every commodity they consume has been grown or manufactured and distributed using generated power. These objectors are happy to benefit from this power generation but want to live well away from it. Living near power generation is something that unnamed 'others' should have to put up with. Here, there is always the unvoiced assumption that power should be generated anywhere other than where the objector happens to live.

The assumption is that those who have chosen to live in a rural location, unlike those living in cities, have a permanent entitlement to be spared from all urban-industrial construction. Such constructions should be located well away from human habitation (the Waubra Foundation's Sarah Laurie says wind turbines should be at least 10 kilometres from any house), or in or near urban areas. Rural areas, the argument runs, should never be considered for developments like windfarms. People who were born in, or who choose to move to, these areas apparently have an inalienable right to be free of any 'unnatural' development. But rural Australia has long been a highly modified landscape, looking very little like it did prior to European settlement. The roads, powerlines, sheds, irrigation infrastructure, fences, dams, introduced trees and monoculture crops are not 'natural' developments.

Anti-windfarm groups regularly have apoplexy about even a single decommissioned wind turbine that is not immediately dismantled and removed. Yet a 2017 report from the Australian Institute estimated that there were approximately 60,000 abandoned mines in Australia, some

33 Warren, Lumsden, O'Dowd and Birnie 2005.

dating as far back as the 19th-century gold rushes, and that very few had ever been rehabilitated or cleaned up.[34]

Sydney radio announcer Alan Jones took this argument to its rhetorical nadir in November 2016:

> There's evidence everywhere of the impact of these infrasound vibrations. As I said, if they weren't a risk to health, why not put them on Bondi Beach? Put them down Macquarie Street, George Street, Brisbane, Collins Street, Melbourne, plenty of wind there. I know, wouldn't do that, because they know they're injurious to health.[35]

Where should one begin with this nonsense? Yes, Jones' named sites are heavily populated, but they are also exceptionally expensive and iconic sites, where all passing traffic and public amenity would be obstructed by turbine construction. In his rhetorical fervour, Jones also appears to have overlooked that the existing noise levels in these places would far exceed that of a wind turbine, and the noise being emitted by the breaking waves on Bondi Beach would similarly put that from a wind turbine well into its wake. Meanwhile, although all these sites would have some wind, it would not compare to that available in the sites carefully chosen after wind measurements have been taken. Property owners interested in hosting a windfarm invite wind companies to make these assessments, and many applications do not proceed because of sub-optimal wind conditions. Just as it would make no sense to grow wheat in a central business district or to drill for oil on Bondi Beach, we don't put wind turbines in the middle of built-up areas where the resource is poor. (There are plenty of European cities that do have decent wind and so have turbines in peri-urban and, in some cases, urban areas.)

Jones' puerile argument shows the quality of debate so often displayed by the opponents of windfarms.

'The energy cost of manufacturing a wind turbine is never recouped in its operational life'

Some windfarm opponents display an obsession with the steel and concrete that make up the turbines' towers and the concrete that keeps

34 Australian Broadcasting Corporation 2017.

35 Jones 2016a.

them firmly upright, helpfully pointing out that turbines require mining, smelting and (mostly) coal-fired heat in their manufacture. By this argument, wind turbines therefore owe their very existence to fossil fuels and mining and so until such time when all energy is derived from renewable sources, windfarms can never 'replace' fossil fuels. One opponent, Roger Sexton, claimed that it would take a windfarm 3580 years to 'pay back' the carbon dioxide embodied just in the concrete foundations of the turbines, a timeframe David Clarke estimates is about 6000 times longer than the real value.[36]

Simon Holmes à Court told us that each of the turbines used by the Hepburn Community Wind Project (both REpower MM82 turbines on 69-metre towers) required 244 cubic metres of concrete for their foundations. A local concrete supply company advised Hepburn that the average house in the area required 40 cubic metres of concrete – i.e. while a local turbine required concrete equivalent to that used to make about six local houses, each turbine is capable of providing annually as much energy as 1000 homes consume.

Construction of 15 much larger turbines at the Blue Creek windfarm in Ohio, USA (these had 100-metre towers and a rotor diameter of 90 metres) required 573 cubic metres of concrete per turbine – about 60 truckloads each.[37] Local geotechnical and wind conditions, plus the larger tower and blade size, explain the greater concrete requirements, and Australian experience has demonstrated that moving to 100-metre towers and 90-metre rotor diameters results in yield improvements of up to 40 percent more energy being captured. Note, however that:

> Relative to the rest of Ohio's power generation fleet, the Blue Creek Windfarm offsets carbon dioxide emissions by approximately 0.72 billion kg per year, which is equivalent to planting an estimated 55,847 hectares of trees, taking 114,000 cars off the road, or not consuming more than 2.1 million barrels of oil. It also avoids the consumption of 1,544 million litres of water per year.[38]

The same desultory, myopic argument of course applies to every manufactured product that uses metals, minerals, fuel or chemicals

36 Clarke 2016.
37 Lafarge 2012.
38 Lafarge 2012.

mined or manufactured by industries which also in turn use such materials. Every house, building and motor vehicle is full of these things. But when it comes to concern about the environmental footprint of building and manufacturing, wind turbines are uniquely singled out by their critics. Presumably only wind turbines made from renewable resources like plantation timber would be acceptable to those making this argument. (By the same logic, it could be argued that the materials for the first car factory were likely transported by horse and cart, yet no one claims that horses are therefore superior.)

A good example of this style of thought came from (now ex-) South Australian Family First Senator Bob Day. On 30 April 2015, Day published a post on his website titled 'Wind turbines' inconvenient truth'.[39] With 'gotcha' exuberance, Day noted that wind turbine motors incorporate rare earths, which are often sourced from heavily polluting mining in environmentally blighted inner Mongolia. Highlighted in bold was an excerpt from a 2011 *Daily Mail* report: 'Whenever we purchase products that contain rare earth metals, we are unknowingly taking part in massive environmental degradation and the destruction of communities.' The subtext was plain: green wind energy supporters are indifferent to the environmental damage and human suffering being caused, and so are massive hypocrites.

A small problem with this accusation is that by far the main use of rare earths is not in wind turbine motors, but in a wide range of electronics that include literally billions of mobile phones and computers, which ex-Senator Day and nearly every Australian use daily.[40] In fact, only a very small subset of wind turbine manufacturers use the permanent magnets that make use of these rare-earth metals. If Day was ignorant of this fact, and somehow convinced that wind turbines were the only market for these rare earths, his blindspot for the evidence that could have been found almost instantly with the most elementary Google search was surely astonishing. Wind turbines produce energy with virtually no emissions after the initial emissions involved in the construction of the turbine and any additional local infrastructure needed to connect the energy generated to the grid. Getting a wind turbine built and operating has an environmental impact, as does all construction. Today's giant wind turbines can stand as high as 230 metres from ground to apex blade tip.[41] They are made

39 Day 2015.

40 See http://www.namibiarareearths.com/rare-earths-industry.asp.

mostly of steel. Depending on the model, they can weigh between 150 and 300 tonnes.[42] Producing the concrete slab that anchors the tower and the fibre-glass blades, and transporting it all to the site, necessarily leaves a carbon footprint.

In its inimitable way, the anti-windfarm website Stop These Things (see Chapter 6), in its anonymous and therefore unaccountable 'Andy's Rant' column, spelt out the whole disastrous folly,[43] although disappointingly failed to provide comparable data on the carbon footprint of a coal-fired power station. Andy's conclusion? Wind turbines 'will incur far more carbon dioxide emissions in their manufacture and installation than what their operational life will ever save.' However, US researchers have 'done the math' and conducted an environmental lifecycle assessment of two 2-megawatt wind turbines being planned for a windfarm. Their 2014 paper in the *International Journal of Sustainable Manufacturing*[44] concluded that a wind turbine with a working life of 20 years will offer a net carbon benefit within just 5.2 to 6.4 months of commencing energy generation. At the time this book went to press, no critiques of this calculation have been published in any peer-reviewed journal.

'Windfarms devalue surrounding properties'

Windfarm opponents routinely assert that property values plummet around windfarms. They often throw this claim around in conjunction with statements about residents having to abandon their homes because of the intolerable noise (see Chapter 3). Who would be foolish enough to buy a house that was constantly bombarded by a noise so sickening that it causes people to walk away from their homes rather than put up with it?

Local opponents' best efforts to publicise the alleged horrors of living near turbines might deter buyers. So the claim that windfarms devalue local properties might be expected to be self-fullfilling, when the same people are fanning buyer concerns. The claim is of course readily testable by comparing housing and land prices near windfarms and in comparable areas nowhere near windfarms. By 2015, the wind-

41 Froese 2016.
42 American Wind Energy Organization n.d.
43 Stop These Things 2014.
44 Haapala and Prempreeda 2014.

energy blogger Mike Barnard had identified nine quality studies that had examined the relationship between windfarms and property value.[45] He summarised their key findings thus:

- The US-based Lawrence Berkeley National Laboratory found no correlation.
- The UK-based Royal Institute of Chartered Surveyors in combination with the Oxford Brookes University found no association.
- The US-based Renewable Energy Policy Project found positive associations between wind turbines and property value increases.
- A University of Illinois Masters in Applied Economics thesis found evidence that fear of an impending windfarm affects property values, but that operating windfarms do not, and that property values near operating windfarms increase faster.
- A New Hampshire study found no correlation between windfarms and property values.
- Fear of wind turbines' impact on property values before the wind turbines are erected and shortly afterward seems to have a short-term impact on property values and sales. If so, anti-wind advocacy groups are complicit in this – arguably intentionally – by publicizing and promoting fear of property value impacts.

What about Australian data? Council minutes from 21 August 2012 for the Pyrenees Council in central Victoria, in which the windfarming township of Waubra is located, make interesting reading. The minutes show that residential house valuations in the Waubra precinct rose more than those in any of the other ten precincts in the council area in the preceding two-year period, 2010–12. The average rise across the ten precincts was 3.62 percent; in Waubra the average increase was 10.1 percent.

Of Australian windfarms, the Waubra farm has received by far the largest number of noise complaints (29 individuals have complained).[46] It has often featured in media reports about the issue, largely thanks to the Waubra Foundation (see Chapter 6). If there was ever going to be a place where negativity about a windfarm affected property values, Waubra would have been it.

45 Barnard 2015.

46 Chapman, St George, Waller and Cakic 2013.

Sub Market Group	Count	% change
Amphitheatre	48	3.8
Avoca	522	-3.0
Beaufort - LDRZ	64	2.8
Beaufort - RLZ	188	4.3
Beaufort Residential	512	3.3
Lexton	94	0.3
Moonambel, Redbank, Landsborough etc.	177	6.8
Snake Valley - RLZ	281	8.1
Snake Valley - RLZ	126	-0.2
Waubra	87	10.1

Table 1.2 Changes in residential property valuations 2010–12, Pyrenees Council, Victoria

'Wind turbines kill many birds and bats'

Claims that wind turbine blades cause the deaths of large numbers of birds and bats are often made by opponents, with turbine rotors often referred to as 'bird choppers'. Claims highlighting the dangers to iconic or rare birds, especially raptors, have attracted a lot of attention. On several occasions, we've had people agree that there is poor evidence that windfarms harm human health, but earnestly inform us that they've read that the turbines kill lots of birds.

Birds and bats are indeed killed by turbine blades, but their contribution to total bird deaths is extremely low. Three recent studies illustrate this. A 2009 study using US and European data estimated the number of birds killed per kilowatt hour generated for wind electricity, fossil-fuel, and nuclear power systems.[47] The author concluded that 'wind farms and nuclear power stations are responsible each for between 0.3 and 0.4 fatalities per gigawatt hour (GWh) of electricity while fossil-fuelled power stations are responsible for about 5.2 fatalities per GWh' – nearly 15 times more. From this, the author

47 Sovaccol 2009.

estimated that 'wind farms killed approximately 7,000 birds in the United States in 2006 but nuclear plants killed about 327,000 and fossil-fuelled power plants 14.5 million.' In other words, for every one bird killed by a wind turbine, nuclear and fossil fuel powered plants kill 2118 birds.

A Spanish study involving daily inspections of the ground around 20 Andalusian windfarms with 252 turbines in the four years between 2005 and 2008 found 596 dead birds. The turbines in the sample had been operational for between 11 and 34 months, with the average annual number of fatalities per turbine being just 1.33. The authors noted that this was one of the highest collision rates reported in the world research literature on this subject. Raptor collisions accounted for 36 percent of total bird deaths (214 deaths), most of which were griffon vultures (138 birds, or 23 percent of deaths). The study area was in the southernmost area of Spain near Gibraltar, which is a migratory zone for birds into Spain from Morocco.[48]

Perhaps the most comprehensive report was published in the journal *Avian Conservation and Ecology* in 2013 by scientists from the Wildlife Research Division of Environment Canada.[49] Their report sought to quantify causes of human-related avian deaths, drawing together data from many diverse sources that included both traumatic deaths by feral and domestic cats, bird collisions with and electrocution by man-made structures, oil spills, mining and agricultural deaths (including pesticide poisonings and harvester deaths), and hunting. Table 1.3 shows selected causes of bird death out of an annual total of 186,429,553 estimated deaths caused by human activity.

In 2013, Loss et al. reviewed available data on bird deaths caused by wind turbines in the USA.[50] They noted that earlier estimates of between 10,000 and 573,000 annual deaths were often based on collisions with multi-barred 'lattice' towers rather than the monopole towers that are now the vast majority of wind turbine masts. Their revised estimate was 240,000 annual deaths across the USA. The American Wind Energy Association declared that at the end of 2016 there were more than 52,000 turbines operating in the USA, meaning that on average just short of five birds are killed per turbine per year.[51]

48 Ferrer, de Lucas and Janss 2012.
49 Calvert et al. 2013.
50 Loss, Will and Marra 2013.
51 American Wind Energy Association 2017.

Cause of bird death	All birds	Contribution to total human-related bird deaths
Cats – feral	79,600,000	1 in 2.3
Cats – domestic	54,880,000	1 in 3.4
Power line collisions	16,810,000	1 in 11.1
Buildings – houses	16,390,000	1 in 11.4
Road vehicle collisions	9,814,000	1 in 19
Harvest – game birds	2,817,000	1 in 66.2
Buildings – low, mid and high rise	1,317,130	1 in 141.5
Commercial forestry	887,835	1 in 210
Power electrocutions	184,300	1 in 1,011.6
Agriculture – haying and mowing	135,400	1 in 1,376.9
Communication tower collisions	101,500	1 in 1,836.7
Wind energy collisions	13,060	1 in 14,275
All other	3,479,328	1 in 53.6
Total	186,429,553	100

Table 1.3 Annual human-related causes of avian deaths, Canada. Adapted from Calvert et al. 2013

Mark Duchamp, the 'president' of Save the Eagles International, is probably the most prominent alarmist on windfarm bird deaths. Here's a typical statement from him:

> The average per turbine comes down to 333 to 1000 deaths annually which is a far cry from the 2–4 birds claimed by the American wind industry or the 400,000 birds a year estimated by the American Bird Conservancy for the whole of the United States, which has about twice as many turbines as Spain.

Such claims always allude to massive national conspiracies to cover up the true size of the carnage ('Mark has long been claiming that it was foolish to allow environmental impact assessments to be directed and controlled by wind farm developers.')[52]

In Australia in 2006 a proposal for a 52-turbine windfarm on Victoria's southern coast at Bald Hills (now completed) was overruled by the then federal environment minister, Ian Campbell, who cited concerns about the future of the endangered orange-bellied parrot (*Neophema chrysogaster*), a migratory bird said to be at risk of extinction within 50 years. The Tarwin Valley Coastal Guardians had been opposing the proposed development. Perhaps the highest-profile objector was the former federal health minister Michael Wooldridge, also a founding director of the Waubra Foundation (see Chapter 6), whose family has an estate nearby.

This endangered bird has regularly been used by interest groups seeking to halt developments,[53] including a chemical storage facility and a boating marina.[54] The proposed Westernport marina also happened to be near an important wetland, 'but the parrot copped the blame, even though it had not been seen there for 25 years', wrote a cynical professor in biodiversity and sustainability.[55] The *Age* reported that modelling 'suggested a wind farm at Bald Hills alone would result in one parrot being killed every 667 years in the worst case, and 1097 years in the best case.' [56]

The Victorian government's planning minister at the time, Rob Hulls, described the windfarm decision as blatantly political, arguing that the conservative federal government had been lobbied by fossil-fuel interests to curtail renewable energy developments. Hulls said there had been 'some historical sightings, and also some potential foraging sites between 10 and 35 kilometres from the Bald Hills windfarm site that may or may not have been used by the orange-bellied parrot.'[57]

Meanwhile, the British Royal Society for the Protection of Birds built a wind turbine at its headquarters because it recognised that wind power is more beneficial to birds than it is harmful.[58]

---

52 Save the Eagles International 2012.
53 Garnett 2013.
54 Marks 2012.
55 Garnett 2013.
56 Topsfield 2006.
57 Hogan 2006.
58 Royal Society for the Protection of Birds n.d.

What of opponents' claims that many bats are killed by turbines? A 2010 review of published and unpublished reports on bat mortality at windfarms in north-western Europe found the estimated number of bats killed per turbine annually was low (0–3) on flat, open farmland away from the coast, higher (2–5) in more complex agricultural landscapes, and highest (5–20) at the coast and on forested hills and ridges.[59] The species killed almost exclusively (98 percent) belonged to a group adapted for open-air foraging.

The authors concluded that other than the open-air foraging group, bats are 'usually not at risk at wind turbines, because they fly below the rotors, but are still killed occasionally'.

'Wind turbines are a danger to aircraft'

Opponents argue that wind turbines pose a grave risk to low-flying light aircraft such as crop dusters. Every day crop-dusting pilots fly near countless trees, power poles and wires as they go about their work, but wind turbines are argued to somehow pose an unacceptable risk. This is an odd argument because compared to trees, power poles and wires, wind turbines are far less common, tend to be clustered together in obvious 'farms', and are much taller and more noticeable than trees and power poles. We do not hear of efforts by agricultural pilots to rid crop lands of all trees and power lines. And we rarely hear from pilots singling out wind turbines as a concern either.

Collisions to date have been extremely rare. In April 2014, a light plane hit a turbine during a major blizzard in South Dakota, killing four, in what was described as a 'freak collision'.[60] But light aircraft often crash into natural hazards like mountains and trees. Australia has guidelines for the siting of wind turbines and other large structures near airports.[61] Figure 1.8 shows a water-bombing aircraft in fires near the Waterloo windfarm in South Australian in 2017.

'Wind turbines are a fire hazard'

Windfarm opponents get excited on the very rare occasions when fires occur in the nacelles of turbines. Photographs of these rare events are

59 Rydell et al. 2010.

60 Desai 2014.

61 Department of Infrastructure and Regional Development n.d.

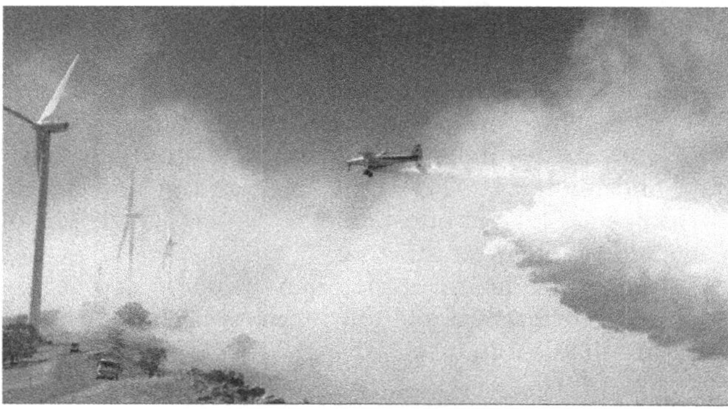

Figure 1.8 Water-bombing aircraft at Waterloo windfarm in South Australia. Source: Waterloo windfarm.

recycled in social media with dire warnings about the grave threat burning turbines pose in dry bush country. They argue that wind turbines may be located in hard-to-reach terrain on the ridges of hills, where wind can be optimal, and that they may there catch fire. This is of course nonsense. Wind turbines are always built with extremely good accessibility, which is needed from the outset for the road transportation of the huge towers and thereafter for maintenance access. Moreover, windfarm companies often construct access roads in order to put turbines in optimal areas. These roads can then be used by maintenance staff and landowners. They can also provide valuable access routes to bush fires for rural fire fighters, who would not have these routes were it not for the wind-turbine construction.

Any type of construction in fire-prone areas can of course be fingered as a potential fire hazard. Fires can be caused by electrical faults, kitchen accidents, discarded cigarettes and other negligent actions by residents. Given there are hundreds of thousands more houses than there are wind turbines throughout Australia (or in any nation which has windfarms), and many more fires caused by these other causes than by wind turbines, we might ask why windfarm opponents do not raise concerns about *any* building in rural areas, or even any human presence in the countryside. Their zero tolerance of wind turbines but their presumed acceptance of rural residences and other buildings clearly exposes their unbridled irrationality on this issue.

There have been three fires in wind turbines in Australia, at Lake Bonney (2006), Cathedral Rocks (2009) and Starfish Hill (2010). None resulted in a bushfire, although one caused a few spot fires that were easily controlled.[62] Turbines have not hindered aerial firefighting efforts and no inquiry into the cause of major fire disasters has ever mentioned wind turbines as a hazard. Three state rural fire authorities (New South Wales, Victoria and South Australia) told the 2015 Senate inquiry into wind turbines that turbines were not seen as an obstacle to aerial firefighting any more than the various other potential hazards navigated by competent aircraft pilots, such as 'power lines, transmission towers, mountains and valleys'.[63] For example, the Country Fire Authority stated that 'here are a lot of other, higher-risk areas, like power lines and the like, over wind towers. They are quite visible and they do not cause the aircraft any concern in aviation operations for CFA'.

But the senators who signed the majority report just could not help themselves, stating 'rural fire services across the country have not properly considered these issues' before quoting speculation by turbine opponents that turbines, had they existed near past fires, *might* have caused a problem for firefighters.

In this chapter, we reviewed a range of non-health objections to wind turbines that are commonly made by their opponents. In the next chapter, we move on to consider the entry into the mix of claims that the turbines are a direct cause of health problems in some of those exposed to them.

62 Clarke 2017.
63 Commonwealth of Australia 2015b.

2

The advent of noise and health complaints

Modern windfarms have operated since the early 1980s, and noise complaints from a small number of families concerning one turbine in North Carolina are on record from around that time.[1] Details of this episode appear to have escaped the attention of the anti-windfarm movement for nearly 30 years, until a report resurfaced in 2013[2] and began to attract excitement on anti-windfarm websites as evidence both that the noise problem had been around for a long time and that the wind sector, government and NASA had conspired to suppress the information in the intervening years, despite the turbine being an experimental 'downwind' design that is not representative of current technology turbines. But with that one exception, there were no documented noise or health complaints throughout the late 1980s and 1990s. Noise and health concerns began to emerge in 2003, as we shall shortly describe. As we summarised in Chapter 1, early opposition to windfarms in Australia and elsewhere concentrated almost entirely on NIMBYist 'we don't like the sight of them' concerns, ideological recoil by climate-science deniers (for whom turbines were totemic reminders of green values), and confected alarm about the deaths of even small numbers of non-endangered birds and bats.

Health concerns were either non-existent or entirely marginal in these early years. We looked in vain for any pre-2004 Australian references to health and noise concerns in the parliamentary

1 Kelley et al. 1985.
2 Martin 2013.

submissions and blog posts of anti-wind groups. There were 37 windfarms operating in Australia in 2010 when Peter Mitchell set up the Waubra Foundation (see Chapter 6) and began to spread alarm about health issues. At only two of these farms were there any previous records of complaints about noise or health: at Toora in 2004, which we describe in detail below, and at Windy Hill in far north Queensland, which received a complaint from one person in 2001. If there had been more complaints in this era, anti-windfarm advocates would surely have done all they could to amplify these early examples in an effort to stress that noise had been an issue for residents living near windfarms for many years.

A list of 78 international 'professionals' who have made statements about their concerns about windfarms appears to confirm this pattern. The list, reproduced on several anti-windfarm websites around the world, shows the year in which each of the 78 first voiced their concerns.[3] The earliest dates on the list are Amanda Harry and David Iser (see below), who first expressed concern about wind turbines in, respectively, 2002 and 2004. Of the 78 professionals, 69 (88.5 percent) are from English-speaking nations (Canada, the USA, New Zealand, Ireland and the UK), with the remainder being from six European nations. Wind turbines and health issues have apparently drawn little interest in nations that don't speak English (see more on this in Chapter 3).

The Harry report

An unpublished report written by an English doctor, Amanda Harry, is frequently described by wind turbine opponents as the first known report of health ill-effects from wind turbines. The report describes data gathered in 2003 on self-reported symptoms in 39 residents living near unnamed English windfarms. Curiously, the report does not appear to have been produced until 2007, four years after the data were collected.[4] The Daylesford and Districts Landscape Guardians in Victoria were then quick off the mark, referring to Harry's report in a 2007 submission opposing a windfarm at Leonards Hill.[5] It is unsurprising

3 European Platform Against Wind Farms n.d.
4 Harry 2007.
5 Wild 2007.

that this abject report was never published. It has nothing even resembling a study design that would reach even the lowest standard of evidence acceptable in science. Harry's description of her research methods consists of this simple statement:

> All people involved in this survey were contacted either by phone or in writing. Questionnaires were completed for all cases. Questionnaires were sent to people already known to be suffering from problems which they felt was due to their proximity to wind turbines. The identity of the people questioned has been withheld in order to maintain confidentiality. The respondents were from a number of sites in the UK – Wales, Cornwall and the north of England.

The report then consists of tables listing the subjects' responses to a simple questionnaire. Eighty-one percent of her sample reported health problems that they attributed to the turbines. The most frequently reported health problems were migraine (26 percent), depression (24 percent), tinnitus (22 percent), hearing loss (18 percent), and palpitations (16 percent). As we will discuss in Chapter 5, each of these problems is very common in all communities, regardless of whether they are located near a windfarm or not.

We are told nothing about how Harry located her informants, but can only assume that there must have been some network of people opposed to windfarms that she accessed or perhaps may have been affiliated with herself. She gives no explanation of what motivated or stimulated her to write her report. She did not interview any comparison group of people living near windfarms who did not attribute common problems like hearing loss or sleep disturbance to wind turbines, nor did she interview people who did not live anywhere near a windfarm to assess the prevalence of these conditions among them. These elementary omissions prevent any speculation about whether her respondents had a higher prevalence of the named health problems than others.

In a remarkable 'pot calling a kettle black' statement, Harry wrote in her conclusion that:

> acoustic experts have made statements categorically saying that the low frequency noise from turbines does not have an effect on health.

> I feel that these comments are made outside their area of expertise and should be ignored.

Harry, a general practitioner with no acoustic expertise, wrote this statement just one paragraph after stating categorically, 'I think it is clearly evident from these cases that there are people living near turbines who are genuinely suffering from health effects from the noise produced by wind turbines.'

The Waubra Foundation website headlines Harry's report as 'ground-breaking', a word windfarm opponents are very fond of using.

The Toora report

In Australia, David Iser, a doctor practising in the Foster-Toora district east of Melbourne, produced an unpublished report[6] in April 2004 after distributing 25 questionnaires to households within two kilometres of the local 12-turbine, 21 MW Toora windfarm, which had commenced operation in October 2002. Nineteen questionnaires were returned, with 11 respondents reporting no health problems. Iser's report consists of just two paragraphs and three dot points summarising his findings. Three respondents reported what Iser classified as 'major health problems, including sleep disturbances, stress and dizziness'. The remaining five reported what Iser categorised as 'mild problems', which included the decidedly unorthodox health problem of 'concern about property values'. Iser forwarded copies of his report to the local shire council and to several Victorian politicians.

Like that of Harry, Iser's report provides no details as to how the sample was selected, whether written or verbal information accompanying the delivery of the questionnaire may have primed respondents to make a connection between the wind turbines and health issues, whether those who reported ill effects had previous histories of the reported health problems, nor whether the self-reported prevalence of these common problems was different from that which would be found in any age-matched population in a similar rural community nowhere near a windfarm.

6 Iser 2004.

In the ten years between the commencement of operation of the first Esperance windfarm in Western Australia and the end of 2003, when the Harry and Toora reports began to be highlighted by windfarm opposition groups, 12 more windfarms commenced operation in Australia. In that decade, besides the two complainants from Toora, we are aware of only one other person, living near the north Queensland Windy Hill windfarm, who complained of noise and later health problems soon after operation commenced in 2000. Importantly in that decade, five large-turbine windfarms at Albany, Challicum Hills, Codrington, Starfish Hill and Woollnorth Bluff Point commenced operation but never received any complaints. An aside in a press report from September 2004 noted that 'some objectors [to windfarms] have done themselves few favours by playing up dubious claims about reflecting sunlight, mental health effects and stress to cattle.'[7] In 2006, a windfarm in Wonthaggi, Victoria, received some ten complaints (but has received none since). With these exceptions, all other health and noise complainants (n=116) first complained after March 2009. As we will discuss in Chapter 5, the nocebo and 'communicated disease' hypotheses would predict this changed pattern and 'contagion' of complaints, driven by increasing community concern. Sixty-nine percent of windfarms began operating before 2009, yet the majority of complaints (90 percent) until 2013 were recorded after this date. So what happened from 2009 to make noise and health complaints escalate?

Nina Pierpont declares 'wind turbine syndrome'

The increase from 2009 (see Figure 2.1) in internet mentions of 'wind turbine syndrome' followed publicity given to a self-published book titled *Wind turbine syndrome: a report on a natural experiment* by a US paediatrician, Nina Pierpont. The book was published by K-Selected Books, a vanity press run by Pierpont and her husband, Calvin Luther Martin (see below), who edited the book.[8] K-Selected Books appears to have only two other titles in its stable, both of them by Martin.[9]

7 van Tiggelen 2004.
8 Pierpont 2009a.
9 See https://kselected.com/.

Pierpont and Martin had generated publicity for the alleged effects of wind turbines prior to her book being published. In August 2005 a local newspaper in upstate New York reported that the Noble Environmental Power Company was complaining that Pierpont and Martin were misleading the public. The pair had addressed a meeting at which they had made statements about low frequency noise being linked to mad cow disease (i.e. bovine spongiform encephalopathy or BSE). BSE is caused by cattle being fed a protein supplement made from meat and bone meal. They were also publicising the claims of a Wisconsin farmer who alleged that 'stray voltage' from a windfarm was killing his cattle. Martin told the reporter, 'within five or six months of the wind turbine coming in, 14 cows died of cancer. Autopsies showed they had black livers … heifers were born with monstrous heads and no eyes … his neighbour lost 350 cows'.[10]

Pierpont's reputation among her followers as an authority on 'wind turbine syndrome' derives from her book, in which she describes wind turbine syndrome as including:

> sleep disturbance, headache, tinnitus, ear pressure, dizziness, vertigo, nausea, visual blurring, tachycardia, irritability, problems with concentration and memory, and panic episodes associated with sensations of internal pulsation or quivering when awake or asleep.[11]

It is not clear whether a person needs to experience all of these symptoms, most of them, or only some to be a candidate for the condition.

Pierpont describes the health problems of just ten families (38 people, including 21 adults and 17 children) living in five different countries who once lived near wind turbines and who were convinced the turbines had made them ill. She interviewed 23 of these people, who provided proxy reports for those in their families whom she did not interview. With approximately 314,000 turbines[12] worldwide today and uncounted hundreds of thousands of people living around these, her sample is tiny, before we even get to the many elementary problems with how she selected them and how she conducted her research.

10 Raymo 2005.
11 Pierpont 2009a, 18.
12 Global Wind Energy Council 2016.

So what are some of the problems with her research that any even basically competent independent reviewer would raise? First, there's the glaring problem of subject selection bias. Pierpont says nothing in the book about how the families she interviewed were selected. She writes, 'I chose a cluster of the most severely affected and most articulate subjects I could find'. So how were these people found? Were they obtained via networks of anti-wind groups that already blamed windfarms for their health problems? We are not told.

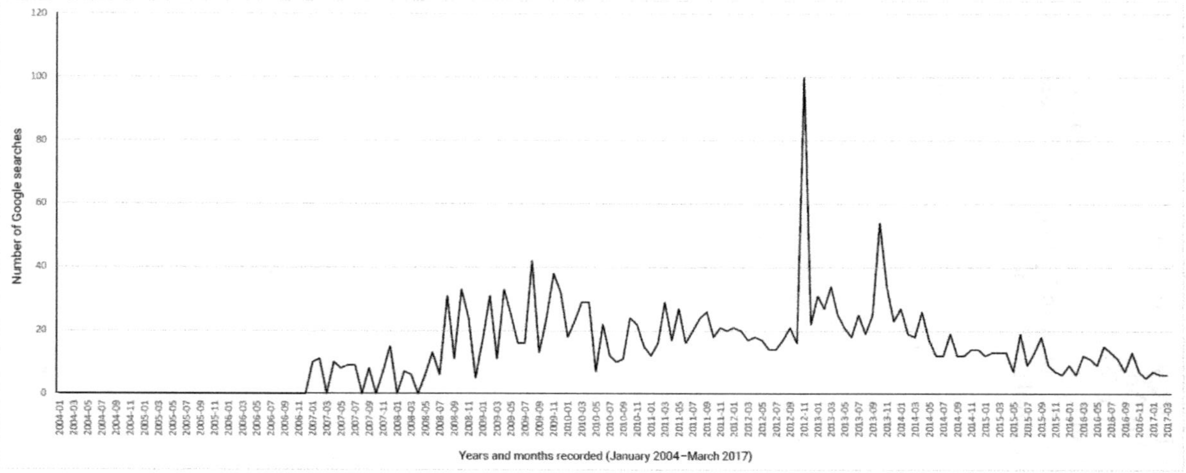

Figure 2.1a Google Trend worldwide data 'wind turbine syndrome', 8 March 2017.

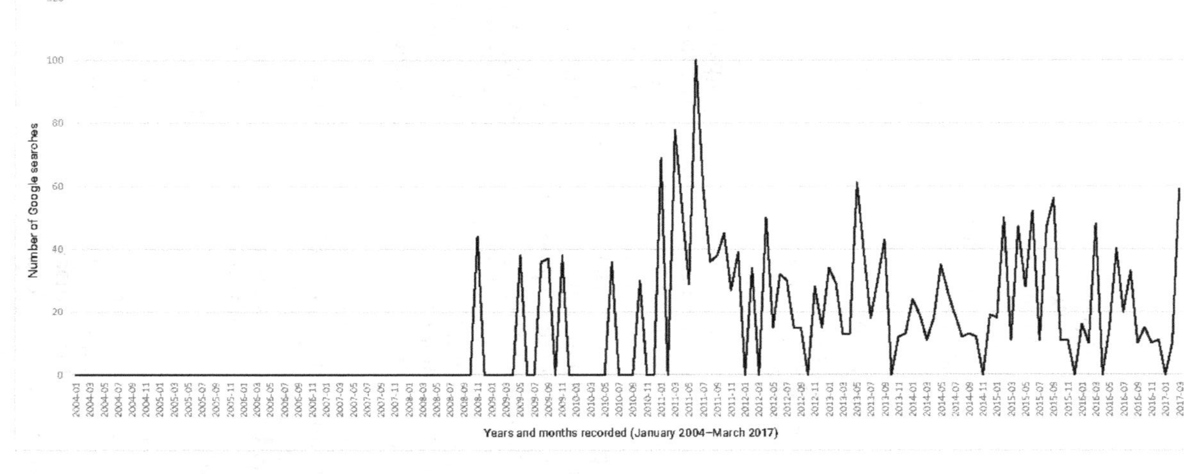

Figure 2.1b Google Trend Australian data for‘wind turbine syndrome’, 8 March 2017.

However, we know that Pierpont spread word about her study through anti-windfarm websites, where she advertised specifically for people who attributed their health problems to windfarms. This meant that her informants were self-selected people who were seeking out and perhaps actively participating in online anti-windfarm forums. They were people who already believed that they were being harmed by wind turbines and so would understandably have had antipathy toward them.

Moreover, her recruitment notice let them know that she was conducting the study with a foregone conclusion in mind: 'one of the purposes of the study is to influence public policy, around the world, to ensure the proper medically responsible siting of wind turbines.' Her study was never going to report anything other than the voices of people who *knew* that the symptoms they experienced were all down to living near windfarms.

Laughably, the notice stated that her study 'will be published in a leading clinical journal in the next 12 months'. No paper from her study has ever been published in any 'leading' journal, nor, as far as we have been able to tell, in *any* journal.

Why did she choose 'articulate', self-nominating subjects and not randomly selected residents living near windfarms? More fundamentally, why did she not make any attempt to investigate controls (people also living near turbines who do not report any illness or symptoms they attribute to turbines, and others experiencing similar symptoms who did not live anywhere near a windfarm)?

Amazingly, she interviewed all her informants by phone and so did not medically examine any of them. Only four families provided medical records for some of their members. However, these are not explicitly referenced in her book. When family members gave proxy reports about others in their family, she does not explain which family members she interviewed, nor consider questions of accuracy in the accounts given by highly motivated informants who were opposed to windfarms. Indeed, she blithely notes that she rejected one informant because she suspected the person of having an ulterior motive for doubting the negative effects of wind turbines ('In other families, excluded from the analysis, one spouse was clearly committed to staying in the house and minimized what the other spouse said.') Only those singing from the same song sheet were included, apparently.

Pierpont provides pages of information on her informants' claims about their own and their families' health while living near turbines.

She also provides summaries of the prevalence of various health problems in these families prior to the arrival of the turbines. These are revealing. A third of the adults had current or past mental illness and a quarter had pre-existing migraine and/or permanent hearing impairment. Six had pre-existing continuous tinnitus. Eighteen had a history of motion sickness. One even had Alzheimer's disease, in addition to an unspecified mental illness.

All this suggests an absence of even the most rudimentary understanding of the design of disease-investigation studies. Her 'study' purports to be a scientific report on human subjects. Nowhere in her book is there any mention of her work having been reviewed or accredited by any human ethics committee. Any researcher in an accredited academic institution doing what she did without such authorisation would be disciplined and probably dismissed. No respectable research journal would ever consider publishing a study without such ethics authorisation.

In summary, her entire 'study' was based on accounts provided to an investigator who was already committed to the view that wind turbine exposure caused health problems. She interviewed aggravated informants selected by an unknown process, and excluded at least one respondent who 'minimized' accounts of symptoms given by another in their family. Her informants were firmly convinced that wind turbines were harming them, speaking to a researcher who was of the same view.

Her book states that her research was peer-reviewed. We discover that this means she sent her manuscript to people she selected and then published some of their responses in the book, including a four-word 'review' by the University of Oxford's Lord Robert May ('Impressive. Interesting. And important.').[13] May's subsequent public silence on the issue may suggest he had second thoughts afterwards. Predictably, all of the quoted reviewers said her study was important (one tends not to publish negative reviews in a self-published book). But as a 'peer review' process this is frankly laughable. It is peer review in the way that publishers add selected glowing snippets about a book to the back-cover blurb. If only independent peer review was simply a matter of authors selecting their own reviewers and publishing those that were most complimentary!

13 Pierpont 2009a.

Calvin Luther Martin

Pierpont's husband, Calvin Luther Martin, is a former academic historian who is aggressively opposed to windfarms, to put it mildly. In an outline for a planned book on fighting the wind industry published five months before Pierpont's own book, he extolled the tactics of Martin Luther King, Jr.[14] Martin never seems to have written the book he outlined, but the lengthy document provides many extraordinary insights into his disposition. He commences by stating, 'I've been fighting the wind bastards well over four years. Four years devoted to almost nothing else.' Far from being detached observers and analysts, the Pierpont-Martin household was a hotbed of seething contempt for wind turbines and the industry.

Martin continues:

> I am no longer an academic. I'm a writer. Writers write to convey something in the most appropriate language for the matter at hand. For wind energy, the most appropriate language is profanity, vulgarity, and obscenity. The louder the better. These are not honourable people. Wind energy is not an honourable enterprise. Big Wind is obscene, profane, and vulgar.

A couple of chapter outlines give a good sense of his disposition:

> Chapter 3. Real evidence doesn't work. The wind sharks fabricate their own, using whorish little companies to perform noise measurements and do environmental impact studies, including bird and bat studies. Companies often consisting of four guys with sweaty balls and BS degrees from nondescript bullshit state colleges, from which they graduated three years ago. But they've got a website and stationery and PO Box – and they're rarin' to get those permits for Big Wind. Give me a break! …
>
> Chapter 7: Wind energy is bullshit. Nitwits who begin their case by telling the local newspaper, 'Well, Gee, we fully support renewable energy, including wind energy, and we feel wind turbines are marvellous so long as they're placed in the right spot' – nitwits who start off their campaign with this are doomed. Wind energy, folks,

14 Martin 2009.

> is horseshit. From beginning to end. Fairy Godmother economics. Right up there with the Easter Bunny. This is 4.5 years of reading thousands of documents, yes, much of it on the physics and economics of wind energy. (By the way, my BA is in science and I did several years of graduate training in hard-core science. Science doesn't scare me.) Wind energy, when subjected to Physics 101, falls apart. It's laughable. Buy a textbook in introductory physics. Start reading.

Eight years after the publication of Pierpont's book, her concocted 'disease' has received no recognition in international medicine. It has never been recognised by any authoritative health or medical agency. It appears nowhere in the International Classification of Diseases and, most tellingly, there appear to be no examples of case reports of the alleged syndrome in any reputable indexed, peer-reviewed medical journal (see Chapter 3).

'Vibroacoustic disease'

After wind turbine syndrome, 'vibroacoustic disease' (or VAD) is probably a very close silver medallist in the race for the weakest evidence. Like wind turbine syndrome and 'visceral vibratory vestibular disturbance' (what Pierpont describes as 'a sensation of internal quivering, vibration, or pulsation accompanied by agitation, anxiety, alarm, irritability, rapid heartbeat, nausea, and sleep disturbance'), VAD is not recognised by any accredited or reputable global health agency and is nowhere to be found in the International Classification of Diseases.

But if you go hunting in cyberspace for VAD, you will find plenty of anxiety-provoking material. In 2012 when I was researching the issue for a paper described below,[15] Google returned 24,700 hits for 'VAD and wind turbines'. There is also a small scientific literature on the topic, overwhelmingly dominated by the work of a small Lisbon-based research group. Two of these authors describe vibroacoustic disease as 'a whole-body, systemic pathology, characterized by the abnormal

15 Chapman and St George 2013. This section has been adapted from this 2013 paper.

proliferation of extra-cellular matrices, and caused by excessive exposure to low frequency noise.'[16] The group argues that VAD is found in occupations routinely exposed to low frequency noise such as aircraft technicians, commercial and military pilots and cabin crewmembers, ship machinists, restaurant workers, and disc jockeys.

In the research paper I wrote with my colleague Alexis St George, we investigated the extent to which vibroacoustic disease and its alleged association with wind turbine exposure had received scientific attention, the quality of that association, and how the claimed association gained traction among windfarm opponents.[17] Our search of the scientific literature located 35 research papers on VAD, with precisely – wait for it – *none* of them reporting on any association between VAD and wind turbines. Of the 35 papers we located at the time on VAD, 34 had a first author from the same Portuguese research group. Seventy-four percent of citations of these papers were self-citations (where the members of the research team re-cited their own work over and over again). Citing one's own work is acceptable and often important and unavoidable in science. But average self-citation rates in science are around 7 percent of a paper's references. So the 'disease' of VAD has received virtually no scientific recognition beyond the group who coined and promoted the concept. With none of the papers containing any reference to wind turbines, we then set out to hunt down the origins of the claim. We found it had first been asserted in a May 2007 press release by the same Lisbon group about a conference paper they were to give at a conference in Istanbul that month. So what was the evidence they produced?

The Lisbon researchers wrote about a 12-year-old boy who lived (along with many others in the vicinity) near a windfarm and who had 'memory and attention skill' problems in school and 'tiredness' during physical education activities. These are of course both very common problems in school children the world over. They are problems which may be caused by a very wide variety of factors. The measured infrasound levels in the boy's house were said to be high. The authors concluded unequivocally that the boy's family 'will also develop VAD should they continue to remain in their home.' Their press release stated that their findings '*irrefutably demonstrate* that wind turbines in the proximity of residential areas produce acoustical environments that

16 Branco and Alves-Pereira 2004.
17 Chapman and St George 2013.

can lead to the development of VAD in nearby home-dwellers' (our emphasis).

It is impossible to understate the abject quality of this unpublished 'study', which was delivered at a conference but has never surfaced in a peer-reviewed journal. There was no control group, just one 'sick' subject, no apparent medical examination of the boy, and no consideration given to any other possible cause of his tiredness.

Factoids are questionable or spurious statements presented as facts, but which have no veracity. They attain popular acceptance as facts because of their repetition, not because of their truth. With some 24,700 mentions in cyberspace, the connection between VAD and wind turbines went viral and stoked the confirmation biases of those utterly committed to the view that turbines are harmful. VAD is now commonly included in submissions to governments by anti-windfarm activists. The term 'vibroacoustic disease' resonates with a portentousness that may foment nocebo effects (see Chapter 5) among those who hear about it and assume it to be an established disease classification acknowledged by medicine. The relationship between VAD and wind-turbine exposure is thus a classic example of a contemporary health factoid, unleashed by a press release on the basis of an uncontrolled case study, then megaphoned through cyberspace. By naming and publicising such questionable 'diseases', windfarm opponents seek to pull what are often extremely common symptoms, such as fatigue, inattention, sleeping problems, high blood pressure and mental health problems, into a memorable, quasi-scientific-sounding 'non-disease'. Vibroacoustic disease is a prime example.[18]

In October 2016, the Sydney radio broadcaster Alan Jones (see Chapter 6) interviewed one of the Portuguese group, Dr Mariana Alves-Pereira, about her work on VAD and wind turbines.[19] Jones commented of her research papers that 'none of them have been disputed', to which Alves-Pereira rapidly concurred, 'No, they haven't,' and stated that her findings were 'indisputable'. Perhaps she had forgotten our critique[20] and those of others. We cited some of the latter when we replied[21] to a letter defending her work that she co-authored in the *Australian and New Zealand Journal of Public Health*,[22] which had published our

---

18 Smith 2002.
19 Jones 2016b.
20 Chapman and St George 2013.
21 Chapman 2014a.

original critique of VAD. For example, in his review of their work, Geoff Leventhall wrote: 'The evidence which has been offered [by the Lisbon group] is so weak that a prudent researcher would not have made it public'[23]; H.E. von Gierke observed that: '"vibroacoustic disease" remains an unproven theory belonging to a small group of authors and has not found acceptance in the medical literature'[24]; and the UK's Health Protection Agency noted that the 'disease itself has not gained clinical recognition'.[25]

Leventhall concluded his review thus:

> One is left with a very uncomfortable feeling that the work of the VAD group, as related to the effects of low levels of infrasound and low frequency noise exposure, is on an extremely shaky basis and not yet ready for dissemination. The work has been severely criticised when it has been presented at conferences. It is not backed by peer reviewed publications and is available only as conference papers which have not been independently evaluated prior to presentation.[26]

One more try?

We've described the lack of recognition that wind turbine syndrome and vibroacoustic disease have been met with since their advocates began pushing for their recognition. Apparently undeterred, two activists against windfarms have attempted to have another high falutin', scientific-sounding name adopted for the same phenomenon: 'adverse health effects in the environs of industrial wind turbines', or AHE/IWT.

Two doyens of the anti-windfarm movement, Robert McMurtry and Carmen Krogh, have attempted valiantly to promote diagnostic criteria for AHE/IWT, first in a non-indexed journal in 2011[27] and twice again in 2014.[28] As of 6 May 2017, interest in McMurtry's 2011

---

22 Alves-Pereira and Branco 2014.
23 Leventhall 2009b.
24 von Gierke 2002.
25 Health Protection Agency 2010.
26 Leventhall 2009b.
27 McMurtry 2011.
28 Jeffery, Krogh and Horner 2014; McMurtry and Krogh 2014.

paper had generated a whole nine downloads in the 68 months since it was published (see Figure 3.6).

Their sweeping 'catch-all' criteria have been severely criticised by others.[29] The case definition allows at least 3264 and up to 400,000 possibilities for meeting second- and third-order criteria, once the limited first-order criteria are met. Institute of Medicine guidelines for clinical case definitions were not followed. The case definition has virtually no specificity and lacks scientific support from peer-reviewed literature. If applied as proposed, its application will lead to substantial potential for false-positive assessments and missed diagnoses. Virtually any new illness that develops or any prevalent illness that worsens after the installation of wind turbines within 10 kilometres of a residence could be considered AHE/IWT if the patient feels better away from home.

Silent and sickening? Infrasound

> No medically plausible link or pathway has been found between infrasound exposure and any of the 200-plus illnesses claimed. The elephant in the room is that the level of infrasonic exposure in ship engine rooms, driving a car with the windows down, or living near a surf beach are vastly greater, yet there is no 'surf coast syndrome'. In other words, the claimed dose / response makes no sense at all. This is homeopathy come to acoustics.—*Roly Roper*[30]

As we wrote in the Introduction, if you have ever been up close to a windfarm and you have not already taken a dislike to them, the sound they emit is neither significant nor offensive. Anyone without an anti-windfarm agenda who has been near a windfarm or single turbine will have found the sound utterly unremarkable. In an amateur video made by a German girl for a school project, we have an elegantly simple demonstration of the sound of a wind turbine compared with sounds she encounters every day in her township.[31] When compared with the range of noises most of us encounter every day of our lives, audible windfarm noise is an utter non-event. If someone said to you, 'Hear

29 McCunney, Morfeld, Colby and Mundt 2015.
30 Roper 2015.
31 See player.vimeo.com/video/63965931.

the sound of that wind turbine? It's unbearable. It's infuriating. It's impossibly loud,' you would think you were in the presence of a very precious petal. Indeed, in Chapter 5 we describe research that shows that those who complain about even micro wind turbines tend to have 'negative', complaining personalities. If they react this way to the gentle, barely noticeable whoosh-whoosh of a turbine, how would they react if they lived, as do billions of the world's population, surrounded by the ever-present din of a city, or to the soundscape of the many occupations in which the noise levels make those near windfarms sound like the silence of a library reading room? However, while anti-windfarm writings frequently refer to the intolerable audible sound of wind turbines (see Chapter 3 for examples of some of the florid language commonly used), they more often demonise sub-audible infrasound as the silently sickening factor responsible for the tsunami of symptoms and diseases set out in Appendix 1.

These efforts find fertile ground in a long history in popular culture and science of animating examples of the dangers of unusual sounds. Steve Goodman's 2012 book *Sonic warfare: sound, affect, and the ecology of fear* catalogues many examples of how sound has been used to create sonic 'weapons'. As the publisher's blurb states:

> Sound can be deployed to produce discomfort, express a threat, or create an ambience of fear or dread – to produce a bad vibe. Sonic weapons of this sort include the 'psychoacoustic correction' aimed at Panama's Manuel Noriega by the US Army and at the Branch Davidians in Waco by the FBI, sonic booms (or 'sound bombs') over the Gaza Strip, and high-frequency rat repellents used against teenagers in malls.

The idea that something you can't hear, constructed by avaricious faceless transnational corporations, is silently eroding your health ticks many boxes for those bewildered by the pace of modern life. Fragments of half-remembered news about the ability of infrasound to terrorise exposed crowds and shake buildings feeds the idea that infrasound from windfarms may well do the same thing.

Infrasound (the 'infra' prefix means 'below', so here indicates sound below audible levels) generated as turbine blades turn in the wind is at the centre of the allegations about windfarms. It is therefore important to understand what it is and the claims being made about it.

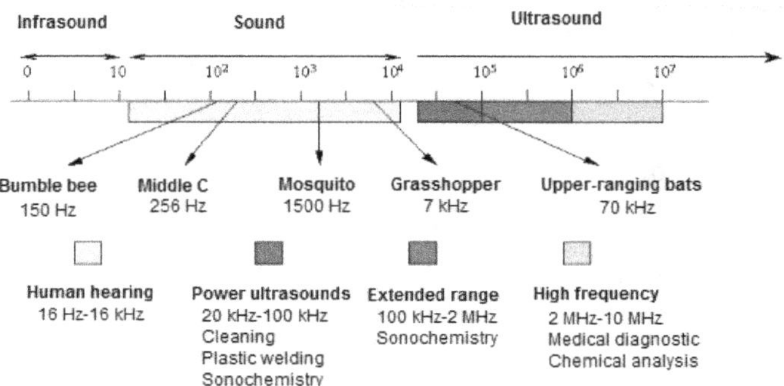

Figure 2.2 Spectrum of sound by frequency (Hz to kHz). Source: Atav 2013.

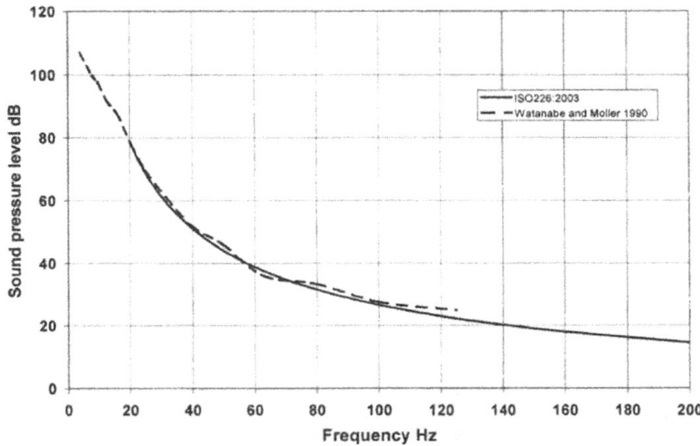

Figure 2.3 Hearing thresholds for a young adult. Source: Leventhall 2009.

Decibels and hertz

First, a brief summary of how acousticians talk about sound. Two terms are always found in discussions about sound: decibels (dB) and hertz (Hz). Decibel numbers refer to the loudness (or pressure) of sounds:

the higher the decibel, the louder the sound. A whisper is around 30 dB while a loud motorbike can be between 100 and 110 dB. You can download free decibel-meter apps for mobile phones and tablets that will allow you to measure the decibel levels of any sound in your environment. As I type this, I am listening to music being played softly on my desk which is between 60 and 70 dB. If I turn the volume up to its maximum, my decibel meter shows 110 dB, which is unpleasant except when I might purposefully seek it out, such as at a rock venue. In a silent kitchen, my refrigerator rates between 45 and 50 dB when its motor switches on to stabilise its temperature.

All sounds also have a certain pitch or frequency. This is measured by the number of waves or cycles that a sound makes per second (cps), measured in hertz (Hz). Figure 2.2 shows the spectrum of sound, showing human inaudible infra- and ultra-sound at either end of the scale, with the sound range audible to humans in-between. Figure 2.3 shows hearing thresholds (standardised for a young adult).

Infrasound is sound between 1 and 20 Hz, which as can be seen from Figure 2.2 is inaudible except at very high volume. People would very rarely be exposed to infrasound at such volume (exceptions might include a volcanic eruption, a violent electrical storm, or at very close exposure to a very loud engine). Infrasound is generated by a variety of mechanical sources, of which wind turbines are just one. Others include power stations, industry generally, motor vehicle and other engines, compressors, aircraft, ventilation and air-conditioning units, and loudspeaker systems.[32] Everyone living in an urban environment is bathed in infrasound daily for most of their lives. Typically, urban residents are exposed to 50 to 65 dB(G) of infrasound most of the time due to traffic, air conditioning, heating fans, subways and air traffic. If they live near airports, they can be exposed to far more. As I sit at my inner-Sydney desk writing this book I'm exposed to both audible noise and infrasound from the planes that pass some 200 to 300 metres over my house, sometimes many times an hour, on their way in and out of Sydney's airport; the sound of passing road traffic on a quite busy road 100 metres from our house; the sounds of trains passing some 200 metres further than the road; and the sub-woofer in the music system I listen to as I write.

Infrasound is also generated by natural phenomena. Human heartbeat, breathing and coughing produce infrasound,[33] so we all live

32 Berglund, Hassmen and Job 1996.

through every day of our lives constantly exposed to it. Other natural sources include rare occurrences like volcanoes and earthquakes that most of us will never experience, but also very common sources like ocean waves, surf and air turbulence (i.e. wind itself) that countless millions, if not billions, are exposed to on most days. Anyone living close to the sea is subjected to constant infrasound from ocean waves. Surf sounds 75 metres from the beach are about 75 dB(G), yet tens of millions of residents living near the sea do not experience symptoms of illness from this exposure. Indeed, many deliberately holiday near beaches partly for the love of the sound of the sea at night. Coastal real estate trades at a premium worldwide. Riding in a car with the windows down exposes occupants to infrasound, and a child on a swing may experience infrasound around 0.5 Hz at 110 dB.[34] This level is much higher than that emitted by wind turbines. Table 2.1 shows a range of data published by the Ministry for the Environment, Climate and Energy of the German state of Baden-Württemberg collected between 2013 and 2016 on low frequency noise and infrasound from six different wind turbines and other commonly encountered noise sources. It can be seen that many common, everyday sounds are comparable and sometimes greater than those recorded for wind turbines (e.g. street noise heard from a balcony, the interiors of cars, and beaches).

Source/ situation	**G-weighted (audible sound) level in dB(G)***	**Infrasound 3rd octave level 20 Hz in dB***	**Low-frequency 3rd octave levels 25-80 Hz in dB***
Wind turbines	**Wind turbine on/ off**	**Wind turbine on**	**Wind turbine off**
WT1	700 m: 55–75/ 50–75 150 m: 65–75/50–70	150 m: 55–70	150 m: 50–55
WT2	240 m: 60–75/ 60–75 120 m: 60–80/60–75	120 m: 60–75	120 m: 50–55

33 Salt and Hullar 2010.

34 Leventhall 2007.

Source/ situation	**G-weighted (audible sound) level in dB(G)***	**Infrasound 3rd octave level 20 Hz in dB***	**Low-frequency 3rd octave levels 25-80 Hz in dB***
WT3	300 m: 55–80/ 50–75 180 m: 55–75/50–75	180 m: 50–70	180 m: 45–50
WT4	650 m: 50–65/ 50–65 180 m: 55–65/50–65	180 m: 45–55	180 m:40–45
WT5	650 m: 60–70/ 55–65 185 m: 60–70/55–65	185 m: 50–65	185 m: 45–50
WT6	705 m: 55–65/ 55–60 192 m:60–75/55–65	192 m: 55–65	192 m: 45–50
Road traffic			
Würzburg urban balcony	50–75	35–65	55–75
Würzburg urban living room	40–65	20–55	35–55
Motorway A5, 80 m	75	55–60	60–70
Motorway A5, 260 m	70	55–60	55–60
Interior car, 130 km/h	105	90–95	75–95
Interior minibus, 130 km/h	100	85–90	80–90
Urban background			
Museum roof	50–65	35–55	Up to 60
Friedrichsplatz	50–65	35–50	Up to 60
Interior	45–60	20–45	Up to 55
Residences			
Washing machine	50–85	25–75	10–75

Source/ situation	G-weighted (audible sound) level in dB(G)*	Infrasound 3rd octave level 20 Hz in dB*	Low-frequency 3rd octave levels 25-80 Hz in dB*
Heating (oil & gas)	60–70	40–70	25v60
Refrigerator	60	30–50	15–35
Rural with wind 6 m and 10 m per second			
Open field, 130 m from forest	50–65 / 55–65	40–70 / 45–75	35–40 / 40–45
Edge of forest	50–60 / 50–60	35–50 / 45–75	35–40 / 40–45
Forest	50–60 / 50–60	35–50 / 40–45	35–50 / 35–40
Sea surf			
Beach, 25 m away	75	55–70	Not reported
Rock cliff, 250 m away	70	55-65	Not reported

Table 2.1 Wind turbine and other sources of infrasound and low frequency noise. Source: Landesanstalt für Umwelt, 2016. *G-weighting measures infrasound, and A-weighting measures audible sound. The G-weighted level is that given by a sound level meter with a G-weighting filter in it.

The fact that wind itself generates infrasound is of particular significance to claims made that infrasound generated by wind turbines is noxious. In a Polish research paper published in 2014, the authors set out to measure infrasound from wind turbines and to compare that with naturally occurring infrasound from wind in trees near houses and from the sound of the sea in and around a house near the seaside.[35] The researchers used the average G-weighted level(L_{Geq}) over the measurement period. This is the standardised measurement of infrasound and approximately follows the hearing threshold below 20 Hz and cuts off sharply above 20 Hz. The infrasound levels recorded near 25 100-metre high wind turbines ranged from 66.9 to 88.8 L_{Geq}

35 Ingielewicz and Zagubień 2014.

across different recordings, while those recording infrasound in noise from wind in a forest near houses ranged from 59.1 to 87.8 L_{Geq} and the recordings of sea noise near seaside houses ranged from 64.3 to 89.1 L_{Geq}. Infrasound levels were thus very similar across the three locations. The peak 88.8 L_{Geq} was recorded very close to the turbines – virtually directly under the blades. The lower 66.9 L_{Geq} was 500 metres away, which is more like the distances experienced by the nearest residences to turbines. Similarly, for the other sources of infrasound, the highest levels were recorded nearest to the source.

Wind is of course a prerequisite for wind turbines to turn. Here, the Polish authors noted that 'natural noise sources … always accompany the work of wind turbines and in such cases, they constitute an acoustic background, impossible to eliminate during noise measurement of wind turbines.' This is a fundamentally important point: wherever there are wind turbines generating infrasound, there is also wind itself generating infrasound, and it is impossible to disentangle the two. Indeed, every time I've been near wind turbines, easily the most dominant sound has been that of the wind buffeting my ears.

A South Australian study reported that infrasound measured near the ears of a person walking was 'similar in dominant frequency to that measured at the houses near wind farms'.[36] The infrasound near the walker's ears was 'significantly higher in level, with levels measured to be 10 dB higher than the highest levels measured near windfarms at 1.5 kilometres away where residences may be located.' In 2013, the South Australian government's Environmental Protection Authority and Resonate Acoustics measured infrasound in a variety of urban and rural settings. The latter included locations near and well away from windfarms. They reported that in urban settings, measured infrasound ranged between 60 and 70 dB. In fact, at two locations, the EPA's own offices and an office with a low frequency noise complaint, building air-conditioning systems were identified as significant sources of infrasound. These locations exhibited some of the highest levels of infrasound measured during the study.

The authors concluded:

> This study concludes that the level of infrasound at houses near the wind turbines assessed is no greater than that experienced in other urban and rural environments, and that the contribution of

36 Stead, Cooper and Evans 2014.

> wind turbines to the measured infrasound levels is insignificant in comparison with the background level of infrasound in the environment.[37]

To summarise, while prolonged exposure to extreme levels of infrasound can have deleterious effects on humans when it is very loud and very prolonged, wind turbines generate far less than other sources are known to make. The evidence remains the same: some people near wind turbines find the audible noise annoying, some of them find it stressful, and some of them lose sleep due to stress.

247 symptoms and diseases, and counting

While it went nowhere fast in the health and medical fields, Pierpont's book precipitated an avalanche of claims about symptoms and diseases being caused or aggravated by wind turbines. From the time I first became interested in this phenomenon, I began to notice a wide variety of such claims on the internet. I was curious to see how many I could find and in January 2012 I set out to compile a list, including sources, most of which were the websites of opponents of windfarms and submissions they had made to governments. Within an hour or two of searching I had found nearly 50 and today the number has grown to an astonishing 247, which are listed in Appendix 1.

The Australian cartoonist 'First Dog on the Moon' found the list the perfect stimulation for a giant cartoon illustrating 244 of these horrors.[38] He then wrote and recited an ode to them for his then weekly radio slot on ABC Radio National.[39] Opponents of wind turbines, however, have reacted badly to the list, which as of September 2017 had been viewed 5700 times on the University of Sydney's eScholarship repository. These opponents argue that by publishing the list and regularly updating it with new claims as they are found, I am 'ridiculing' people who say they are ill. This is a peculiar charge, as it suggests that those who actively publicise these alleged problems want to have it both ways. They continue to publicise the allegations because they wish to promote awareness about the supposed harms being caused.

37 Evans, Cooper and Lenchine 2013.
38 First Dog on the Moon 2015a.
39 First Dog on the Moon 2015b.

Yet they say that it is disgraceful to compile a list of these complaints as I have done, because it invites ridicule. However, the list is simply a compendium of claims made by others: it is not a list I have somehow 'made up'. When you read it, you may ask whether you can recall a more diverse collection of threats to humanity. Old Testament accounts of pestilence and plague seem mild compared to the manifold problems attributed to wind turbines. Almost every conceivable health problem has been attributed to windfarms at one time or another – yet many European countries have numerous windfarms without experiencing an epidemic of these symptoms.

Curiously, many of the symptoms on the list are common to similar lists promoted by victims of other highly questionable non-diseases. For example, an article on the frequently described non-disease 'pyroluria' lists 72 symptoms including difficulty remembering dreams, inability to think clearly, emotional instability and 'severe inner tension', with the author noting that most symptoms are 'vague, ambiguous and non-descript and could be attributed to virtually any trivial or serious illness'.[40] Wi-fi phobics and self-identifying 'electrosensitives' also promote very similar symptom lists, with cognitive decline, fatigue, heart palpitations, sleep problems and headaches commonly mentioned.[41] What many of these symptoms have in common is that they are common expressions of anxiety. We explore this further in Chapter 5. Of all the doomsday claims we've heard about the consequences of living near windfarms, an October 2012 submission by the Buddhist Tharpaland International Retreat Centre in Scotland to the Australian Senate committee convened by John Madigan must take first prize.[42] It spells out the full extent of the apocalypse that the authors believe threatens any nation embracing wind power:

- A decline in general public health and wellbeing, including a major increase in cancer, heart disease and immune-deficiency related diseases, entailing illness, suicide and violent crime, adding a further burden on the health system.
- A decline in standards throughout the educational system, due to a degeneration of learning ability, which depends upon the ability to develop concentration.

40 Sakula 2016.
41 Johnson n.d.
42 Tharpaland International Retreat Centre 2012.

- The main economic sector within the Scottish economy – tourism – could be wiped out.
- Spiritual centres and communities could be forced to close and disperse.

I do not believe I have ever read a more all-inclusive statement of the alleged perils of windfarms to the very fabric of a nation. I have worked in public health since the mid 1970s. In all this time, I have never encountered anything in the history of disease across the millennia that has been said to cause even a fraction of the problems attributed to windfarms. Other than perhaps the aftermath of a nuclear blast, there is nothing known to medicine that comes close to the morbid apocalypse described by anti-wind groups. Wind power is blamed for 'numerous serious illnesses and, yes, many deaths, mainly from unusual cancers',[43] which have oddly enough never come to the attention of any coroner. Did you know that wind turbines can cause lung cancer, leukaemia, diabetes, herpes, 'electromagnetic spasms in the skull', infertility and the ghastly sounding 'loss of bowels'? Any very common problem known to affect literally millions if not billions of people across the world (sleep problems, high blood pressure, lack of concentration, forgetfulness, poor performance at school, nosebleeds, muscle twitches) can be explained by exposure to wind turbines. But there are some benefits, too. Those who are overweight can lose kilograms through exposure to wind turbines – while the excessively slim can gain weight! Is this magic? All of these claims can be found in Appendix 1. As my collecting efforts rolled on, I amused myself by googling random health problems. One day I entered 'haemorrhoids', and sure enough, there it was too.

> People living near wind turbines have been shown to suffer from VAD [vibroacoustic disease] as a result of their exposure to the noise. Stage III is severe and occurs with over 10 years of exposure to LFN. It causes psychiatric disturbances, haemorrhages of nasal, digestive and conjunctive mucosa, nose bleeds, varicose veins and haemorrhoids, duodenal ulcers, spastic colitis, decrease in visual acuity, headaches, severe joint pain, intense muscular pain, and neurological disturbances.[44]

43 Whisson 2011.
44 Noisegirl 2014.

Animals too

It's not just humans that are affected. The ever-expanding collection of diseases and symptoms attributed to wind turbines (see Appendix 1) includes many affecting domestic and wild animals. Almost every known malformation in birds and farm animals has been laid at the feet of wind turbines by their critics.

Did you know that 'seagulls no longer follow the plough in areas near wind turbines … the seagulls have learned that the worms have all been driven away … They must go elsewhere for their food.' This can happen as far as 18 kilometres from a turbine! Whales have their sonar systems disrupted, chickens won't lay, and sheep's wool is poorer in quality. Tragically, a 'peahen refused to go near a peacock' and dogs 'stare blankly at walls', ignoring their owners.

Other more interesting reports include the extinction of bees; a farmer opining that echidnas (Australia's iconic spiked monotreme) are disoriented by turbines, causing them to 'dig up more soil looking for food than before', and that they could 'pinpoint the location of their food source much more accurately back then [before turbines were installed]'; and the death in 2009 of 'more than 400 goats' from 'exhaustion' on an unnamed, outlying Taiwanese island[45] – a report still unquestioningly displayed today on the Waubra Foundation website. Four hundred is a nice big round number for dead goats and, oddly enough, it's the same big round number of goats that allegedly also 'dropped dead' in New Zealand.[46]

In 2013 in Nova Scotia, the Canadian Atlantic province where midwinter temperatures fall to -20 degrees Celsius, a small emu farm closed down. There's nothing unusual about this. Investment in emu farming was an ill-fated get-rich-quick bubble that burst in Canada over a decade ago. It has been described as a 'failed industry'.[47] But what made this sad story even sadder was that the husband and wife team behind it blamed the closure on wind turbines, saying they had seen many of their birds lose weight and die of 'stress'. Tellingly, no necropsies were performed on the 20 birds that died, prompting one commenter to write, 'So they didn't have necropsies performed on any of the animals? That is extremely irresponsible farming. The

45 Anon. 2009.

46 Raferty 2012.

47 Turvey and Sparling 2002.

department of Agriculture should be called in to inspect for animal cruelty.'[48] In emus' native home of Australia, they don't tend to be kept in pens and fed on pellets. The birds roam freely around turbines, among sheep and cattle, and never in -20 degrees Celsius weather. Anti-windfarm websites are awash with these astonishing claims that seem to have escaped the relevant authorities. Such catastrophic events would always attract huge attention from government authorities concerned about the possibility of a serious disease outbreak that might threaten a nation's livestock. As anyone with even a passing familiarity with farming knows, mass or unusual deaths in livestock are of intense interest to governments because of concerns about infectious diseases with the potential to devastate the farming sector, export trade or even animal to human transmission. Concern about diseases like brucellosis, avian influenza and the Hendra virus see authorities swiftly isolate farms and destroy all remaining stock. Massive publicity follows. But when 400 goats unaccountably 'drop dead' or a farmer reports decimation of their flock of emus, these same government authorities are nowhere to be seen. Try to find news about government action on such incidents and instead you will only find unverified anecdotes. Try searching for any official corroboration and you'll be looking for a long time. It must be an international conspiracy of silence, engineered by the wind industry!

'Wind turbine syndrome' symptoms are common in all communities

All of the human health problems windfarm opponents attribute to wind turbines occur in *every* community, regardless of whether they are near windfarms or not. Forty-five percent of people report symptoms of insomnia at least once a week.[49] Anxiety and depression are widespread. Getting old? Is your hair turning grey or receding? Perhaps your eyesight, hearing, or balance problems are increasing with age? Are you gaining or losing weight? As we saw earlier (and in Appendix 1), all of these very common 'problems' are among those said to be caused by wind turbines. Many of the claims about animals fall into the same category. Yolkless eggs and those without shells are phenomena known to every bird breeder.[50] But when such eggs are laid by chickens

48 Canadian Broadcasting Corporation 2013.
49 Wilsmore et al. 2013

belonging to someone who doesn't like windfarms, they can only have been caused by the dastardly turbines. Dogs, horses, sheep or cattle getting listless, skittish, off their food … or anything, really: wind turbines are to blame if you don't like windfarms. Every day in every country, thousands of people are diagnosed for the first time with one of countless health problems. Most live nowhere near a windfarm. They weren't having the symptoms that drove them to the doctor a few months ago, and once they have a diagnosis, they start thinking about what might have caused it. If they don't like the look of windfarms, or if they have been exposed to scary tales about all the things that wind turbines can do, and if they happen to live near a windfarm, then the *post hoc ergo propter hoc* ('after therefore because of') fallacy can powerfully kick in to make sense of their new problem. We explore this further in Chapter 5.

Florid language

Clues about the likely veracity of the claims being made by windfarm opponents can be found in the words they use to describe their experiences. As one wades through claims about the alleged harms caused by wind turbines, it is impossible not to be struck by the propensity of opponents to use language that immediately makes you say, 'Uh-oh, what's going on here?' Let's consider some examples.

How loud?

If you have a spare couple of hours and the fortitude to watch all 117 minutes of *Pandora's pinwheels*, the 2011 home movie made by the open opponent of windfarms Lilli-Anne Green, who gave evidence to the 2015 Senate inquiry about her 'research' on windfarms,[51] you will hear many truly bizarre statements. The film includes interviews with windfarm opponents in New Zealand and the Waubra district of Victoria. Nobody interviewed has a good word to say about wind energy. There are endless examples of florid language, such as:

50 See for example https://www.beautyofbirds.com/eggproblems.html.
51 Green 2015.

> 'It was continually like a 737 [jet] about to take off and [it] never did and [it] went on for hour after hour after hour.'
> 'Like a train going over a bridge.'
> 'A plane that won't go away.'
> 'Someone hiding a bumble bee in your ear.'
> 'Sometimes it's like a jet plane has parked itself above.'
> 'Windfarms are tuning forks glued to a hill ... they vibrate the ground.'

A witness who gave evidence to the Senate inquiry on 19 June 2015, Charles Barber, stated: 'I visited them on a very, very windy day; I was out of the car, and within half an hour I felt like I had been at the Rolling Stones for four hours.'[52] I spoke with Mr Barber outside the Senate hearings at Sydney's Parliament House on 29 June 2015 and told him I was curious about his Rolling Stones comparison, as I'd seen them three times, including once from the mosh pit of their February 2003 gig at Sydney's 2200-capacity art deco Enmore Theatre.

'Have you ever been to a Rolling Stones gig?' I asked him. He confirmed he had. But he was unshifting in his comparison. I smiled at him, giving him permission to confess he had used a little rhetorical licence in his testimony. But Mr Barber was not for turning. Having been to hundreds of rock gigs, and having sung in a loud covers band myself for ten years, it was hard for me to know where to go next in such a conversation.

How painful?

Ann Gardner, a prominent opponent living near the AGL-owned Macarthur windfarm in Victoria, drew on some unique experiences to explain how painful the effects of wind turbines can be. She has apparently experienced being inside a microwave oven when it is turned on: she told radio broadcaster Alan Jones on 21 August 2015, 'I feel like my body's been cooked in a microwave.'[53] Meanwhile her husband apparently knows what it feels like to be repeatedly hit in the head with an axe ('All of sudden he's hit by this bolt of pressure as if someone's chopping him in the back of the head with an axe').[54]

52 Commonwealth of Australia 2015b.
53 Sky News 2015.
54 Fair Dinkum Radio 2014.

Jan Hetherington, another prominent windfarm objector from Victoria, also seems to have had some very violent experiences that she can draw on in describing the sensation.

> **Alan Jones:** You said to me early this morning, 'I woke up at 4.35 with a very sharp ice pick stabbing on the top of my head …'
> **Jan Hetherington:** Oh yes.
> **Alan Jones:** '… behind my right ear.'
> **Jan Hetherington:** Yes.
> **Alan Jones:** 'This was followed by vibration running through my body, then came the headache in my right temple and right eye. I just had to get out of bed. Unfortunately, there's no running away from this infrasound. Nothing can stop it.'
> **Jan Hetherington:** That's right, that's right, it is terrible … oh it's hard to talk about it because it's so, it's so real, it happens.[55]

Heartfelt testimonies like these from people claiming to be suffering health problems can never be a substitute for evidence-based assessment of their claims. These accounts can only be an important start to the process of assessing what is going on. And for all the fervour of these personal accounts, one very inconvenient problem quickly emerges. There is no body of case reports – not even a small one – to be found in the medical research literature (see Chapter 3).

We have all at one time or another suspected or believed that a particular symptom is likely to have been caused by something we have eaten or been exposed to, or by some activity we have engaged in. But we are often mistaken. The history of medicine is littered with sometimes highly entrenched, widely accepted beliefs about the cause of particular symptoms that were subsequently discarded when alternative explanations arose from new evidence. When someone tells you passionately and in great detail that they are ill, the social expectation is that we should be empathic, sympathetic, and accept their account. If their account raises doubts or questions, we may be reluctant to forcefully or even tactfully try to repudiate their beliefs about the cause of their illness. Medical sociologists have for decades noted that adopting the 'sick role' can confer social advantages on those who say that they are ill.[56] These can range from being treated with

---

55 Stop These Things 2015a.
56 Mechanic and Volkart 1961.

extra consideration and care by those around you to being exempted from normal family, social and work obligations and even receiving compensation.

When we see people making often highly emotional statements in the media about how much they are suffering, it can be awkward to publicly question whether the accounts they give should be taken at face value. It is bad manners to cast doubt on whether an alleged victim is indeed ill. Questioning a person's claim that they are being made ill by windfarms is likely to be taken as an affront. They may get angry and claim that they are not being 'respected'. But concern about being considered insensitive should never cause such questioning to be abandoned. Claims by individuals that they are being made ill from windfarms can be considered from two perspectives. First, we can ask whether those making the claims are genuinely suffering the symptoms they say they are suffering. Second, if we are satisfied that they are, we can ask how reasonable is their explanation that their symptoms are caused by exposure to wind turbines.

In the next chapters, we consider the evidence – or lack of it – for the claims made by windfarm opponents, and look at what the most recent major review of the evidence on windfarms and health says.

3

Core problems with health claims about windfarms

Those who claim that wind turbines are harmful to human and animal health argue that the infrasound and low-frequency noise generated by the turbines turning are *direct* causes of the symptoms experienced by those who report problems. They passionately reject the suggestion that their negative experiences are in any way mediated by personal or social factors like antipathy toward windfarms, anxiety about the possible effects of exposure, a general disposition toward complaining, noise 'sensitivity', or any wider motivation to discredit windfarms.

As we saw in Chapter 2, windfarms existed in Australia long before these health complaints began to surface. The elephant in the room is this: if wind turbines *did* cause immediate effects in a proportion of people as claimed, why were there no clinical or even media reports of these problems between 1993 and 2004, when David Iser's unpublished study about Toora emerged?[1] If the claims are to be believed, why are there no records of the alleged problems in news media, wind-company records, or case reports published in medical journals? In this chapter and the next, we will consider some of the immediately obvious problems that arise for arguments that wind turbines are the direct cause of health problems in those exposed to them. We consider problems arising from claims that turbines cause rapid, acute effects; the idea that only those who are 'susceptible' suffer; and the mystery of why there are no case reports published in the medical literature about people suffering from health problems caused by wind turbines.

---

1 Iser 2004.

We will then examine the proposition that it is only large, new turbines that might cause problems; the peculiar phenomenon of wind turbine health complaints being a disease that seems to occur mainly in English-speaking nations; an interesting antidote for health problems caused by wind turbines (the drug 'money'); and finally the frequently made claims about windfarms causing people to 'abandon' their homes. We conclude the chapter by looking at the proposition that wind turbines are 'the new tobacco'.

In the chapter following, we will then give a critical account of several of the windfarm opponents' most often cited studies, which they seem to believe make a strong case for direct adverse effects of wind turbines on health.

Acute effects from wind turbine exposure

> After a period of about one hour, which time had been spent setting up instrumentation in the basement and using a laptop computer in the kitchen, the author began to feel a significant sense of lethargy. As further time passed this progressed to difficulty in concentration accompanied by nausea, so that around the three-hour mark, he was feeling distinctly unwell.
>
> He thought back over the day, to remember what food he had eaten and whether he might have undertaken any other action that might bring about this effect. He had light meals of cereal for breakfast and salad for lunch, so it seemed unlikely that either could have been responsible ... It was only after about 3.5 hours that it suddenly struck home that these symptoms were being brought about by the wind turbines.—*Malcolm Swinbanks, windfarm opponent and acoustic engineer*[2]

Windfarm opponents repeatedly argue that turbines cause both acute, rapid-onset effects and chronic, long-gestation health problems. The claim about acute effects in particular creates major problems for their argument.

It is common to read accounts like that above of people having been adversely affected within hours or even minutes of being exposed

2 Swinbanks 2015.

to turbines. The anti-windfarm film *Pandora's pinwheels* provides many examples of opponents talking about such acute, immediate effects experienced when wind turbines are turning.[3] They claim that when the turbines start up when the wind blows, the problems commence, but when the turbines stop turning or the sufferer spends time away from home, all is well and their symptoms reduce or stop. A seven-minute video promoted by the Waubra Foundation also shows several victims making these points.[4]

An unpublished Canadian report described a visit to turbine-exposed houses where the researchers involved in the study claim to have become affected almost immediately: 'The onset of adverse health effects was swift, within twenty minutes, and persisted for some time after leaving the study area'.[5] Apparently in all seriousness, Sarah Laurie from the Waubra Foundation told an April 2012 meeting of anti-turbine protestors in the Victorian town of Mortlake that one night in a house in proximity to a wind turbine saw 'just about everybody … every five or ten minutes needing to go to the toilet'.[6] So, let's assume the residents went to bed at 11 pm and got up at 7 am. If we take Laurie at her word, that would mean over 60 visits to the toilet for each person during the night. Perhaps her claim was nothing more than rhetorical hyperbole for her supporters, common in motivational talks. Perhaps all she intended to say was that the people in the house went to the toilet more than usual that night. Perhaps her audience wondered whether those in the house had been drinking a lot. Did many among them have prostate problems that might have added to their need to urinate so often? And perhaps they might have wondered why, if it were true that those present had collectively experienced a sudden Niagara of urination, did this bizarre phenomenon apparently go unreported to medical authorities?

If I were in a house with multiple occupants and 'just about everybody' came down with repeated bouts of the same symptoms throughout the night, I would expect that those present might find the experience disturbing and formally report it. This would almost certainly occur with food poisoning or exposure to some unidentified environmental pathogen. But as we will see, a mysteriously large

3 PR Resources Inc. 2011.
4 Waubra Foundation 2011a.
5 Benedetti, Durando and Vighetti 2014.
6 Unpublished transcript received by the authors.

number of hand-on-heart claims about the serious health problems caused by windfarms never come to the attention of the doctors of those who make them.

If it was the case that wind turbines caused rapid-onset, acute health effects, a big problem immediately arises for those making this claim. Windfarms existed in Australia long before the first claims about health ever surfaced. Australia's first, the Ten Mile Lagoon windfarm near Esperance, Western Australia, started generating power in 1993 so has been operational for 24 years. There have been no recorded health or noise complaints from any of the residents living within ten kilometres of the windfarm (ten kilometres is a distance commonly argued by opponents as the distance within which people are affected). Victoria's first windfarm, Codrington, has been operating since June 2001, and has 14 turbines, each capable of producing 1.3 MW. There's nothing new about large wind turbines in Australia. And yet health complaints are relatively recent, with the few in Codrington occuring after a visit to the area by a vocal opponent with an interest in spreading anxiety.

Only the 'susceptible' suffer

Windfarm opponents are well aware that a very small minority of people in any given community will report symptoms that they attribute to windfarms. Nor do they argue that the many health problems listed in Appendix 1 are unique to those exposed to turbines, but only that turbines can cause or aggravate these problems in 'susceptible' people. This is like saying that the only people affected are those who are affected.

They nonetheless need to advance some explanation of why most people are unaffected. Here, they point to other exposures that affect people differently. Most people can eat particular foods (e.g. those containing gluten or peanut) and experience no ill-effects whatsoever. Others have adverse reactions which can be swift and sometimes very serious, even life-threatening. Some suffer motion sickness in cars, boats or aircraft while others do not. And some, they argue, react badly to noise, including the sound emitted from wind turbines.

We all understand that infectious pathogens like viruses and bacteria can have a wide range of infectivity: only a proportion of people exposed to these agents acquire those diseases. But there is a thundering great rhino in the room that rather wrecks this quaint analogy when it is applied to windfarms.

Every community exposed to infectious or toxic agents like influenza, Legionella, Ebola, very high air pollution particle counts, salmonella in food, and so on will report 'incident' (i.e. new) cases following those exposures. *Every* community will have members who are susceptible to motion sickness. But there are *no* recorded instances of cholera being found in a local water supply where no one was stricken with cholera.

With windfarms, a very large number have never attracted any health or noise complaints from nearby residents. For example, when we searched for evidence of health or noise complaints in all of Australia in 2012, we found that 33 out of 51 (64.7 percent) of Australian windfarms, including 18 of 33 (54.5 percent) with turbine sizes larger than 1 MW, had never been subject to noise or health complaints.[7] These 33 farms had an estimated 21,633 residents living within a five-kilometre radius and had operated complaint-free for a cumulative 267 years. Western Australia and Tasmania had seen no complaints. There is no remotely plausible explanation why, in these 33 areas, there was no one apparently 'susceptible' to the alleged ill effects of windfarms. Why were there no susceptible people in two whole states? Are Western Australians and Tasmanians made of sterner stuff than their eastern counterparts? There is also a problem of inconsistency with the motion sickness analogy. In a video posted by Stop These Things, several members of a family describe being badly affected by wind turbines.[8] The argument appears to be that the alleged effects of turbine noise affect all or most of those in a house. But motion sickness typically does not 'run in families': we generally see situations where perhaps only one person in a family gets car or sea sick, rather than most or all. If turbine noise is affecting most occupants in a small proportion of houses near turbines, problems immediately arise for the 'individual susceptibility' hypothesis. An alternative explanation, that the adverse reaction is *socially* 'contagious' within communicative environments where the turbines are disliked and provoke anxiety, is very plausible. We discuss this in Chapter 5.

Opponents also repeatedly say that animals such as sheep, cattle, dogs and poultry are badly affected, with problems like malformations,

---

7 Chapman, St George, Waller and Cakic 2013.
8 Stop These Things 2013c.

sudden death, sterility and yolkless eggs being common (see Appendix 1). Against this, on any trip to a windfarm region, one can find hundreds of livestock grazing contentedly around the turbines. In Tasmania there is a poultry farm at Sassafras with a wind turbine at the front gate, very near the poultry barns, that helps power the farm.[9] Is the argument here that only some animals are 'susceptible' too?

A disease that only speaks English?

The 'individual susceptibility' argument faces its biggest test when we look at the international pattern of complaints. It has been frequently noted that complaining about wind turbines is very obviously an Anglophone phenomenon. Modern multi-megawatt wind turbines have operated since 1978 in the USA and Europe. Today, there are an estimated 314,000 turbines in operation globally.[10] European nations with windfarms include Belgium, Cyprus, Denmark, England, France, Germany, Greece, Ireland, Italy, Lithuania, the Netherlands, Poland, Portugal, Romania, Scotland, Spain, and Sweden. The turbines are often located very near cities, towns and villages (see Figures 3.1 and 3.2), thus exposing a huge number of people across Europe to their putative sickening sound emissions on a daily basis. Anyone who has spent time in these nations will have seen many of them.[11]

Yet windfarm health complaints have nearly all occurred in English-speaking nations. In Canada, parts of English-speaking Ontario have experienced many complaints while neighbouring Francophone Quebec sees little opposition. In Australia, complaints have been concentrated around farms targeted by anti-windfarm groups, suggesting the phenomenon is a 'communicated disease'.[12]

Since I became interested in windfarms and the problems they allegedly cause, I've gone out of my way to ask my international colleagues when I see them whether this is a 'problem' in their countries. European and Asian public health colleagues tend to ask me to repeat the question, as if they were confused about what I was asking.

---

9 Kelley 2014.

10 Global Wind Energy Council 2016.

11 For a map showing the location of turbines in Europe, see http://bit.ly/2ij8FwM.

12 Chapman, St George, Waller and Cakic 2013.

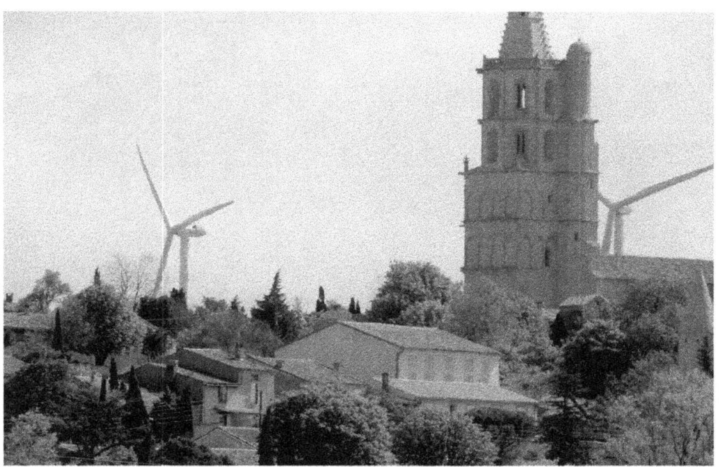

Figure 3.1 The village of Avignonet-Lauragais in the commune of Haute-Garonne in south-western France. Source: Simon Chapman.

They then nearly always say that they have never even heard of the issue.

I once asked two friends, one of whom was a former health and medical reporter for the *Sydney Morning Herald*, if they would ask local residents about the issue as they undertook a six-week walk in northern Spain, where there are many windfarms. When they returned home they said, 'Look, we asked quite a few people about it in the first few days when we were walking near windfarms. But people always looked at us as if we were some sort of weirdos, asking about that. No one we spoke with had ever heard of it. So we just stopped asking after a while.'

I stressed this point in my submission to the 2015 Australian Senate inquiry into windfarms.[13] In their final report, the committee stated:

> Professor Chapman has argued that complaints of adverse health effects from wind turbines tend to be limited to Anglophone nations. However, the committee has received written and oral evidence from several sources directly contradicting this view. The German Medical

13 Chapman 2015b.

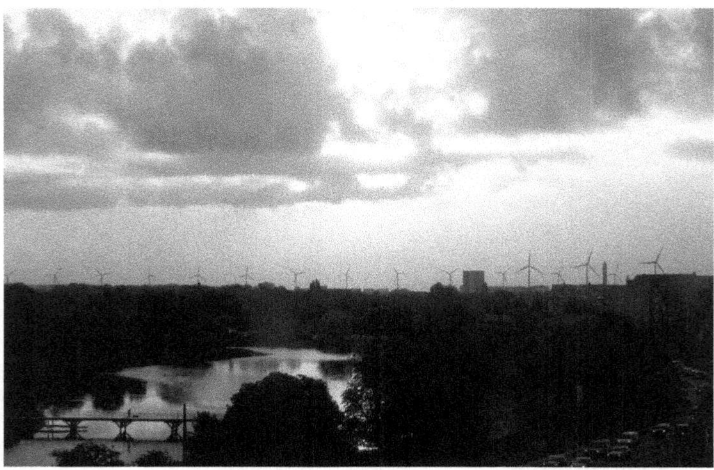

Figure 3.2 Wind turbines surrounding suburban Copenhagen, Denmark. Source: Simon Chapman.

Assembly recently submitted a motion to the executive board of the German Medical Association calling for the German government to provide the necessary funding to research adverse health effects. This would not have happened in the absence of community concern. Moreover, Dr Bruce Rapley has argued that in terms of the limited number – and concentrated nature – of windfarm complaints:

'It is the reporting which is largely at fault. The fact is that people are affected by this, and the numbers are in the thousands. I only have to look at the emails that cross my desk from all over the world. I get bombarded from the UK, Ireland, France, Canada, the United States, Australia, Germany. There are tonnes of these things out there but, because the system does not understand the problem, nor does it have a strategy, many of those complaints go unlisted.'[14]

Unlike Rapley, with his excited and vacuous talk of being 'bombarded' by 'thousands' and 'tonnes' of complainants but no record of having made these publicly available, I took the trouble to transparently

14 Commonwealth of Australia 2015b.

attempt to quantify estimates of complainants in Australia and submit these to a peer-reviewed journal, where they were published.[15] As to the claim that the German Medical Association was representing 'community concern', enquiries revealed that it was simply passing on the concerns of just one of its thousands of members.

The Senate committee declared that it had received submissions that 'contradicted' my point about Anglophone nations dominating complaints. These included one from Lilli-Anne Green, whom they described as 'the Chief Executive Officer of a healthcare consulting firm in the United States'. When questioned about the name of her company by Senator Urquhart, Green replied, 'I do not want that on the record … I am speaking as a private citizen.'[16] She later stated, 'I am the only employee at this point in time.' She affirmed that '300,000 physicians have undertaken training' through her company. Green is also an active member of Wind Wise Massachusetts, an anti-windfarm group. Green stated in evidence that in 2012 she and her husband had interviewed people complaining about windfarms in 'France, Germany, Holland, Denmark and Sweden – who either needed an interpreter to speak with us or who spoke broken English.' Her submitted evidence also stated that she had interviewed people in China and Portugal. When Senator Urquhart said to her, 'I could not find any of the transcripts, either in your submission or online. I am sorry if I have missed them,' Ms Green replied: 'You have not missed them. In the company we are still in the process of editing the films. It is a huge undertaking of many months, at huge expense. There is a lot of information that is still being edited.'

> **Senator Urquhart:** Are you able to provide copies of the transcripts and the full names of the people you interviewed?
> **Ms Green:** No. It is on film; it is videotaped interviews, and the film is being edited.

Even David Leyonhjelm noted, with great understatement, 'I appreciate we are not pretending this is a gold-plated, statistical survey.'

Green's submission to the committee consisted of a set of slides about her interviews with windfarm opponents.[17] They contain no data at all. It was beyond belief that the committee could cite this amateur

15 Chapman, Joshi and Fry 2014; Chapman, St George, Waller and Cakic 2013.
16 Commonwealth of Australia 2015a.
17 Green 2015.

'study' as evidence of anything other than Green being someone totally immersed in the global anti-windfarm network and committed to its objectives. There is not a single piece of data in the submission, despite it purporting to be the 'findings' of Green's global investigations. This epitomised the scientific illiteracy of the committee's majority report. The committee also cited three Danish submissions of a similarly woeful quality, containing bald data-free statements like 'there are health problems at many places'.[18] One was from a mink farmer who lived near turbines and claimed that in one year, 'There were over 2000 dead mink whelps … And the third part of them was seriously deformed.' He also claimed to have had heart pains, and that 'The doctors told me after the examination that there was nothing wrong with my heart.'[19] Another of the Danish submissions stated:

> There has never been conducted any medical research in these problems in DK [Denmark], even if the complaints have been increasing since the 1980s. The complaints are dismissed everywhere and no statistics are available from the wt [wind turbine] producers/ manufacturers, all state authorities and all local/communal authorities. The sufferers are asked to speak with their doctors, but these have never got ANY information from health or other authorities. The *Danish Medical Journal* has never published anything about health risks for wt neighbors.[20]

Presumably, this is all a national conspiracy to cover up case reports of victims.

It looks like whoever wrote the Senate report was told to 'find some submissions from non-English-speaking countries that we can throw back at Chapman' and never bothered to actually read them.

The European Platform Against Windfarms website, run by activist Mark Duchamp (see Chapter 2), today lists 1276 organisations in 31 European countries allegedly opposed to windfarms. This is an increase since 2012, when the site listed 554 from 24 nations. Ketan Joshi took the trouble to look at a lot of those listed. His hilarious blog on his findings is worth reading. For example:

---

18 Gallandy-Jakobson 2015.
19 Olesen 2015.
20 Johansson 2015.

> France serves as a great case study. Of the 201 signatories listed for France only 54 included links to websites. Of the 54 URLs listed, there were seven dead links, a link to a wiki page, a link to a website about the ocean (they provide 'rentals, watersports, scuba diving, windsurf, kite, sailing, snorkelling, brokers, marinas, provisioning, ship chandlers, schools, boatyards etc.'), and a website about horses (an organisation that seemingly once opposed a nearby wind development).[21]

One link to an Italian site (Comitato Monte dei Cucchi) took you to a Japanese site on the best ways to cook rice.

Case reports

Most claims about the alleged health impacts of wind turbines come either from those who say they are being harmed, or from a small, often internationally networked group of dedicated windfarm opponents whose personal identities are often strongly bound up in their mission to 'defeat' the scourge of 'industrial windfarms'. We will profile some of the latter group's most prominent Australian members in Chapter 6. Here, we consider the role of those who believe they are suffering wind turbine syndrome, and the importance of case reports in assessing their claims.

Victims of diseases and health problems have had a long and often vitally important role in the evolution of the identification, understanding, treatment and prevention of disease. Indeed, our understanding of disease always starts with people who are affected coming to the attention of those in the health professions for the first time. Case reports of newly identified health problems have always been published in medical journals and in the writings of the ancient precursors of today's physicians and other medical specialists. Today, newly identified and new strains of infectious and vector-borne diseases continue to occur (HIV, Ebola and Zika are three well-known examples from recent decades), and likewise whole new areas of complex disease aetiology have also emerged. Metabolic syndrome,[22]

---

21 Joshi 2012b.

22 Rodriguez-Monforte, Sanchez, Barrio, Costa and Flores-Mateo 2016.

the exponential rise in type-2 diabetes,[23] and rapidly emerging concerns about endocrine-disrupting chemicals[24] are just three examples. As further case studies come to light and are either reported in clinical journals or brought to the attention of health authorities for formal investigation, principles of disease investigation are used to address basic questions that include the quality of evidence, whether a relationship between a putative cause and a disease outcome is a mere statistical association or whether and to what extent criteria for establishing causality (such as the Bradford-Hill criteria[25]) are satisfied by the evidence available. As studies accumulate, systematic review and meta-analytic protocols are applied to the body of evidence to try to determine what conclusions can be drawn. Case reports are always the start of any process that leads to health authorities declaring that an agent, environmental exposure or behaviour causes a health problem. However, such case reports are only the very first step in what needs to happen before such causal conclusions can be drawn.

We have looked in vain for any clinical reports published in non-junk, peer-reviewed journals about the health problems said to be caused by exposure to wind turbines. Such clinical reports are common when doctors encounter unusual health problems with hitherto unreported possible aetiology. The closest we found was a 2013 news report mentioning a Massachusetts vestibular specialist, Steven Rauch, who had a patient referred to him by Nina Pierpont (who coined the term 'wind turbine syndrome').[26] Rauch said he was 'unwilling' to rule out wind turbine syndrome as a real medical condition, and that it was a 'plausible' explanation. No report of the case was found in any medical journal. If this was a phenomenon with any substance, we would by now surely have seen a long series of such reports published. Strangely, none of the three medical vanguards of windfarm-caused 'disease' whom we discussed in Chapter 2 – Amanda Harry, David Iser and Nina Pierpont – appears to have published any such case reports in the peer-reviewed literature, in spite of the obvious importance to their concerns of doing so.

As we saw earlier, the nearest we have to such a report is the case report of one individual publicised at a conference by a group

23 Fazeli Farsani, van der Aa, van der Vorst, Knibbe and de Boer 2013.
24 Giulivo, Lopez de Alda, Capri and Barcelo 2016.
25 Fedak, Bernal, Capshaw and Gross 2015.
26 James 2013.

promoting the unrecognised 'vibro-acoustic disease'.[27] This research has never been published in any indexed peer-reviewed journal. Indeed, it would be an interesting exercise to survey medical practitioners working in townships near windfarms in the attempt to find anyone who has ever formally diagnosed even a single case of 'wind turbine syndrome' in Australia or elsewhere. If any such cases emerged from such a study, all (de-identified) relevant case notes could be made available to a panel of specialised doctors appointed by the Royal Australasian College of Physicians. Consent would of course be needed from the patients concerned, but as they would be entirely confident that their diagnosis was real, they would surely leap at the opportunity to have this corroborated by an independent, expert assessment process.

Past medical records of complainants

Another way of considering the veracity of health claims about turbines would be for those making the complaints to consent to having their past medical records examined. Such records from both before and after the operation of the suspect windfarm could settle the question both of whether the complaints were sufficiently serious to have been given medical attention, and whether the complainants had these problems before the windfarm commenced operation. In Canada in 2012, the Ontario Environmental Review Tribunal called for a group of 'wind action' plaintiffs to produce such records. Tellingly, they declined, and their case fell over.[28] They then complained that these medical records would have been too onerous to obtain:

> It is clear that it will not be possible to obtain and organize documents for witnesses prior to the start date of the Zephyr appeal, which is currently scheduled for March 7th. While we have an impressive staff, they cannot perform a Biblical miracle – i.e., produce in 6 days all the 23 witnesses' medical records for the past 10 years.[29]

---

27 Alves-Pereira and Branco 2007; Chapman and St George 2013.

28 Farber 2012; Environmental Review Tribunal of Ontario 2012.

29 Ontario Highlands Friends of Wind Power 2012.

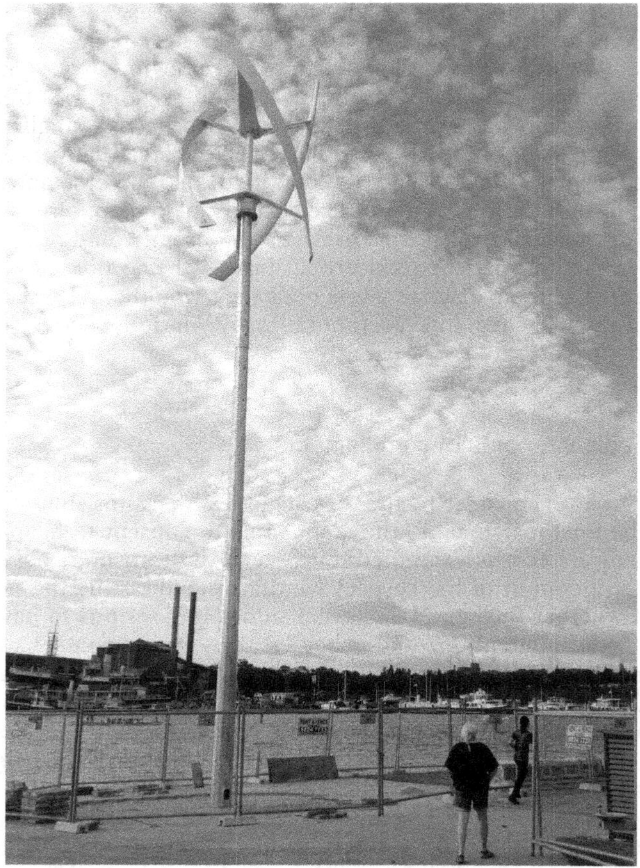

Figure 3.3 A micro-turbine in Jubilee Park in the inner Sydney surburb of Glebe, New South Wales. Photograph by Stephan Ridgway via Flickr, CC BY 2.0: http://bit.ly/2gVkTeQ.

This is a questionable claim: my GP can produce my records instantly onscreen, going back nearly 20 years. Canada has an advanced health care system, and producing medical records is highly unlikely to have been problematic.

Small turbines not noxious?

When it is pointed out that wind turbines existed in Australia long before health concerns emerged, one stock response from opponents is that in the years before health complaints were reported, the turbines operating were much smaller than those that are standard today. The implication is that only the very large turbines cause health complaints.

There are two problems with this answer. First, as mentioned, there were large wind turbines operating in Australia well before complaints started. These included those in Albany, Western Australia from October 2001 (1.9 MW turbines); Codrington, Victoria from 2003 (1.3 MW); Callicum Hills, Victoria from 2003 (1.5 MW); and Starfish Hill, South Australia, from 2003 (1.5 MW).

Second, a research paper from England examining residents' perception of the noise emanating from small or micro wind turbines 'showed individuals with a more negative attitude to wind turbines perceive more noise from a turbine located close to their dwelling and those perceiving more noise report increased levels of general symptoms.'[30] Even tiny micro turbines like the one in Jubilee Park in the inner Sydney suburb of Glebe (see Figure 3.3) are likely to draw negative responses from local people who don't like them. So where are all the complaints in Australia about the many small turbines that have been operating for years?

Is money an antidote to windfarm complaints?

> 'It's absolutely black and white. There's sort of half a dozen landowners who are supportive [i.e. those being paid to host turbines] who are blind and deaf to any contrary view. And there's virtually all of the rest of the community who are opposed to it.'—
> *Murray Martin, Palmerston, New Zealand*[31]

Wind turbine hosts almost never complain about the turbines that directly benefit them financially. This has been noted in several studies. For example, in 2014, Health Canada published a summary of the

30 Taylor, Eastwick, Lawrence and Wilson 2013.

31 PR Resources Inc. 2011.

results of a much-awaited $2.1 million investigation into the health effects of windfarms. The report noted: 'Annoyance was significantly lower among the 110 participants who received personal benefit, which could include rent, payments or other indirect benefits of having wind turbines in the area.'[32] Some have remarked that the 'money drug' must therefore be a very effective antidote to the onset of any health complaints. Below, we describe the only two known cases in Australia of complaints from people who were benefitting financially from wind turbines. There are no known complaints in Australia by current or past windfarm employees, who are daily exposed both point-blank and at larger distances to wind turbine sound emissions and vibrations.

A stock response to this observation from those opposing windfarms is to argue that there are many examples of landowners who agree to host wind turbines on their land and then suffer in silence without being able to speak out. The claim is made that they are 'gagged' by clauses in their contracts with wind companies forbidding them from complaining publicly about their experiences. They instead suffer silently, with all the subtexts of injustice and corporate bullying that go along with such a claim.

I raised this issue with the 2015 Madigan-chaired Senate committee, who fired back in their report that 'there have been several Australian windfarm hosts who have made submissions to this inquiry complaining of adverse health effects.' Several? A footnote in the report directs readers to four submissions where this is said to be documented.[33]

Submission 118, at page 3, refers only to a court case during which a wind energy company called two witnesses who hosted turbines on their properties and were 'bound by contracts not to speak against turbines'.[34] There is no evidence that these two people had complaints themselves and were suppressing them under duress. Submission 356, at page 2, states:

> Hosting property owners for the Capital Wind Farm have themselves stated they hear noise and have shadow flicker from the turbines, however they are able to sacrifices [sic] this for the income derived from hosting the turbines ... [35]

32 Health Canada 2014.

33 Australian Senate 2015.

34 Quinn 2015.

This unsubstantiated statement clearly provides no evidence of any host complaining. Submission 165 was authored by a person who initially signed a contract to host turbines at the planned Robertstown windfarm, which was never built. So it too is not an example of a host who has complained about operating turbines.[36]

This leaves two known turbine hosts throughout Australia who have complained about the turbines on their property. We consider these two cases below.

A tale of two turbine hosts

The first example is the Gares (Clive and Trina), who host 19 turbines on the AGL-owned North Brown Hill (Hallet 4) windfarm 17 kilometres from Jamestown in South Australia. The 2015 Senate report states that the Gares have earned $2 million over five years for hosting the 19 turbines: $400,000 per year, or an average of $21,053 per year per turbine. Their house has been soundproofed by the wind company.

Clive Gare told the Senate committee that he suffers 'sleep interruption, mild headaches, agitation and a general feeling of unease … only when the towers are turning, depending on the wind direction and wind strength.' His work requires him to work among the turbines so he suffers 'the full impacts of noise for days at a time without relief.' He said he would not buy a house within 20 kilometres of a windfarm, despite already living in such a house. I was intrigued about this and so asked around some contacts I had in the wind industry. This is what I was told.

When the windfarm was being planned, the Gares' property was considered as a possible location for the farm's electricity substation, which would have earned them considerable extra money if they had agreed to sell a parcel of land to the company. In the event, a decision was made to locate the substation on the property of a neighbour who was willing to sell a similar small parcel of land. Sources within AGL told me that this decision caused some tension between the Gares and the company. This context may be relevant to understanding why the Gares chose to raise their complaints to the Senate committee.

35 Martin 2015.

36 Schaefer 2015.

The second turbine host who has complained is David Mortimer. He lives near Millicent in South Australia, and is one of Australia's highest-profile critics of windfarms. Mortimer derives rental income from two turbines, which are part of the Lake Bonney windfarm. Mortimer bought a property in 1987 and agreed to the turbines being erected from 2004. In the ten years to May 2013, the Wattle Range Shire council had never received a health complaint from any resident. In the same period, Mortimer did not make a complaint to the windfarm operator, Infigen. Mortimer, however, has been a long-standing and vocal critic, claiming that he and his wife have been made ill by their exposure to the two turbines from around 2006 (although he did not make his claims public until 2012).

In about 2006 the Mortimers moved into a newly built house in the area with an expansive view, vacating their house on their property with the two turbines. In 2010, at a public consultation about the Woakine windfarm proposal, he learned that he would be able to see the proposed turbines from his new house. In his written submission to the planning process, he complained about the impact of the proposed Woakine development on his view and property values but did not mention health concerns.

Mortimer attended an anti-windfarm meeting at Mount Gambier on 27 March 2012, at which Senators Madigan and Xenophon spoke. There he heard for the first time allegations that windfarms make people sick. He claims that he then realised that windfarms were making him and his wife sick.[37] In his presentation to a community forum on King Island in Tasmania he noted that his doctor had not found a connection between the turbines and his maladies. Further, in submissions, Mortimer has reported that he has worked with fibreglass at home, a pastime that exposes him to toxic chemicals. He has also reported that he spent a significant portion of his naval career exposed to loud artillery noises. On 4 June 2012 he appeared on the television program *Today Tonight* describing his health problems.[38] He has since been interviewed on Sydney Radio 2GB by Alan Jones (January 2015)[39] and Steve Price (March 2013)[40] and has been covered extensively by the anonymously authored Stop These Things website (see Chapter 6). At a

37 Stop These Things 2013e.
38 Seven Network Pty Ltd 2012a.
39 Jones 2015.
40 Price 2015.

Stop These Things rally on 18 June 2013 he told the small audience that 'somewhere during the night it [turbine noise] is going to wake me up and I am going to find myself halfway down the passageway, trying to get away from scorpions and snakes and whatever the hell frightens the hell out of me.'[41]

On 18 June 2013 Mortimer spoke at a poorly attended anti-windfarm rally on the front lawn of Parliament House in Canberra, chaired by Alan Jones (see Chapter 6).[42] Here is part of what he said, with my emphasis in italics:

> Now, not terribly long ago, earlier this year, we went for a bit of a tour up around north of Adelaide, etc., *and we happened to turn up at [Mary Morris'] place, and we stayed the night there. Now we could look all around us, and we couldn't see a turbine within coo-ee, and so we thought there are no turbines around.* Now, we went to sleep about ten o'clock that night in our little camper, which is parked down the road, and we had been in bed for about ten minutes, I suppose, and I rolled over and said to my wife, I said, 'You know, you're not going to believe this', and she said, 'Yeah, I can hear it too.' Well, you know, I didn't prompt anything. In the back of our head we could feel it, the same pulsing sensation, the same deep rumbling, down inside our head, that disturbs our sleep. You can't block it out with ear plugs or ear muffs.
>
> We had an absolute terrible night's sleep. Now we expected to have a good night's sleep, as we always do when we go away from home. We can sleep next to a parking bay, as we did on Saturday night. Trucks going past all night. When the trucks are not there, the silence inside our head is absolutely like a vacuum. It is profound. While we're home, it's just a constant pulsing turmoil. You don't get any sleep.
>
> *But anyway, we asked Mary next morning, 'Are there any turbines around?' and she pointed up the range, she said, 'Seventeen kilometres up that way.' Seventeen kilometres, and we could still pick it up.*

So, David Mortimer drove with his wife some 475 kilometres from his house near Millicent to near the town of Waterloo, where he 'happened to turn up' at Mary Morris' place. Mortimer and Mary Morris are

41 Mortimer 2014.
42 Aston 2013.

known to each other as active opponents of the windfarms near where they live. By claiming to have asked Mary Morris the next morning, 'Are there any turbines around?' and writing that he 'had no idea until next day that there were turbines in our vicinity', Mortimer was suggesting that he was unaware that she lived near the Waterloo windfarm, when in fact she has often written and spoken about its effects on those living in the district. So is this 'Well, I never!' account one that a reasonable person should accept?

Earlier in the year, Mortimer and his wife had travelled to King Island in Tasmania, where Mortimer spoke to a meeting of residents about a proposed development. The *King Island Courier* ran an account of his speech, in which he described his neighbours as 'all being alcoholics', charmingly adding that 'if my house was on fire and I wasn't threatened, I'd let them burn'. In his speech to the Parliament House rally Mortimer referred to this visit (emphasis added):

> Now we went down to King Island, in Tasmania, to tell those poor silly fools down there that they're not going to have an island left to live on, if they get these some 200 to 600 turbines on their place. We got taken to a little bed and breakfast that night, somewhere after midnight. We had no idea of our surroundings, and we had no idea what the island was like. We got into bed about, heading on towards midnight I suppose, and we once again had a terrible night's sleep, with this same pulsing, rumbling sensation inside our head, the same sense of anxiety in our chest.
>
> *We went for a drive the next morning, and on our way into Currie, the little town there, about four kilometres away from where we were staying, was five ruddy great big wind turbines. Part of their local wind, their local power plant.* Now those were about 1-megawatt units. The next night the wind was blowing straight across those turbines and we had an absolute shit of a night's sleep. Now once again, we'd expected to have a damn good night's sleep. We were sleeping next to the coast, the ocean was calm, so there was no noise coming from there.[43]

Mortimer had been invited to King Island to address a meeting of residents about the proposed new windfarm on the island. In his words above he suggests that through all his preparations for the visit, and

43 Chapman 2013b.

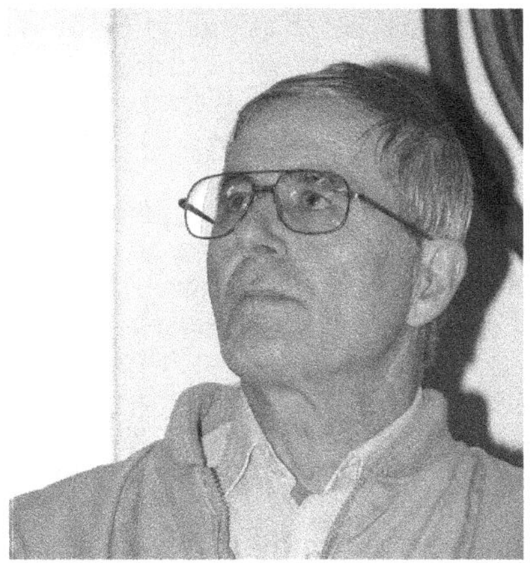

Figure 3.4 David Mortimer as pictured in the *King Island Courier* in April 2013.

during his conversations with those who had brought him there, he remained completely unaware that the tiny community of King Island already had a windfarm in place that had been operating for 15 years. The fact that the island already had wind turbines just never came up?

The owner of the guest house in which the Mortimers stayed has said, 'We built the house in 2004 and lived there for a year before renting it out as tourist accommodation since then. No one else, apart from David Mortimer, has complained about any problems at the Ettrick house.'[44]

On 7 October 2013, Mortimer posted a comment on an ABC blog post in which he returned to the same issues. He wrote:

> neither my wife nor I have sleep problems when we are significantly removed from turbines but do so when we are home or in the vicinity of turbines such as we have been 17km from Waterloo SA, 4km from King Island.[45]

44 Chapman 2013b.
45 Wilson 2013.

The cases of the Mortimers and the Gages provide an obvious response to those who claim that unhappy wind turbine hosts are contractually gagged from speaking out. They have contracts with wind energy companies and yet they *have* complained, and have not been penalised for breach of contract.

I have been shown numerous examples of *pro forma* windfarm hosting contracts from Australia. They do contain clauses about confidentiality. But these nearly always relate to the financial arrangements that have been made between the landowners and the wind companies. The reasons for such confidentiality should be obvious to anyone with any commercial experience. Some wind companies negotiate rental terms with potential turbine hosts that reflect the different electricity-generating potential of different topographical conditions. Some locations are worth more than others, and accordingly there can sometimes be variations in the rental offers that are made to different landowners. As with any commercial transaction, the parties concerned seek to maximise their self-interest. Landowners seek to maximise the rent they can get, and wind companies seek to minimise it. Once a price has been negotiated, companies naturally hope to keep these details confidential so that other landowners do not assume that they will get the same figure.

When the gag clause accusations first began to be made, I spoke with lawyers I know. The unanimous view was that, even if some wind companies did require their contracted turbine hosts to sign gag clauses about ill effects, these would be unenforceable: no contract can override common law rights to redress from negligence.

Michael Holcroft, president of the Law Institute of Victoria, in 2011 told the ABC that courts consider the public interest when ruling on contracts:

> They could certainly put it into a contract but whether it's enforceable or not is another issue … Normally when courts consider whether they will enforce contracts they take into account a public purpose and public interest component, so if a contract so offended the public interest, they probably wouldn't enforce it.[46]

In March 2013, the Clean Energy Council published a statement endorsed by 12 wind-energy companies. As can be seen, this public

46 Australian Broadcasting Corporation 2011.

statement repudiated any suggestion that turbine hosts were not free to talk as publicly as they wished about health or noise concerns. Windfarm opponents never refer to this statement.

> WIND INDUSTRY STATEMENT ON CONFIDENTIALITY CLAUSES IN LANDOWNER CONTRACTS:
> As responsible wind farm developers, we have never intended to restrict landowners from raising concerns they may have in relation to alleged potential health impacts of wind farms.
>
> All landowners, who are business partners in the wind farm project, may freely discuss such matters with their doctors, government agencies and in public.
>
> In order to avoid any confusion, the wind industry is in the process of clarifying this with landowners directly.
>
> The industry strives to provide open communication with landholders and we would encourage anyone with concerns about potential health impacts to contact the relevant company.
>
> Like any other commercial contract, our landholder contracts do contain some confidentiality clauses, which are designed to protect the interests of both parties. These are only intended to be concerned with the commercial terms of our contracts, and are not meant to restrict landowners from discussing any concerns they may have.[47]

The problem of falling and stagnant real estate prices in many of Australia's rural areas is well known. When landowners with low-value property that would be hard to sell see a wealthy energy company moving into an area and paying significant sums in lease payments, it is not surprising that some might see potential for being 'bought out' by such companies. Mining companies regularly buy out landowners. When this happens, word can spread fast through the community. I have heard accounts of hopeful complainants giving energy companies lavish 'shopping lists' of demands to pay for renovation or relocation. Tellingly, four allegedly unliveable houses near Waubra, where complaining residents were bought out, now house non-complaining occupants. When anti-windfarm leaders move around communities, sometimes with entrepreneurial lawyers, spreading anxiety that the turbines can harm heath, we see a potent combination: poorly

47 Clean Energy Council 2013.

informed, worried and angry residents are seeded with the idea that their protests might lead to a payout.

Other complainants appear to see the turbines as symbols of values and movements that they despise: totems of green politics, modernity and urban artifice. I have received many heated emails suggesting I should host a turbine in my inner-city backyard. As I noted earlier in the book, the irony is that for 26 years I've lived 300 metres under the main flight path into Sydney airport, 30 metres from a busy road and 200 metres from a railway line. The combined noise is incomparably louder than hundreds of wind turbines. I rather think I wear my fair share of community noise. But some in the bush believe that it is their birthright to be sheltered from any intrusion into their pristine surrounds, the ultimate in NIMBYism. Fortunately, anti-windfarm voices in the bush are in a small minority, as a 2012 CSIRO study shows.[48]

Abandoned homes and 'windfarm refugees'

One of the most enduring claims made by anti-windfarm activists is that families have had to 'abandon their homes' near windfarms because of the insufferable effects on their health.[49] Details are rarely provided but a powerful image remains of lives so desperate that people have walked away from their homes.

I began noticing this claim in my earliest days of following this issue. The Waubra Foundation stated in June 2011 that:

> The Foundation is aware of *over 20 families* [my emphasis] in Australia who have abandoned their homes because of serious ill health experienced since the turbines commenced operating near their homes. Most recently, five households from Waterloo in South Australia have relocated … [50]

This was repeated in November 2011 by Max Rheese, then executive officer of the Australian Environment Foundation, an anti-windfarm,

48 Hall, Ashworth and Shaw 2012.

49 This section is an edited version of Chapman 2014c.

50 Waubra Foundation 2011b.

climate-change denialist group established by the right-wing Institute of Public Affairs. He wrote, '*More than 20 homes* have been abandoned in western Victoria because of Wind Turbine Syndrome' (my emphasis).[51] Rheese later went on to become a senior staff member to Senator David Leyonhjelm, another trenchant enemy of windfarms. By September 2011, Sarah Laurie from the Waubra Foundation had started using stronger language: 'There are now *well over 20* rural families in Australia [my emphasis] who have been forced to leave their homes because of serious health problems they have developed since the turbines commenced operating.'[52] A year later, Laurie bumped the number right up, stating in a letter to a NSW politician that 'wind turbine refugee families now number *more than 40*'.[53]

When I saw this sudden leap I immediately wondered if I might be starting to smell the deep fragrance of factoid: a likely baseless claim that if repeated often enough comes to be accepted as true.

So, curious, I wrote to Laurie on 16 November 2012 asking her to send a list of the addresses of these abandoned homes. I wanted to start enquiries in each location to corroborate her claim. I planned to get in touch with local contacts like real-estate agents or the windfarm companies operating the turbines to seek corroboration of each claim about home abandonment.

Laurie replied that she had sent the information in a confidential submission to the Labor senator Doug Cameron, who was chairing the 2012 Senate inquiry into windfarms. Over the phone, a staff member in Cameron's office confirmed to me that a submission had been received from Laurie, that its contents were confidential, but that the submission contained no names or identifying details of anyone claimed to have abandoned their house.

In an email, Laurie shut down the conversation by writing, 'As the information was provided to me in confidence, I will not be providing it to you, so please do not ask me again.' Her claims were thus not open to any scrutiny, often a tell-tale sign of factoid status.

So I set out to try to corroborate her claim that 'more than 40 families' have abandoned their homes in Australia because of windfarms.

---

51 Rheese 2011.

52 Laurie 2011b.

53 Laurie 2012a.

How did I check?

Six sources were used to search for evidence of claims about abandoned homes. First, I reviewed 2394 submissions made to three parliamentary inquiries on windfarms for any statement from or about people either 'abandoning' their homes, moving temporarily or selling up because they had been distressed or made ill by the presence of a windfarm.[54] I also searched the anonymously authored, aggressively anti-windfarm website Stop These Things for any account of or reference to abandoned homes or windfarm refugees. This website publishes profiles of people claiming to have been harmed or annoyed by wind-turbine exposure and daily comments from dedicated opponents of windfarms. Publicising emotive profiles of 'refugees', if they existed, would be irresistible to the authors of this site. I also emailed 18 known Australian opponents of windfarms and invited them to send any information about allegedly abandoned homes. I then repeated this request to senators Nick Xenophon, John Madigan and Chris Back, who had each publicly referred to home abandonments or 'refugees'. I searched the Factiva news media database on 23 October 2012 using the search string 'wind AND farms AND [abandon* OR refugee*]' for all Australian news sources. Finally, I put word out to a network of colleagues and associates with interest and expertise in windfarms including acousticians, wind industry employees, rural health specialists and environmentalists, that I was seeking to corroborate the abandonment claim and asking for any information about instances of homes being abandoned in Australia. The information obtained from this process consisted of (1) people who had already been publicly identified – generally by their own publicity efforts, and (2) various descriptions of unnamed people said to have abandoned their houses, with information about the windfarm that was said to have prompted them to flee. In the latter cases, I sought to find additional information by contacting the relevant wind company. Below I discuss these cases of so-called home abandonment. Where this information has previously been made public via websites or media coverage, identifiable details

54 The NSW Department of Planning and Infrastructure's 2012 call for submissions regarding its *Draft Planning Guidelines: Wind Farms* (http://bit.ly/2zQmniz); the 2012 Senate Inquiry into the Social and Economic Impact of Rural Wind Farms (http://bit.ly/2y5Qtl2); and the 2012 Senate Inquiry into the Renewable Energy (Electricity) Amendment (Excessive Noise from Wind Farms) Bill (http://bit.ly/2xnFbEj).

are provided. Where information relates to cases that have not been made public, I have kept all identifying information confidential.

What did I find?

Twenty-one emails were sent to known opponents of windfarms, including Senators Xenophon, Madigan and Back. None of the senators replied, despite follow-up emails. One abusive reply was received from an activist who co-ordinates opposition to a planned windfarm, and one reply was received that supplied details about a property whose owners had moved out because of nearby turbines. Table 3.1 summarises all 12 known claims of home 'abandonment' due to windfarms in Australia obtained from the six sources described.

Twelve cases (seven in Waubra and five in Toora) where windfarm companies had purchased houses from their owners were not counted as examples of houses being 'abandoned'. These owners negotiated to sell their properties, sometimes to windfarm developers, in five cases prior to the commencement of the operation of the farms; several of these houses are now used as accommodation for windfarm personnel. One much publicised case at Waubra is that of the Godfreys.[55] It is understood that the developer made technical errors in the amenity assessment and an agreed financial settlement was reached after the windfarm began to operate.

In addition, anti-windfarm activist George Papadopoulos (see Chapter 6), who lives 35 kilometres away from the nearest windfarm at Gunning in New South Wales, has claimed sometimes to sleep in his car to escape turbines noise.[56] He has also claimed to be able to hear wind turbines from 'up to 100 kilometres' away.[57] If this were possible, all of the population of Canberra (340,000), Adelaide (1.2 million) and Melbourne (4 million) might be able to hear wind turbine noise[58] because of the windfarms within 100 kilometres of these cities (see Figure 6.5). I regarded this claim as sufficiently extreme to not take it seriously. So, using six potential sources of information, I was able to find only 12 examples of families living near seven of Australia's then 51 windfarms who claimed to have left their homes either permanently

55 Morris 2010.
56 Papadopoulos 2013.
57 Papadopoulos 2012b.
58 Joshi 2012a.

Location and family name (where public)	Comments
Cape Bridgewater, Victoria Kermond, Ware and Nicholson	'Not being able to live in our own home is debilitating.' (Kermond n.d.) '80 percent of our neighbours have left.' (Stop These Things 2013d)
Oaklands Hill, Victoria Anon.	These departures were confirmed by correspondence from the family and corroboration by the wind company.
Leonards Hill, Victoria Mitric-Andjic	'I was living … only 1.5 kilometres away from industrial turbines. I myself, my family and most neighbours are experiencing the same cluster of symptoms from the same time since the turbines started operating [in June 2011]. As a result of this our family had to move.' (Mitric-Andjic 2012).
Macarthur, Victoria Gardner and Hetherington (both temporary 'abandonments')	'We, and others are forced to leave our property for at least two days and two nights every week.' (Gardner 2013) Gardner is the public officer of a local anti-windfarm group and had been so for several years before construction of the windfarm. She 'regularly travels to Melbourne and Port Fairy to stay with relatives and escape the symptoms she experiences at home.' (Parnell and Akerman 2014)
Toora, Victoria Garitto	'We have been out of our house for two years now, having tried to stay there for eight months.' (Anon. 2005) The house was eventually sold.
Waterloo, South Australia Marciniak (two families)	'My brother got so bad that he moved from his house that just he spent over $100,000 to renovate, to the next town and stays in a caravan, he comes here only for a short time and goes again because the turbines make him so ill that he can't bare [sic] to be here anymore.' (Marciniak 2012b) Wind industry sources have reported that two other families also moved from the same area.

Location and family name (where public)	**Comments**
Waubra, Victoria Stepnell	'My wife and I got so ill after only one night of sleeping in our home [of 35 years] with turbines operating all around us, we left and had not lived in the house since.' (Stop These Things 2013g) 'We had to move.' (Stop These Things 2013a)

Table 3.1 Cases of claimed permanent (*n*=10) and temporary (*n*=2) home 'abandonment' near windfarms in Australia

or occasionally because of the proximity of windfarms and without any financial settlement or compensation from windfarm companies. Of these, none appears to be a case of true 'abandonment' in the sense that the families concerned 'fled' their house, unable to sell it. Nine appear to be examples of owners deciding to move out of the house completely or for extended periods, but retaining ownership. In two cases, the owners return to their properties for work during the day, but reside elsewhere.

However, important questions arise about some of these. One informant with many years' experience in the wind industry remarked that 'there is almost always more to these stories'. Some may be trying to bring negative publicity to the wind companies concerned in an effort to leverage more lucrative financial settlements. It is common knowledge that when large companies (mining, housing or industrial development) show interest in developing a major project, they can sometimes attract ambit or speculative claims and resort to purchasing properties rather than risk potentially protracted complaints from objectors. Where a property owner would ordinarily have little prospect of selling in a depressed market or because a run-down house is unsalable, the temptation to complain in the hope of being bought out might be predictable.

Many economically struggling rural towns and hamlets have properties like this, with real-estate agents' windows advertising many long-term unsold properties. The small town of Waterloo in South Australia, for example, is said by windfarm opponents to be a hotbed of abandoned homes. It is. But not for the reasons claimed. Waterloo is a small settlement that is looking very tired. Climate change–denying journalist James Delingpole described it thus in the *Australian*:

> Waterloo felt like a ghost town: shuttered houses and a dust-blown aura of sinister unease, as in a horror movie when something dreadful has happened to a previously ordinary, happy settlement.[59]

Such towns typically have few if any shops or services, and little employment. Many children on leaving school move away. In such environments, when a large wind-energy company establishes a local windfarm and stories spread of 'drought-proofing' lease payments being paid to turbine hosts, it is conceivable that a minority may pursue a strategy of vexatious complaints in order to procure improvements to their property or even an otherwise unlikely sale. Moving away from a house may be a strategy designed to leverage such settlements.

In at least two cases, those who had 'abandoned' their houses citing health complaints had histories of medical problems pre-dating the construction of the windfarms. One had been on a disability pension for several years, and another had made a public statement about a serious ongoing brain injury unrelated to and pre-dating the windfarm. One 'refugee' is known by those in the community to have moved to a town that has medical facilities needed by a family member. Another family member has since moved into the 'abandoned' home after the owner unsuccessfully sought a settlement beyond the market value of the house.

One of those listed in the table as having moved has only part-time work in the area. Most of this person's work is outside the area and the person is known to have other houses. In this particular case, there are more than 50 houses closer to the windfarm that have not claimed 'refugee' status or complained. It is likely that there were other reasons for this family to have left this home.

Another 'refugee' has a history of antagonism toward the relevant wind company after his commercial services were declined during the construction of the windfarm. Still another has recently moved back into the windfarm district, building a new house. A frequently complaining couple sold their home on the open market and attributed their departure to their dislike for the windfarm. However, they cannot be said to have 'abandoned' the house, having sold it. The new owner

59 Delingpole 2012.

is enthusiastic about living near the windfarm and turned down the windfarm developer's offer to plant trees on the property because she enjoys seeing the turbines through her kitchen window.

In addition to the 12 families shown in Table 3.1, Sarah Laurie has referred to 'numerous families' having abandoned their houses near the Toora windfarm in Victoria.[60] One house was demolished near the Toora farm and two others were sold on the open market. It is inconceivable that a windfarm company would demolish a house it did not own, so this claim could not refer to an 'abandoned' house but to a purchased one. Claims have also been made of other 'refugees' in the Macarthur area. However, attempts to corroborate these claims were unsuccessful. It might be argued that despite my being unable to find evidence for any more than 12 families claiming to have abandoned their houses, many more exist but have not made public complaints or sought publicity. How plausible is this? Imagine that your home was subject to some environmental assault so egregious and relentless that you had no option but to abandon your home: walk away from it without sale, because no one would be foolish enough to buy it when they saw what you were enduring. And then try to imagine that, under these circumstances, you never publicly identified yourself. Never protested about what you were experiencing. Never made yourself known to those causing the problem. Never called in the media to report the unfair conditions under which you lived. Never mentioned it in a submission to parliament.

While the first is possible to imagine, the second would be hard to fathom. People at the end of their tether tend to be angry. They have awful stories to tell. They welcome arc lights thrown on their situation so that the injustice might be stopped. Yet this is the situation we are being asked to accept when it comes to claims that Australian windfarms have allegedly driven 'more than 40' families to abandon their homes and become 'windfarm refugees'.

If this were true it would be reasonable to expect that many of the people would not have sought anonymity, but quite the opposite. The injustice of having to leave one's home without selling it, or being penalised for breaking a lease, could attract media and political attention and perhaps trigger compensation. None of the anti-windfarm activists contacted provided any information about abandoned homes when given the opportunity to do so. If more such

60 Laurie 2012b.

cases exist, they would provide important publicity in aid of the anti-windfarm cause.

Industrial developments like highway construction, new airport runways, tunnels and the re-zoning of residential areas for industrial use often attract virulent protest from local residents. Those most affected write complaints, picket councils and parliaments, are interviewed by the media, put signs on their fences and front lawns, and sometimes engage in civil disobedience. They have strong reasons to complain and the last thing they'd want to do is to be timid, seek anonymity and not raise hell.

Here a blog comment I found is apposite, comparing residents openly protesting in Melbourne about the construction of a major road tunnel with claims that 'more than 40' families have abandoned houses because of wind turbines:

> It seems strange that people are happy to voice their discontent when being disenfranchised courtesy of a proposed road tunnel in Melbourne while others apparently remain mute because of wind farm projects. It's more than a little odd that the anti-tunnel people grab media attention at every chance and happily have their names publicised yet people who claim to be adversely affected by wind farm projects … [are allegedly] afraid to be named or provide evidence to support their claims.[61]

I concluded that claims about 'more than 20', let alone 'over 40' home abandonments in Australia are not open to any scrutiny, are highly likely to be without foundation, and should be regarded as factoids until validated. The Waubra Foundation has been a major proponent of this contagious factoid. The foundation even publicised a 'respite' program, offering affected residents temporary accommodation elsewhere, an initiative that appears to have now disappeared from its website. A credible hypothesis is that the anti-wind lobby has embellished and inflated the actual number of people leaving homes in order to support their lobbying efforts to frustrate the development of windfarms.

Of particular concern is the way the word 'refugee' was used in the service of this issue. Three Senators (Back,[62] Madigan[63] and

61 Donaldson 2013.

62 Back 2012.

63 Seven Network Pty Ltd 2012b.

Xenophon[64]), while not repeating the '40' figure, publicly used the expressions 'abandoned home' or 'refugees'. Refugees are people who risk their lives to escape death, persecution and war. The appropriation of this term as an emotive rhetorical device, with the numbers involved exaggerated to increase attention, is frankly odious. If the members of the 2015 Senate inquiry did have 'confidential knowledge' of many more people abandoning their homes than I have been able to find evidence for, the matter could be investigated by a judicial investigator such as a retired judge. Such a person could be appointed to investigate the veracity of these claims. Questions to be asked would include whether those who had moved had any other reasons for moving, such as seeking work, eviction from a rented property, or a need to be near medical facilities. The judge could investigate whether any complainants were property owners whose applications to host lucrative turbines were declined because of unsuitable topography, and who then began resenting neighbours whose land was suitable.

Those claiming to have to regularly leave their house for respite from the turbines should of course have no objection to making their home telephone records available to corroborate that no calls were made or taken during the many periods when they claim to have been away. They should also be willing to provide receipts for hotel accommodation or statutory declarations from family and friends who might have put them up on all of these alleged occasions.

Are windfarms the new tobacco, asbestos or thalidomide?

One of the most brutally flogged tropes in contemporary debates about alleged new health risks is the idea that some heinous new agent may turn out to be the new tobacco, asbestos or thalidomide. This argument has three core ingredients.

First, there's the idea that few ever suspected that these nasties were anything but benign; they were used by many for years to no apparent ill effect, but some intrepid investigators knew better.

Next comes the narrative of the brave whistle-blower, following in the path trodden by Copernicus and later Galileo, who endured the wrath of the church when they challenged the Ptolemaic doctrine

64 Seven Network Pty Ltd 2012b.

of a geocentric, earth-centred universe. These pioneers of true understanding weathered the taunts and ridicule and their truths finally won out. Those highlighting the risks of some new agent see themselves as equally heroic, revolutionary and unappreciated. They are trying to tell us the truth and disbelievers are either myopic conservatives or the running dogs of corporate liars.

Finally, there's the near-universal contempt for the industries that did all they could to deny that their products were harmful, and an assertion that the new industry is no better: 'Tobacco and asbestos companies denied the health risks of smoking for decades. We're seeing the same thing happening now with [insert new problem like windfarms here].'

On 19 May 2015, Liberal Democratic Senator David Leyonhjelm gave the argument a heavy workout in the Senate inquiry into windfarms, amazingly the third such inquiry in four years. Questioning Andrew Bray of the Australian Wind Alliance, Leyonhjelm got into stride:

> **Leyonhjelm:** Not everybody who smoked cigarettes got lung cancer. Not everybody who was exposed to asbestos got mesothelioma. Are you saying that, because somebody can live next to a wind turbine and not suffer adverse effects, nobody does?
> **Bray:** That is not what I am saying. I am saying that, if you were to take a study of people all around a wind turbine, you would find that the incidence of health problems is not high. I think you need to take that into account.
> **Leyonhjelm:** With cigarettes, the incidence of lung cancer was not high either.[65]

It is difficult to know where to begin here. Leyonhjelm's party has taken 'tens of thousands' of dollars from tobacco transnational Philip Morris,[66] a company whose products kill up to two-thirds of long-term users. In 2015–16, his Liberal Democrat Party declared a $20,000 donation from Philip Morris Ltd and $90,000 from the Australian Alliance of Retailers,[67] a lobbying organisation set up by three tobacco companies.[68] With Philip Morris coming in second only to the Chinese

65 Hansard 2015.
66 Bourke and Cox 2014.
67 Gartrell 2017.

National Tobacco Monopoly in annual sales, they win the all-comers silver medal for the company whose products cause the most deaths globally. Leyonhjelm, a caring champion of those claiming to have been harmed by windfarms, is happy to take what has often been called big tobacco's blood money. Lung cancer is apparently OK, but anxiety about a wind turbine is not. Is that the message here? The association of smoking with disease can be traced back to as early as 1912, when Isaac Adler published what historians recognise as the first strong connection between lung cancer and smoking.[69] It was not until the early 1950s, when the first serious case-control studies of smoking were published in the USA[70] and England,[71] that the association rapidly came to be acknowledged as causal, ten years later. Twenty-six years ago, in 1990, the US surgeon-general said: 'It is safe to say that smoking represents the most extensively documented cause of disease ever investigated in the history of biomedical research.'[72] The World Health Organization reports that between 1995 and 2007, 92,253 deaths from asbestos-caused mesothelioma were reported in 83 nations. In Australia in 2014, there were 641 mesothelioma deaths, with deaths predicted to continue to rise until 2021. The prevalence of Australians living with the disease is put at some 18,000.[73]

By comparison, the evidence that windfarms cause direct harm to anyone is of homeopathic strength. There are no documented instances or coronial reports of anyone ever dying from exposure to a wind turbine, other than rare industrial accidents during turbine construction. As the prominent Australian science and health commentator Karl Kruszelnicki succinctly put it, 'the science is absolutely clear that the only health effects of wind turbines is that if they fall on you.'

In June 2015 Leyonhjelm wrote in the *Australian*, 'there is already quite a lot of evidence [about the health effects of windfarms] and it is building.'[74] This is utter nonsense. As we will consider in the next chapter, there have now been 25 reviews of the evidence on whether

68 Tobacco Tactics n.d.

69 Adler 1912.

70 Wynder and Graham 1950.

71 Doll and Hill 1950.

72 Novello 1990.

73 Mauney 2017.

74 Leyonhjelm 2015b.

windfarms harm health.[75] All conclude that the evidence is very poor for any direct relationship. Most conclude that people who do not like windfarms, or who have been exposed to frightening stories, or who are consumed with anger about neighbours getting big money for hosting turbines when they cannot, can worry themselves sick. Sickeningly, such people are being used as pawns by ideologues opposed to renewable energy. Leyonhjelm is a man totally inexperienced in any area of health or medical research. He is a man who infamously believes that armed citizens can prevent the sort of gun violence that we see in one of the most heavily armed societies on earth: the USA.[76] His understanding of the history of tobacco industry denials is just as absurd. The tobacco and asbestos industries denied the health problems of their products for many decades after the science was clear that smoking and asbestos killed. The wind industry denies that its turbines directly harm people because, as 25 reviews have confirmed since 2003, there's no good evidence that they do. That's a fundamental difference. Any Logic 101 undergraduate understands that it does not follow that any company disagreeing with accusations that their products are harmful are mendacious liars.

Windfarm opponents have grasped the straw that the evidence that wind turbines are dangerous is poor, and argue that we therefore need to invest in research that they just *know* will eventually prove their point. There's also 'poor evidence' that UFOs, the Loch Ness monster and leprechauns exist, but no serious scientific body thinks investing research in such claims is sensible, other than the politically pressured NHMRC, which in 2015 allocated $2.5 million into wind and health research.[77]

---

75 Chapman and Simonetti 2015.

76 Leyonhjelm 2015a.

77 Chapman 2015d.

4
The best evidence opponents have to offer

In this chapter, we will take a critical look at some of the windfarm opponents' favourite research papers that are regularly highlighted in their advocacy. We will look at what judges and tribunal bodies have said about some of the expert witnesses that these groups have used or tried to use to support their cases. We will then summarise the very latest independent reviews of the evidence, highlighting the 2015 Australian National Health and Medical Research Council's systematic review,[1] as well as the single most important study in this field: a longitudinal study of the health of people living near windfarms in two Canadian provinces, Ontario and Prince Edward Island. This study was conspicuously ignored by the authors of the majority report of the 2015 Australian Senate Committee on Wind Turbines.[2]

Early data on annoyance

Opponents try to walk on both sides of the street with this argument, as their megaphoning of a report about a very early turbine in the USA illustrates. In 2013, anti-windfarm networks got very excited when they unearthed a 1985 report that had been presented at a 1987 US conference by Neil Kelley, a staff member of the Solar Energy Resarch

1 National Health and Medical Research Council 2015.
2 Australian Senate 2015.

Institute.[3] Kelley's work was stimulated by complaints made by 'about a dozen families' living within a three-kilometre radius of a single wind turbine near the town of Boone in North Carolina. These families represented 'a very small fraction of over 1000 families' living within the same radius.

The investigations found that very low frequency noise (including infrasound) generated by the turbine was the cause of the 'annoyance' reported by these families. This annoyance included 'sensations', 'a sense of uneasiness', and 'booming or thumping pulsations'. These sensations were experienced worst in bedrooms. The authors concluded that the low frequency noise was amplified by the complainants' homes. The field work took place between 1979 and 1981. The turbine being tested was a downwind turbine of a type that no longer exists today. One of the reasons they no longer exist today is that the downwind design had noise issues that did not occur with upwind designs.

Indeed, this was confirmed in another report on an upwind turbine (MOD-2) by Kelley in 1988, in which he concluded:

> We determined from our analysis of both the high- and low-frequency-range acoustic data that annoyance to the community from the 1983 configuration of the MOD-2 turbine can be considered very unlikely at distances greater than 1 km from the rotor plane.[4]

Predictably, while lionising Kelley's findings on the now long-redundant turbine, windfarm opponents have been utterly silent on his 'unhelpful' findings about the upwind turbine.

If a report on the noise or emissions levels of cars built in the late 1970s was presented today as evidence about the noise or emission footprints of modern vehicles, people would understandably laugh because of the huge progress that has been made with emission controls in the last 40 years. But this has not stopped anti-windfarm groups from doing just that when it comes to wind turbines. Russell Marsh, then director of the Clean Energy Council, commented appositely that the relevance of this old study today was 'the equivalent of taking a study about Ataris [game consoles] and applying it to the latest iPads.'[5]

3 Kelley et al. 1985.
4 Kelley et al. 1988.

This didn't stop the 2015 Senate inquiry, chaired by Madigan, from describing Kelley's research as 'ground-breaking'.[6] This is just one example of the questionable research promoted by windfarm opponents. Next, we will consider some of their other favourites.

Alec Salt's work on rodent cochlea outer hair cells

Alec Salt, PhD is an inner-ear-fluid physiologist and professor in the Department of Otolaryngology at Washington University in Saint Louis. He maintains a web page about his research into the effects of infrasound, particularly as he believes it applies to infrasound emanating from windfarms.[7] He is listed as a scientific advisor to the Society for Wind Vigilance,[8] a group comprising a who's who of individuals who are openly hostile to windfarms. His work is almost invariably referenced in submissions to governments by windfarm opponents who want to point to physiological evidence for their assertions. He has also made numerous submissions himself.

Salt has published research on what happens to the ears of laboratory guinea pigs and chinchillas when they are exposed to experimentally generated infrasound.[9] His and others' work has demonstrated that in guinea pigs the outer hair cells of the cochlea are stimulated by low-frequency sounds at levels much lower than are the inner cochlea hair cells. On the basis of this work Salt has speculated about whether infrasound from wind turbines might cause some of the symptoms typically associated with 'wind turbine syndrome'. While on his web page his language is less circumspect ('Wind turbines *can be* hazardous to human health' – our emphasis), in his scientific writing Salt is guarded on this possibility, writing (our emphasis):

> The fact that some inner ear components (such as the OHC) *may respond* to infrasound at the frequencies and levels generated by wind turbines *does not necessarily mean that they will be perceived or disturb function in any way.* On the contrary though, if infrasound

5 Lloyd 2013.
6 Australian Senate 2015.
7 Salt 2016.
8 Society for Wind Vigilance n.d.
9 Harding, Bohne, Lee and Salt 2007; Salt and DeMott 1999.

> is affecting cells and structures at levels that cannot be heard this leads to the possibility that wind turbine noise *could be* influencing function or causing unfamiliar sensations. Long term stimulation of position-stabilizing or fluid homeostasis systems *could result* in changes that disturb the individual *in some way that remains to be established.*[10]

Note here that Salt and his co-author take care to stress that their speculations refer to *long-term* stimulation by wind turbines. In the previous chapter, we reviewed claims by opponents that exposure to wind turbine infrasound could cause disturbances within minutes of exposure. It is notable that Salt has not himself published original research on humans exposed to wind turbine infrasound and low frequency noise.

Swedish acoustical researchers have dismissed Salt's speculations:

> Salt and Hullar (2010) hypothesized from previous research that the outer hair cells are particularly sensitive to infrasound even at levels below the threshold of perception. In their article, the last paragraph mentions that wind turbines generate high levels of infrasound, with reference to three articles, two of which are not relevant to exposure in residential environments (Jung and Cheung 2008) ... No references were made to published compilations of knowledge that indicates that the infrasound to which humans are exposed to by wind turbines is moderate and not higher than what many people are exposed to daily, in the subway and buses or at the workplace (Jakobsen J 2005). It is therefore hard to see that Salt and Hullar's results are relevant for risk assessment of wind turbine noise in particular.[11]

Nissenbaum, Hanning and Aramini's sleep disturbance study

Michael Nissenbaum and Christopher Hanning are board members and Jeff Aramini is a scientific advisor with the anti-windfarm Society for Wind Vigilance.[12] In 2012 they published a study in which they

10 Salt and Hullar 2010.

11 Bolin, Bluhm, Eriksson and Nilsson 2011.

compared validated sleep questionnaires from cross-sectional samples of 38 people who lived between 375 and 1400 metres away from an Ontario windfarm with those of 41 people who lived between 3.3 and 6.6 kilometres from turbines.[13] Their abstract declares that those living nearer the turbines:

> had worse sleep, were sleepier during the day, and had worse SF36 Mental Component Scores compared to those living further than 1.4 km away and that significant dose response relationships were identified between these outcomes and distance from turbines.

This finding is frequently highlighted by windfarm opponents. The study was savaged in two letters later published in the same journal, where it was pointed out that the authors did not report any actual sound data in their paper, but instead used *post hoc* 'visually obtained' data.[14] This was said to be 'not scientifically defensible' and an astonishing omission, given the centrality of the sound data to their claims about the dose-response relationships of distance (as a proxy for sound) and sleep and mental health outcomes. The critics also noted that 'The authors did not provide the r^2 values [the core sleep outcome results] for any of the three figures nor did they present the slope equations for these lines.' They also noted that with the ESS scale the study used to rate sleep, a score of 10 or more is considered sleepy and a score of 18 or more is considered very sleepy. In the study, those living near turbines had significantly different ESS sleep scores than those in the far group (7.8 vs. 5.7)

But these scores do not indicate any serious sleep problems. The percentage with ESS scores greater than 10 was not statistically different between the two groups. They also noted that between 10 and 20 percent of the general population report having ESS scores greater than ten.

Despite their involvement with the oppositional Society for Wind Vigilance, the three authors made no declaration of competing interests and even thanked two other society members, Rick James and Carl Phillips (see later in this chapter), for their advice on the manuscript.

---

12 The Society for Wind Vigilance n.d.

13 Nissenbaum, Aramini and Hanning 2012.

14 Barnard 2013; Ollson, Knopper, McCallum and Whitfield-Aslund 2013.

Daniel Shepherd and the Makara Valley sleep study

Daniel Shepherd is a psycho-acoustician from Auckland University of Technology. He has published several studies and commentaries about wind turbines. In one critical commentary[15] on a Polish study,[16] he writes of the omission of a relevant competing interest statement from the paper: 'The fact that this relationship was not disclosed in the section dedicated to "Conflicts of Interest" is indeed the most astonishing omission of all.' Yet Shepherd then fails to disclose his own role as a listed scientific advisor to the Society for Wind Vigilance.[17]

Another, in the non-indexed *Bulletin of Science, Technology and Society* (see later in this chapter), is an opinion piece about his views on the siting of wind turbines near communities.[18] A third is a study, frequently cited by windfarm opponents, which they claim presents important evidence about the effects on sleep quality of residents living around a New Zealand windfarm at Makara, some ten kilometres to the west of Wellington.[19] The trouble is, it doesn't.

The study was cross-sectional and used a control group consisting of people who lived at least eight kilometres away from the Makara windfarm. It used what is called 'non-equivalent group design', where intact (i.e. pre-existing) groups are compared, which lacks the advantage of random selection: although the research may rest on an assumption that the groups are comparable, they may differ from one another in some significant way. In this case, the sample of people living close to the windfarm was drawn from 56 houses, while the control group was drawn from 250 houses. The researchers did not identify how many participants per household were recruited, but the final sample was made up of only 39 people in the windfarm exposed group and 158 in the control group. The study therefore seems very underpowered.

Shepherd's researchers asked participants to respond to two questions relating to amenity: (a) 'I am satisfied with my neighbourhood/living environment'; and (b) 'my neighbourhood/living environment makes it difficult for me to relax at home'. They

15 Shepherd 2017.
16 Mroczek, Banas, Machowska-Szewczyk and Kurpas 2015.
17 Society for Wind Vigilance n.d.
18 Shepherd and Billington 2011.
19 Shepherd, McBride, Welch, Dirks and Hill 2011.

reported that, compared to those living in a turbine-free area, members of the Makara sample were less satisfied with their living environment and reported that they found it more difficult to relax at home. There were no differences between the groups in terms of self-rated health and current illness. The Makara sample reported lower sleep satisfaction than the comparison group, and the researchers posited that 'the high incidence of annoyance from turbine noise in the turbine group is consistent with the theory that exposure to wind turbine noise is the cause of these differences'.

In addressing this claim, it is important to understand the practical implications of recent findings that it is noise annoyance that mediates the relationship between exposure to windfarm sound and sleep disturbance.[20] There is a relationship between noise annoyance and concern about the health consequences of noise exposure.[21] In short, people annoyed by noise are more likely to evaluate the effects of noise negatively and to have concerns about noise related health issues, such as the possibility of sleep disturbance. As we discuss in depth in Chapter 5, when people are concerned about the health effects of an environmental agent they are inclined to monitor their physiological state and attribute their ordinary experience of symptoms to that environmental agent.[22] Thus people concerned about noise-induced sleep disturbance may begin to monitor their sleep patterns and erroneously attribute any disturbance to noise emitted by wind turbines. Epidemiological studies consistently indicate that sleep disturbance and fatigue are commonly experienced in the community.[23] For instance, evidence has shown 27 percent of New Zealand adults aged 20 to 59 years have a current sleep problem.[24] Beyond a priming effect, where ordinary sleep disturbance is misattributed to windfarms, concern may itself interfere with sleep patterns, given the relationship between anxiety and sleep difficulties, such as insomnia.[25]

Further, concern itself can have an effect on objective and subjective sleep quality. In a double-blind experimental field study in

20 Bakker et al. 2012.
21 Kroesen, Molin and van Wee 2008.
22 Petrie et al. 2005.
23 McAteer, Elliott and Hannaford 2011.
24 Paine, Gander, Harris and Reid 2005.
25 Jansson-Frojmark and Lindblom 2008.

Germany, participants were exposed to sham signals and electromagnetic field signals from an experimental base station while their sleep was monitored in their home environment over 12 nights.[26] There was no evidence that the electromagnetic fields emitted by mobile phone base stations had any direct short-term physiological effects on sleep quality. However, the results indicated a negative impact on objective and subjective sleep quality in subjects who were concerned that their proximity to the base stations might negatively affect their health.

This study has particular relevance for Shepherd's study, as at the time his survey was distributed there had been some negative publicity about the Makara windfarm. For instance, on 4 August 2009 a small number of people experiencing apprehension about the windfarm, such as concerns about sleep disturbance, publicly discussed their concerns on a free-to-air national television program. Media reporting about the adverse impact of environmental factors has been shown to create or exacerbate concern within ostensibly affected communities, even when these concerns are unwarranted.[27] Further, an opposition group, the Makara Guardians, was formed in 1997 and claimed to represent the views of 85 percent of the small community. Its agitation against the windfarm for over ten years would have fomented and consolidated health concerns in the district.[28] Thus, there are a number of reasons why people may attribute sleep disturbance to windfarm noise, without there being a direct relationship between noise exposure and sleep disturbance. It is also very important to be aware that objective and subjective measures of sleep disturbance are only modestly correlated.[29] Therefore subjective measures of sleep disturbance measured in windfarm studies may not reflect actual sleep disturbance. In fact, in Chapter 5, we explore a study comparing objective and subjective measures of sleep disturbance in people living near a new windfarm development in Ontario, Canada.[30] Subjective data, gathered using sleep diaries, showed a deterioration in reported sleep quality after the windfarm began operating. However objective data, collected using polysomnography, revealed the issue was one of perception. In reality there had been no significant change in

26 Danker-Hopfe, Dorn, Bornkessel and Sauter 2010.

27 Jauchem 1992; Page, Petrie and Wessely 2006.

28 See https://en.wikipedia.org/wiki/Makara_Guardians.

29 O'Donoghue, Fox, Heneghan and Hurley 2009.

30 Jalali et al. 2016

sleep parameters following exposure to wind-turbine sound. It is also relevant that Shepherd's 2010 survey was distributed relatively soon after the windfarm began operating in April 2009. For those living in proximity to windfarms, positive attitudes to windfarms have been shown to increase over time.[31] Given the windfarm was a relatively new feature of the landscape, and that there had been adverse publicity about the effects of the windfarm on the living environment, it is unsurprising that, overall, the 39 people who responded to the survey were less satisfied with their living environment than the control group. Importantly, by 2012, complaints about Makara windfarm were fading.[32]

Finally, Shepherd was quoted in 2013 – some two years after publishing his study – as saying that 'he knew of no one in New Zealand who had suffered health problems from wind turbine infrasound' and that 'the issue was hotly contested in the scientific community'. He observed that 'The debate was not "black and white" and scientists needed to research whether infrasound was caused by the "voodoo effect" of bad publicity or the hum.'[33]

Iranian windfarm worker's sleep problems

Graham Lloyd at the *Australian* regularly reports on claims about windfarms in a manner that delights windfarm opponents. The febrile anti-windfarm website Stop These Things cannot get enough of his work:

> Green groups, environmentalists and wind farm supporters say the *Australian*'s coverage of this issue is linked directly to the Murdoch ownership of Cavan, a property near Yass in New South Wales under threat from wind farms.
>
> But anyone who knows environment editor Graham Lloyd would know this man is not for sale. Lloyd has been a consistent and fearless reporter of the other side of the wind industry. He is one of the few, if not the only journalist in the mainstream media to look at this issue dispassionately and beyond the 'group think' that appears to exist at many other media organizations.[34]

31 Warren, Lumsden, O'Dowd and Birnie 2005.
32 Meridian Energy Ltd 2015.
33 Stewart 2013.

In May 2015 Lloyd reported on a study by researchers from Tehran University.[35] The study purported to show that maintenance employees who worked closest to an Iranian windfarm's turbines had poorer sleep patterns than those working in security and administration, further away from the turbines. Lloyd highlighted a quote from the study's abstract in two of his reports: 'despite all the good benefits of wind turbines, it can be stated that this technology has health risks for all those exposed to its sound.'[36] *All* those exposed. Not just some, please note. Ketan Joshi, an experienced analyst of renewable energy policy, took apart this study on his blog on the same day Lloyd's report was published.[37] He noted that the Iranian paper's very opening raised immediate suspicions that we were dealing with a less than well informed group of authors when they stated: 'Noise from wind turbines is one of the most important factors affecting the health, welfare, and human sleep'. As Joshi replied: 'No it isn't. Transportation noise is, by and large, the major cause of sleep loss'. There is no report anywhere that places windfarms as 'one of the most important factors'.

The authors used the Epworth sleepiness scale to measure the impacts of windfarm exposure on sleep in 54 employees of a windfarm.[38] Joshi noted that the study lacked a control group, instead comparing three groups of windfarm employees: mechanics, security personnel and officials, who, the authors noted, worked at different distances from the turbines. Bizarrely, the authors did not say how many people were in each group or provide any data on how far away the security and officials worked from the turbines (for example, did the officials work in a town or city, or in an office near the farm?). There was no plainly highly relevant information about whether the participants had any history of sleep problems or other risk factors for such problems. Even more bizarrely, Joshi noted, the authors also wrote of the Epworth scale that:

> 'A number in the range of 10–24 is recognized abnormal (high sleepiness)'. However, in their results table, there are no average scores higher than 10.5, and seemingly, most staff seem to be under

34 Stop These Things n.d.
35 Abbasi, Monazzam, Akbarzadeh, Zakerian and Ebrahimi 2015.
36 Lloyd 2015b; Lloyd 2015c.
37 Joshi 2015c.
38 Omachi 2011.

> 10. In other words, most scored [at levels] below having sleeping problems.

Joshi concluded:

> For this study to make any sense, the workers sleep next to wind turbines, the security guards sleep at the perimeter fence, and the office workers sleep in their office. This is an unlikely set up.
>
> Why is wind farm noise affecting the sleep of people who work, but don't sleep, at the wind farm? Why wasn't there a control group? The measure of sleep impacts looks at 'daytime sleepiness' – so is the author saying the wind turbines are making them sleepy, or that the wind turbines somehow cause sleep loss later on, like some sort of weird latent magic? And how does looking at wind turbines cause sleep loss? ... All this paper has done is established that people working in different professions have different sleep quality levels.

And what about Australian windfarm employees? In 2013–14, there were 1720 people employed in the wind industry.[39] In a report in Victoria's *Hamilton Spectator* newspaper on 13 April 2013, AGL's wind energy operations manager Brendan Ryan said that absenteeism due to ill health had been very low. 'Site morale is high and engaged, with total hours worked since June 2012 being 36,171 hours. Sick hours during this period is 136 hours – which is less than half of one percent'.[40]

Japanese brains 'cannot achieve a relaxed state' after wind turbine exposure

Graham Lloyd's May 2015 report in the *Australian* also referred to an experimental Japanese study published in an Iranian journal where 15 test subjects were exposed to several sound stimuli, including the recorded aerodynamic noise from a wind turbine and a synthetic periodical sound.[41] The subjects were examined with an electroencephalogram and the authors reported that 'the test subjects cannot keep relaxed and their

39 Australian Bureau of Statistics 2016.

40 Anon. 2013.

41 Inagaki, Li and Nishi 2015.

concentration after hearing the sound stimulus at the frequency band of 20 Hz.' Geoff Leventhall, a vastly experienced acoustician who has often appeared as an expert witness in windfarm court cases, told me that in this study:

> Noise was recorded ten metres from the turbine, which was a small one. The recording was used for lab simulation played through loudspeakers which did not reproduce the infrasound region ... The threshold at 20 Hz is around 78 dB. So it is not at all remarkable that the greatest effect was noted at 20 Hz from 105 dB pulsed tone excitation that bears no relation to wind turbine noise.

Ketan Joshi's take on this study?

> [the study] doesn't control for expectations, and it's very likely that the subjects could perceive the sound = 20 Hz at 92 dB(G), [at] the volume at which the synthesized noise was played, would annoy anyone.

Similar to Leventhal, Joshi compared such levels to the noise that would be experienced right inside a wind turbine nacelle, not hundreds of metres or several kilometres away, and notes that windfarm workers would *never* work inside turbine nacelles when the turbines were turning. Lloyd's report, meanwhile, seemed oblivious to the totally unrealistic sound levels used in the study. One wag I follow on a blog quipped, regarding this study, that given Denmark has the greatest concentration of wind turbines in the world, 'How do Danes survive without being consistently excited by their turbines?'

Brains are again 'excited' by infrasound

In July 2015, the indefatigable Lloyd was at it again, with a front-page story.[42] This time it was yet another 'ground-breaking' study which was 'challenging wind energy proponents' insistence that turbines are not linked to health complaints reported by those living close by'.

42 Lloyd 2015c.

According to Lloyd, a German research group had concluded ominously:

> that exposure to infrasound below the range of hearing could stimulate parts of the brain that warn of danger. It finds that humans can hear sounds lower than had been assumed and the mechanisms of sound perception are much more complex than previously thought.
>
> The researchers do not claim the results are definitive regarding wind turbines and health impacts, and say more work is needed.
>
> But the research builds on recent work in Japan and Iran – and investigations by NASA dating back to the 1980s – that suggests the health science of wind energy is far from decided and would benefit from further inquiry, though it is unlikely to persuade prominent windfarm advocate, Simon Chapman.

In fact the study, presented at a conference, was not about wind turbines at all, but about infrasound generally.[43] But Lloyd was spot on in his prediction: I was anything but persuaded, because as we shall now see, this study was also much ado about nothing. We have already considered Kelley et al.'s NASA/Solar Research Institute study (see Chapter 3), and the Japanese and Iranian studies above. So let us look at what excited Lloyd and windfarm opponents this time.

In the study, subjects were exposed to infrasound and then asked to describe their experience. Their brain responses were measured using magnetoencephalography and functional magnetic resonance imaging. This demonstrated that sounds of 8 Hz could be measured in the brain, a whole octave lower than had been previously assumed, and that excitation of the primary auditory cortex could be detected down to this frequency.[44] All participants said that they had heard something. But these findings were hardly 'ground-breaking'. Earlier work found evidence of very similar auditory cortex stimulation from noise at 12 Hz, only slightly higher than the 8 Hz in this study.[45] The *Australian*'s subeditors ran the headline 'Brains excited by wind turbines study', but it wasn't a wind turbine study at all, and auditory cortex stimulation at 8 Hz (at pressure levels around the threshold of hearing) is meaningless

43 Bauer et al. 2015.
44 Szemerszky, Koteles, Lihi and Bardos 2010.
45 Langford and Wessely 2015.

in the context of wind turbine-generated infrasound, which is well below the threshold of perception.

Moreover, even fake stimuli can precipitate measurable activity in the brain. We know that both placebos and nocebos can increase changes in cerebral metabolic rate when viewed via positron emission tomography (PET) scanning.[46] Expectations do not just affect people's subjective experience of a stimulus (such as exposure to infrasound) but can actually produce measurable changes in brain activity which may or may not be markers of anything clinically significant. Fascinating work from Hungary[47] and Germany[48] on 'electrosensitive' people (for example, those claiming to be made ill by exposure to mobile phones, wi-fi or other 'stray' electricity) has shown that when such individuals are exposed to sham radiation from their feared source while thinking it is real, they experience symptoms. Correlates of these symptoms can be measured in the brain. The Hungarian study exposed both people with 'Idiopathic Environmental Intolerance (IEI) attributed to electromagnetic fields' and control subjects not reporting this condition to sham radiation.[49] Those claiming IEI to electromagnetic frequency radiation both expected and experienced more symptoms. In the German study, subjectively electrosensitive patients and gender-matched healthy controls were also exposed to sham mobile phone radiation and heat as a control condition. The subjects were not aware that the radiation was fake.[50] Both before and during these exposures, increased activations in anterior cingulate and insular cortex as well as fusiform gyrus were seen in the electrosensitive group compared to controls, while heat stimulation led to similar activations in both groups.

As the Hungarian researchers noted, electrosensitivity:

> seems to be formed through a vicious circle of psychosocial factors, such as enhanced perception of risk and expectations, self-monitoring, somatisation and somatosensory amplification, causalization and misattribution.

46 Eknoyan, Hurley and Taber 2013.
47 Szemerszky, Koteles, Lihi and Bardos 2010.
48 Eknoyan, Hurley and Taber 2013.
49 Szemerszky, Koteles, Lihi and Bardos 2010.
50 Landgrebe et al. 2008.

In short, as the old saying goes, you can worry yourself sick. And those who spread fear and worry are arguably an important part of this process.

Lloyd left messages for me to comment on the German research for his story. His report noted that I did not respond. I had zero interest in obligingly playing into what has long been a campaign by the *Australian* to discredit wind energy. The *Australian* has reported on a succession of 'studies' ranging from trivial to terrible, and has published opinion pieces which are exalted by the tiny cells of anti-windfarm activists who are happy to embrace any fragment that furthers their cause.

No reporter from News Corporation has ever reported on any of our now ten papers published in peer-reviewed journals on wind turbines (listed at the end of this book). The News Corporation agenda on wind energy is a travesty of good journalism.

Steven Cooper's windfarm 'signature' study

Steven Cooper is an Australian acoustician whose work is lauded by windfarm opponents. In 2013 he was engaged by the windfarm operator Pacific Hydro (PacHydro) to conduct a study involving residents who had been complaining about noise and vibration from the Cape Bridgewater windfarm in Victoria. Cooper was the acoustician requested by the complainants to conduct the study during 2014, and which was publicly released jointly by Pacific Hydro and Cooper's company on 21 January 2015. Interestingly, one study participant's report of her experiences in the project notes that the project was 'supported directly by Senator Madigan and staff', while another says that the study was 'facilitated by Senator John Madigan'.[51] Madigan is a virulent opponent of windfarms.

Cooper recorded noise data at a total of three houses and the diary entries of six residents living in these houses, situated 650 to 1600 metres from the nearest turbine at the Cape Bridgewater windfarm. Acoustic monitoring of noise and vibration was undertaken, data were provided to Cooper by Pacific Hydro on when the turbines were operating or shut down, and the residents were asked to maintain diaries over eight weeks, noting and rating what Cooper calls

51 Cooper 2015a.

'sensations' they experienced. These included 'headache, pressure in the head, ears or chest, ringing in the ears, heart racing, or a sensation of heaviness'. These sensations were rated by the residents from one to five, with five being the most severe.

Completing the diaries would have imposed an onerous task on the six residents, who 'as far as possible … were asked to provide diary entries on a one to two hourly basis', excluding sleep periods.

In his introduction to the study, Cooper states:

> While the study found for the six residents that there was no direct correlation between the power output of the turbines and the residents' diary observations with respect to noise, it found a trend between high levels of disturbance (severity of 'sensation') and changes in the operating power of the wind farm.[52]

Changes in operating power of course occur when wind conditions change. Turbines visibly slow when the wind dies down and speed up when it lifts. When three families with histories of protesting virulently against the local windfarm are asked to make diary entries for an acoustician whom they requested to conduct the study, it is reasonable to ask whether they may have been cued by these changes in the wind to make their diary entries.

The report does not name the occupants of the three households that took part in the study. However, they were all complainants. Three households that have very publicly objected to the Cape Bridgewater windfarm have been those of Brian and Joanne Kermond,[53] Melissa Ware and Rikki Nicholson,[54] and Sonia Trist[55] and her son Crispin.[56] All three households have co-operated in the publication of video interviews by the coy, nameless operators of Stop These Things.[57] Sonia Trist was named as a study participant in the *Australian*,[58] and Melissa Ware confirmed that she was a participant in her submission to the

52 Cooper 2015a ii.
53 Stop These Things 2013c.
54 Stop These Things 2013d.
55 Stop These Things 2013f.
56 Trist 2015.
57 Stop These Things 2013d, 2013f.
58 Lloyd 2015a.

2015 Senate committee.[59] Brian Kermond told the 2015 Senate committee that

> I moved my family of four from our residence at Cape Bridgewater in 2010 after we had all been subjected to the torture of trying to co-exist near the neighbouring wind facility … We have not been able to return to live at our home for any extended period of time and cannot be there when the conditions of the weather and wind facility are not favourable. This appears to be most of the time the wind facility is online.[60]

Cooper's report states that 'One of the houses [number 87 in the report] is abandoned with the occupants advising they reside elsewhere.' In Appendix A to the report, there are several interior photographs of house 87.[61] Interestingly in the context of claims about home 'abandonment' (see Chapter 3), the house appears to be fully furnished with kitchen equipment, dining tables, decorations and beds. Appendix M of the report details how the owners returned to the house during the daytime during the study to make their diary entries.[62]

Cooper has long argued that wind turbine infrasound has a unique 'signature' that differentiates it from other sources of infrasound, including that generated by wind itself. This idea has enormous appeal to windfarm opponents, as it could potentially allow an argument that infrasound generated by wind turbines, even at sub-audible volumes, unlike infrasound from wind, surf, cars and so on, has unique, exceptional qualities that cause distress and perhaps health problems to those exposed. Cooper emphasises in his report that he has given this breakthrough a name, resplendent with its very own capital letters.[63] A major conclusion from his report was that his study had 'confirmed the results of previous investigations. It demonstrated that there is a unique signature attributed to windfarms … This unique infrasound pattern has been labelled by the author in other investigations as the "Wind Turbine Signature".'

59 Ware 2015.
60 Kermond 2015.
61 Cooper 2015a.
62 Cooper 2015a.
63 Cooper 2015a.

But in bad news for windfarm victims like Ann Gardner and acoustician Les Huson (see Chapter 6) who believe that wind turbines emit noxious infrasound even when turned off (because of the wind whipping off them when the turbines are stationary), Cooper asserts that the bothersome 'signature' only strikes up when the turbines are turning:

> The shut-down testing confirmed that the Wind Turbine Signature is present when the turbines are operating but does not occur in the natural environment (i.e. wind farm shut down).
>
> The investigation identified for the turbines used at Cape Bridgewater that when the turbines were operational there is a distinct frequency generated at 31.5 Hz that exhibits side bands on either side of that frequency (at multiples of blade pass frequency). This pattern confirms the presence of an amplitude modulated signal which is not present in the acoustic environment when the turbines are not operating.[64]

Cooper's report received extensive publicity, not only in Graham Lloyd's front-page write-up in the *Australian*. The report and the publicity it received quickly became the focus of a commentary in *The Conversation*,[65] a detailed evisceration by Ketan Joshi[66] (who was by now a content specialist at the Australian Renewable Energy Agency), a highly critical review by the Association of Australian Acoustical Consultants,[67] and a very public examination by ABC TV's *Media Watch* program.[68] On 16 February 2015, about a month after the report's release, Cooper and PacHydro took the unusual step of issuing a public statement in which they stated unequivocally that:

> the study was not a scientific study … this was not a health study and did not seek or request any particulars as to health impacts. Therefore, we cannot enter into a debate about health issues or health impacts that have been raised in the media and the written questions.[69]

---

64 Cooper 2015a.
65 Hoepner and Grant 2015.
66 Joshi 2015.
67 Association of Australian Acoustical Consultants 2015.
68 Australian Broadcasting Corporation 2015.

This statement sits interestingly alongside others made by Cooper and those who have lauded his report.

In his submission to the 2015 Senate inquiry, Cooper appended a series of effusive letters written by acousticians and others. When he appeared before the Senate committee, Senator Ann Urquhart asked Cooper to answer several questions on notice about his report (Senator Urquhart eventually submitted a dissenting report[70] that differed dramatically from the majority report). The transcript of these exchanges stretches to 30 pages, with Cooper several times showing his irritation. Some of these interactions are extremely notable.

> **Urquhart:** On page 115 of the report it seems to say that all Severity 4 'sensation' reports were excluded from your audio analysis. Does this mean at 441 out of the 522 instances of Severity 4 and Severity 5 reports were left out of the analysis? Given this is close to 85 percent of the data, what was the reason for doing this?

She also asked:

> **Urquhart:** The report goes on to say that of the 81 Severity 5 reports, a further 50 reports were excluded from the analysis, leaving only 31 to be analysed. If I'm reading this correctly, that means only around 6 percent as of the sensation reports were used in the final audio analysis. Is this correct? Is this an adequate proportion of the data to provide confidence in the findings? Why or why not?

The Association of Australian Acoustical Consultants went to the same point in their Senate submission: 'The hypothesis is based on a very limited subset of the data, with any data excluded from the analysis if it did not fit the theory. When all data are considered, the evidence does not support the hypothesis.' [71]

Cooper confirmed that only 'severity 5' data were considered because these were defined as being at the 'worst case scenario' level of severity and so of particular interest. Of the excluded data, he said, 'Whereas some compliance test reports hide or dismiss the failed or

69 Pacific Hydro and the Acoustic Group 2015.
70 Commonwealth of Australia 2015e.
71 Association of Australian Acoustical Consultants 2015.

removed data, page 115 of the report identified the sensation severity 5 data that was excluded from the analysis.'

This response from Cooper was manifestly inadequate. Urquhart's supplementary question was about recorded noise data that were missing for 50 of the 81 (61.7 percent) occasions when 'severity 5' diary entries were entered by the study participants. So here, a large majority of the data were missing or unusable, rending the remaining 38.3 percent of usable data pairings possibly confounded by unknown variables. Missing values are very common in research and different statistical techniques are available to address missing values. Without conducting a missing values bias analysis on a data set with such a large proportion of data missing, there is no way of knowing whether important biases might have influenced the computations.

Urquhart also asked: 'Are you aware how many times a wind turbine signature in your hypothesis occurred and the residents reported no sensations?' Cooper replied with heavy sarcasm, arguing that he could not comment on such occasions because the subjects obviously did not record sensations at such times: missing (unrecorded) diary entries were just that – missing. But this was of course, the whole point of Urquhart's question. Cooper appeared not to understand that Urquhart's question was an invitation for him to look at his wind turbine 'signature' data and predict from it when the severe sensations *should* have occurred (and been reported) if indeed his hypothesis that the 'signature' infrasound moments were associated with intolerable sensations in the residents was correct. In other words, Urquhart's question went to the core issue of whether the hypothesised infrasound 'signature' had any predictive value for the sensations that these residents had long complained about.

Cooper's omission of this key issue underscores the statement in the joint release that the report was 'not scientific'. It is highly unscientific to note only the occasions when the data show an association, but not to consider that with such vast missing data, there may have been many other occasions when the residents felt sensations.

Urquhart also asked:

> On 14 February this year, the *Weekend Australian* reported that your study has established a 'cause-and-effect' existed between windfarms and health impacts on some nearby residents. Would you agree with this statement? Why or why not?

Although Cooper had jointly issued a statement with Pacific Hydro that his study was 'not scientific', he did not hesitate to concur that his work had established the 'fact' that his study had established a 'cause-and-effect' relationship.

> **Cooper:** I agree with Dr Schomer that the study found a cause and effect between the wind farm and the disturbances reported by the specific local residents. That is clearly apparent because that was what we were required to do and satisfying the first part of the brief identified that fact.

Beyond the small echo chamber of his supporters, the reception to Cooper's work has been sceptical. Acoustician Geoff Leventhall delivered a paper to the 7th International Conference on Wind Farm Noise in Rotterdam in May 2017 in which he strongly criticised Cooper's study:

> Cooper was determined to promote infrasound as the cause of problems, presumably because he had developed a prior belief in this, and so failed to take into account the broad research which has been conducted in the area of human response to audible noise … Thus, the potential that resident responses are linked to *audible* noise was neglected in favour of inaudible infrasound, although it is clear from the Cape Bridgewater Report that the wind farm was audible at the residences, as shown by many indications of audibility in residents' diaries. It is also clear from descriptions in the Report that some of the turbines were visible from the residences.
>
> The Cape Bridgewater Report concedes that the measured levels of vibrations are below the levels for human perception, and vibration is accordingly dismissed as a source of impact. However, for consistency, the same conclusion could be made in relation to inaudible infrasound, but it was not.
>
> … the response of the residents at Cape Bridgewater is unlikely to be due to effects from low levels of inaudible infrasound, as the Cape Bridgewater Report claims. Responses are likely to be due to the audible noise which is, of course, produced together with the infrasound. Both are generated by the rotating blades, occur at the same time and cannot be separated.
>
> Stress from low levels of audible noise is associated with a number of somatic sensations, particularly of the heart and stomach.

> Stress from wind turbines, if it arises, is often low level but, in a very small number of persons, the reactions may become intense and overpowering, so that neighbouring wind turbines dominate their lives.[72]

Two authors from the Australian National University wrote in *The Conversation:*

> this study is an exemplary case of what we consider to be bad science and bad science reporting. Far from 'resolving the contentious debate', it's much more likely to inflame an already fractious and fraught situation … It's a study that wouldn't have done very well if put up for peer review – or submitted for assessment in an undergraduate science degree … Giving unfettered and un-reviewed methodological control to someone endorsed by anti-wind-turbine groups is a bit like giving Dracula the keys to the blood bank.[73]

They described some of the key methodological problems in Cooper's report, such as the small sample size, lack of any control group, major study population bias, and motivated reasoning. Moreover, they observed that the total report is remarkable for the complete absence of any form of statistical testing of the associations it posits between the independent variables of noise-recording data and the dependent (or outcome) data of 'sensations' noted in the diaries of the six individuals in the three houses. I concurred with their analysis and in the comments section wrote:

> Nice work! One of the 'findings' from the diaries kept by the six complainants was that their experiences of 'sensations' corresponded with noticeable changes in wind turbine operation (e.g. starting up, speeding up in high wind, slowing down when wind speed fell). Well, hello! Six people with long-term complaining form participating in a study they might hope would do damage to the wind farm concerned rush to their diaries to report 'sensations' when they are cued by audible changes in the sound? No chance of any collusion in such a study when these six would all know of each other, and half actually lived together? If this dog's breakfast of a study means anything, it

---

72 Leventhal 2017.
73 Hoepner and Grant 2015.

provides support for the nocebo hypothesis: those with pre-existing anxiety and antipathy to the turbines, when cued by audible sound from those turbines, record 'sensations' on cue.

In March 2015, Cooper told the television program *Today Tonight* that he had commenced legal action against me over two public criticisms I had made of his study (see Chapter 7).

The *Bulletin of Science, Technology and Society*

In October 2010, the openly oppositional Society for Wind Vigilance held a conference titled 'First International Symposium: The Global Wind Industry and Adverse Health Effects: Loss of Social Justice?' in Picton, Ontario. In September 2011, eight papers from the meeting were published in a special edition of a journal you could be excused from never having encountered. The *Bulletin of Science, Technology and Society* has appeared erratically. It was indexed between 1981 and 1995 by the Web of Science, the international scientific indexing platform which as of September 2014 covered some 12,000 journals worldwide and over 160,000 conference proceedings. But after 1995 it was dropped from the list of journals being indexed by the Web of Science, generally a sign that an indexing service regards a journal as having fallen below an acceptable scientific standard.

A citation search I conducted on 10 October 2011 showed that in the 14 years it was indexed, the journal published 961 papers that had been cited a grand total of 345 times – or an average of 0.36 times per paper. An advanced PubMed search I conducted on 27 February 2017 for any papers published in the journal found just five listed: one from 1992, and four from between 2012 and 2016. PubMed is the indexing service of the US National Library of Medicine. In summary, this journal is not simply a low-ranking scientific publication. At the time of writing, it is more accurately described as an 'unranking' journal. Nonetheless, anti-windfarm websites have jubilantly described it as a 'leading scientific peer-reviewed journal' and the issue as 'ground-breaking'.

Among the eight papers in the collection was one by Carmen Krogh, a retired pharmacist and inveterate opponent of windfarms.[74] In this paper, Krogh explains that she 'began investigating reports of adverse health effects made by individuals living in the environs' of wind turbines in Ontario, Canada 'more than two years' ago. That's it. And this is called peer-reviewed 'research'. The paper contains no explanation of its methods, so it fails to conform to the most basic requirement of scientific reporting: that it contain details of how the research reported was undertaken. This is a fundamental requirement because without it, readers have no way of assessing the adequacy and rigour of any investigation, and whether any results reported and conclusions drawn are justified or not.

Instead of describing her research methods, Krogh mixes up statements apparently made to her by de-identified informants about the negative effects of exposure to turbines with similar examples from other parts of the world, from websites and submission to inquiries by windfarm opponents. We are told nothing about the process by which her informants were interviewed, the questions they were asked, how they were selected, or whether her 'study' was approved by any institutional research ethics committee. This paper would not make first base as a serious scientific investigation. Its findings contain not a single example of an informant reporting anything but adverse effects of exposure to windfarms, when it is widely acknowledged that a large majority of those so exposed neither report adverse effects nor complain about the turbines – and that many even like them!

In an attempt to understand the peer-review process that had been followed, in August 2011 I wrote to the editor of the *Bulletin of Science, Technology and Society*, asking the following questions:

1. Were you approached by those participating in [a 2010 anti-windfarm meeting held in Ontario] to publish these papers? Or did the initiative come from you?
2. Did you personally edit this issue or were guest editors used? If so, can you please describe how they were selected?
3. Was there a charge made to the authors to publish their papers together like this?
4. It is plain that all the papers are openly negative about windfarms, which is curious given that there is a large body of research that demonstrates a very different picture. Did you put out a call for submissions or approach researchers working in this area to submit manuscripts?

---

74 Krogh 2011.

5. Did you approach any authors who did not have affiliations with the anti-windfarm movement?
6. Were all the papers peer reviewed?
7. Did the authors propose their own reviewers and were these the reviewers used?
8. Can signed or de-identified copies of these reviews be made available to others on request?

Over several testy email replies, the editor made the following comments:

> A third party mediated between the organizers of the symposium and myself. We are dealing with a very difficult situation in which there is no balanced approach to begin with. Deep pockets have controlled the research agenda and professional people with impeccable credentials did what they did in this case out of there [sic] own pocket. As far as refereeing is concerned, never has any issue been so over refereed by people with impeccable credentials in anticipation of the kinds of concerns you voice.
>
> I can assure you that this Bulletin is not a front for any special interest group and that I would not have dreamt of publishing this issue had it not been for the questionable conduct of the wind farm industry and government officials. The issue attempts to create a little bit of balance, and show that there are legitimate other voices coming from people with impeccable credentials who are not funded because of their views.

No copies of reviews or reviewers' names were provided. A researcher from the University of Adelaide subsequently wrote directly to the authors and received no reviews back. The principle of open peer reviewing is widely discussed in research publishing and while requests by others to see reviews are unusual, refusal to be transparent can only promote suspicion about the process, particularly when the quality of the papers is considered.

Carl Phillips

Carl Phillips is a former academic who left his last university job in 2009 following criticism of his association with a tobacco company.[75]

He is listed as a scientific advisor to the Society for Wind Vigilance, which in April 2017 was still referring to him as 'professor' despite his having no university affiliation.[76] Phillips gave a presentation titled *The Absence of Health Studies Proves Nothing* at the 2010 conference organised by the Society for Wind Vigilance, and then developed this into a prolix argument for the importance of accepting individuals' accounts of how wind turbines have caused their various health problems in the special issue of the *Bulletin of Science, Technology and Society* discussed above.[77]

In that paper, which contains just eight references to windfarms, Phillips states without blinking that there is 'overwhelming evidence that wind farms cause serious health problems'. His basis for this is the number of 'adverse event reports' collected by groups with an interest in the issue. Here he names the self-published 'scholarly book' by Pierpont with its 38 cases, the unpublished 'study' by Harry with 39 (see Chapter 3 regarding both of these), and another paper that describes 109 cases,[78] a total of 186 cases. Amazingly, from this he continues:

> Since several [unnamed] research groups and non-governmental organisations have collections [of adverse case reports] that number in the three-figure range, it seems safe to conclude that the total number published or collected in some form is in the four-figure range, and it is quite conceivable that the total numbers of adverse event reports are in five figures.

So in a single sentence we are asked to deduce from the existence of 186 cases that it is 'quite conceivable' that there are between 10,000 and 99,999 cases of adverse events caused by wind turbines. And where is this mass carnage occurring? We are not told. Instead of referencing case reports published in clinical journals (admittedly difficult to do, because there aren't any – see Chapter 3), Phillips provides excerpts from three self-published cases that 'his research group' found on the internet.

One of these describes a family with a five-year-old who had sleeping problems and a 13-year-old with 'dramatic behavioural

75 Tobacco Tactics n.d.b.
76 The Society for Wind Vigilance n.d.
77 Phillips 2011.
78 Krogh, Gillis, Kouwen and Aramini 2011.

changes' who was 'spending too much time in her room' and became defiant. Such behaviour has of course only rarely been observed in young children or teenagers![79] But because it started happening after a nearby turbine started operating, Phillips suspends the most elementary principles of scientific scepticism, assuring us that we should treat such case reports with the same urgency and seriousness as we would reports from people in a North African city who 'started sending out messages that government forces are shooting into the crowd'. It's all that simple.

In late 2013, Phillips testified in an Alberta court related to the Bull Creek Wind Project. The final judgment gave him very short shrift over his slap-dash evidence, stating:

> The Commission carefully reviewed the evidence provided by Dr Phillips and finds that his prediction that 3 percent of area residents will experience severe health effects and approximately 50 percent will experience some health effects is not supported by the evidence for the following reasons.
>
> First, Dr Phillips provided little rationale for his predictions regarding the number of people who would experience health effects from the project. Dr Phillips stated he based his prediction that 50 percent of nearby residents will experience health effects on 'things like the Nissenbaum study' but did not elaborate further …
>
> Second, Dr Phillips confirmed that his conclusions were not based upon any particular adverse event reports and, in fact, he had not reviewed any adverse event reports in the preparation of his written evidence. He clarified that the adverse event reports or series that he discussed in his evidence were included just to demonstrate that such reports are out there.
>
> Third, Dr Phillips confirmed that the data he looked at was not organized in a systematic way and that he did not break down the data to determine a dose-response relationship between wind turbine operation and the symptoms he described. In other words, he did not correlate the prevalence or the intensity of the constellation of symptoms he identified with the sound levels at the persons' residences or the distance between the person experiencing the symptoms and the turbine(s) in question.

79 Maughan, Rowe, Messer, Goodman and Meltzer 2004.

> Fourth, Dr Phillips conceded that he had not specifically defined the population upon which his conclusions were based upon.

Phillips is not the only windfarm opponent to have attempted unsuccessfully to have his 'expert' conclusions accepted by a court. Several opponent groups have sought legal injunctions against planned and operational windfarms.[80]

In August 2014 Mike Barnard summarised the outcomes of 49 such cases concluded since 1998 from five English-speaking nations (17 from Canada, ten from Australia, nine from the UK, eight from the USA and seven from New Zealand).[81] He noted that Germany, the Netherlands and Denmark had also seen legal cases brought by objectors dismissed but that these judgments were not available in English. In all but one case,[82] these actions failed in government tribunals or courts. The provinces or states that have seen the most legal actions have been Ontario in Canada (14 cases, all of which failed) and Victoria, Australia (seven cases, all failed). Barnard's report highlights passages from many of the judgments about witnesses attempting to have their proposed expert status accepted by the courts or tribunals. Sixteen individuals are profiled, with several of these noted by the judiciaries as being members of anti-windfarm groups like the Society for Wind Vigilance.

Reviewing the evidence

As of April 2015 there had been a remarkable 25 published reviews of the available evidence about windfarms and health,[83] with the first appearing in 2003.[84] These are reviews of all available studies, not single pieces of research. Taken together, they conclude that wind turbines in some places annoy a minority of those who live in their vicinity, that annoyance can sometimes generate health problems consistent with those associated with stress and anxiety, but that there is no strong evidence of direct health effects from turbine exposure. Moreover, they

80 Alberta Utilities Commission 2014.
81 Barnard 2014.
82 Muse 2013.
83 Chapman and Simonetti 2015.
84 Pedersen and Halmstad 2003.

conclude that pre-existing negative attitudes to windfarms are generally stronger predictors of annoyance than distance from the turbines or recorded levels of noise. In other words, people who don't like windfarms or who are anxious about them can often be annoyed and worried by them as well. As we will review in Chapter 5, some of these people might even worry themselves sick.

The 2015 National Health and Medical Research Council (NHMRC) Review

More recent reviews are of greater interest than earlier efforts because they are of course able to consider more recent evidence as well as a longer body of research. Of these, that published by Australia's National Health and Medical Research Council (NHMRC) in 2015 stands out as the most rigorous because of its highly detailed and transparent strict criteria for study inclusion.[85] The full methods and levels of evidence included in the report are set out in full in a systematic review that was commissioned by the NHMRC.[86]

The two most important conclusions of the 2015 NHMRC report were:

1. There is no consistent evidence that noise from wind turbines – whether estimated in models or using distance as a proxy – is associated with self-reported human health effects. Isolated associations may be due to confounding, bias or chance.
2. There is consistent evidence that noise from wind turbines – whether estimated in models or using distance as a proxy – is associated with annoyance, and reasonable consistency that it is associated with sleep disturbance and poorer sleep quality and quality of life. However, it is unclear whether the observed associations are due to wind turbine noise or plausible confounders.

In its search for evidence, the authors of the review noted that searches of peer-reviewed and 'grey' literature (i.e. that not published in peer-

85 National Health and Medical Research Council 2015.
86 Merlin, Newton, Ellery, Milverton and Farah 2015.

reviewed publications) was conducted and identified 2850 potentially relevant references.[87] The NHMRC also provided 506 documents obtained from public submissions or from other sources. However, only 11 articles – reporting on seven cross-sectional studies that investigated associations between wind turbines and health – met pre-specified eligibility criteria. Windfarm opponents predictably rejected the findings. This was always going to be the case, as a 2013 interview with Sarah Laurie indicated:

> **Sarah Dingle:** If federal and state governments agree to fund the research you're calling for around the country, and it clears wind farms of any adverse impact on human health, would you accept that?
> **Sarah Laurie:** Sarah, the adverse impacts have been shown by a number of studies, both overseas and in Australia.[88]

As a South Australian court judgment stated, Laurie 'rejects all studies … which are not consistent with her theories'. The NHMRC's review would have been acceptable to the opponents only if its conclusions were in lockstep with their own.

The review published in 2015 was undertaken in a highly politicised context. A rapid review of the evidence published by the NHMRC in 2010 had intensely annoyed windfarm opponents because, like all other reviews published before and since, it had not reached conclusions that confirmed their claims.[89] A small number of federal politicians who were virulently opposed to windfarms saw to it that three Senate inquiries into the issue were held between 2012 and 2015. The Abbott Coalition government desperately needed as many cross-bench senators as possible to support its legislation and so indulged four of these (Madigan, Xenophon, Leyonhjelm and Day) with the third Senate inquiry in 2015.

Following the release of the NHMRC report in early 2015, the head of the NHMRC, Professor Warwick Anderson, told a Senate Estimates Committee hearing that $2.5 million was being allocated from existing NHMRC research funds to further research into wind turbines and

87 'Grey' literature is research literature not published in peer-reviewed scientific journals. It can include reports to government or scientific bodies.

88 Dingle 2013.

89 National Health and Medical Research Council 2010.

health.[90] Questioned by Greens Senator Richard Di Natale about why scarce funding was being allocated to the topic when the NHMRC report had found no evidence of a direct effect on health, Anderson explained that the report had shown that the 'science is not good, there's not much of it and it's all poor quality'. The funding was an attempt to fill this gap by producing research of a high standard, he argued.

But Di Natale drew Anderson's attention to a statement from a senior NHMRC official who had written that the decision to allocate funding to wind turbine and health research reflected the 'macro-political environment'.[91] In other words, the NHMRC's decision had been politicised: it was responding to the government's need to soothe the politically powerful crossbench.

Instead of setting up a dedicated research funding pool for windfarm research, Warwick Anderson and the NHMRC should have stated clearly and emphatically that any researcher wanting to investigate windfarms and health was at perfect liberty to submit such a proposal to compete with those being submitted by researchers considering any other topic. Such a proposal would stand or fall on its competitiveness as determined by peer review. There is no dedicated research funding being set aside by the NHMRC to further investigate the known massive risks to human health from fossil-fuel extraction and burning. And it would be unimaginable for the NHMRC to quarantine money for any other non-disease like wi-fi sensitivity, the dangers of smart electricity meters or 'fan death', the widespread folk belief in Korea that sleeping near an electric fan can cause death (see Figure 4.1). Yet this is what it did in allocating special funding to research into windfarms.

The money allocated was a very small proportion of the NHMRC's total budget. But the real damage was that in elevating this issue to privileged research status, the NHMRC greatly encouraged the political apostles of windfarm opposition.

Health Canada study

In 2014, Health Canada published a summary of results of a much awaited $2.1 million investigation into the health effects of windfarms,

90 Australian Greens 2015.

91 Hannam 2015.

가까이에서 오랜시간 사용하지
마십시오.
수면시 밀폐된 공간에서 장시간 사용시
질식사의 우려가 있으며 특히 어린이,
환자, 노약자에겐
더욱 좋지 않습니다.

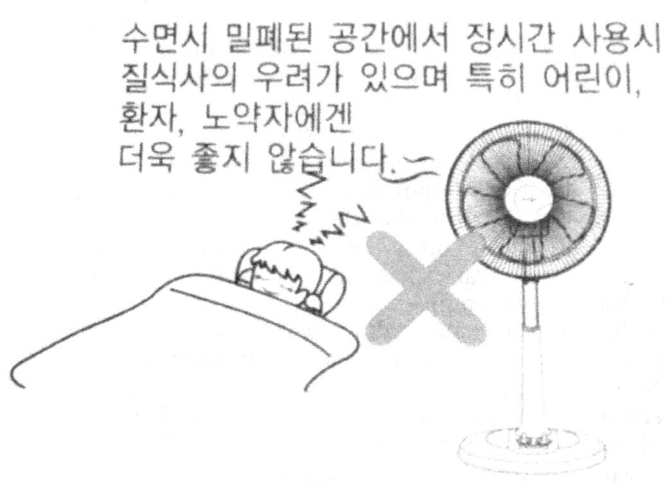

Figure 4.1 Extract from a Korean fan manual warning people not to sleep with the fan running, for fear of 'fan death'. Source: Not Just Kimchi blog, http://bit.ly/2zQmniz.

in the very sort of direct study that opponents had been demanding.[92] The Canadian study data were collected between May and September 2013 from adults aged 18 to 79 (606 males, 632 females), randomly selected from households located between 0.25 and 11.22 kilometres from wind turbines in two Canadian provinces, Ontario and Prince Edward Island.

In March 2015, the Health Canada study group published its full findings in a series of open-access papers in the *Journal of the Acoustical Society of America*,[93] the world's most-cited acoustical research journal,

92 Health Canada 2014.
93 Michaud et al. 2016a; Michaud et al. 2016b; Michaud et al. 2016c; Michaud et al. 2016d.

and in *Sleep*,[94] a leading journal in sleep research. Following is a summary of some of its chief findings.

Sleep disturbance

The researchers assessed self-reported sleep quality over the preceding 30 days using the Pittsburgh Sleep Quality Index, and used a wrist monitor to record the total sleep time and the rate and duration of awakening bouts, for a total of 3772 nights. Averaged over a year, the measured sound of the turbines at the houses reached a maximum of 46 dB(A) with an average of 35.6 dB(A). A volume of 46 dB is about as loud as a dishwasher operating in a kitchen.

The study found that self-reported health effects (migraines, tinnitus, dizziness, etc.), sleep disturbance, sleep disorders, quality of life, and perceived stress were not related to the level of wind turbine noise.[95] Similarly, both self-reported and objectively measured sleep outcomes consistently revealed no apparent pattern or statistically significant relationship to wind turbine noise levels.[96] Unsurprisingly, sleep was affected by whether residents had other health conditions (including sleep disorders), their caffeine consumption, and whether they were personally annoyed by the blinking lights to alert aircraft on the wind turbines. As we have previously emphasised, sleeping problems affect around 29 percent of people in all communities, regardless of whether they are near windfarms or not.[97]

Stress

The researchers used a recognised scale to measure self-reported stress (the perceived stress scale, or PSS) as well as recording hair cortisol concentrations, resting blood pressure, and heart rate.[98] Wind turbine noise exposure had no apparent influence on any of these. Moreover, the majority (between 77 and 89 percent) of the variance in the PSS scores was unaccounted for by differences in these objective measures. Again, the study concluded that the findings did not support an

94 Michaud, Fidell, Pearsons, Campbell and Keith 2007.
95 Michaud et al. 2016b.
96 Michaud et al. 2016a.
97 Petrie, Faasse, Crichton and Grey 2014.
98 Michaud et al. 2016c.

association between exposure to wind turbines and elevated self-reported or objectively defined measures of stress.

Do wind turbines annoy people?

Expressions such as being 'hot and bothered' are well understood. Being annoyed is not a health problem in itself, but chronic annoyance can have health consequences. The Health Canada study reported:

> Visual and auditory perception of wind turbines as reported by respondents increased significantly with increasing wind turbine noise levels as did high annoyance toward several wind turbine features, including the following: noise, blinking lights, shadow flicker, visual impacts, and vibrations … Beyond annoyance, results do not support an association between exposure to wind turbine noise up to 46 dBA and the evaluated health-related endpoints.
>
> The proportion of residents reporting that they were very or extremely annoyed by wind turbine noise was 2.1 percent when sound pressure levels were below 30 dB, and increased to 13.7 percent when the noise was between 40 and 46 dB. Those who found the turbines annoying tended to be those who lived nearer to them.[99]

There is much variation in how people react to noise. A 2014 review of symptoms related to modern technology (including wind turbines) found that those who were more anxious, worried, concerned, or annoyed about a source that they believed to be a health risk more commonly reported symptoms than did those without such beliefs.[100]

While proximity to the turbines was statistically significantly associated with annoyance, the relationship was weak. It was better explained by factors such as holding negative views about the visual impact of the turbines, being able to the see the blinking aircraft warning lights, the perception of vibrations when the turbines were turning, and holding high concerns about physical safety. These are all variables that bothered some but not most people.[101] Less than 10

99 Ellermeier, Eigenstetter and Zimmer 2001.
100 Rubin, Burns and Wessely 2014.
101 Michaud et al. 2016d.

percent of the participants derived personal benefit (such as income) from the turbines. Deriving personal benefit had a modest but statistically significant relationship to not being annoyed. The study authors concluded: 'Annoyance was significantly lower among the 110 participants who received personal benefit, which could include rent, payments or other indirect benefits of having wind turbines in the area.'

Yet again, a study shows that the wonderful drug known as money appears to be a very effective prophylactic against this non-disease. The authors suggested that 'these findings would support initiatives that facilitate direct or indirect personal benefit among participants living within a community in close proximity to wind power projects.' Strategies such as sharing rental incomes across the community, offering free electricity or home improvements, and paying amenity payments may reduce annoyance (see Chapter 8).

There was arguably no greater display of the naked anti-windfarm agenda of the 2015 Senate committee than the total absence from their majority report of any mention of the Canadian study. While no peer-reviewed papers from the study had been published at the time of the Senate committee, the summary results had been public since 30 October 2014. Labor Senator Urquhart's minority report noted that many submissions to the inquiry recognised the great contribution of the Health Canada study to the body of knowledge on the potential impacts of windfarms on human health.[102] The plainly deliberate decision to ignore the Canadian findings marks the Madigan committee as little more than a show trial run by a small group of politicians who had probably made up their minds about what their proceedings would conclude before they started.

In the next chapter, we will move to explore the central thesis of the book: that those experiencing symptoms which they attribute to the direct impact of nearby wind turbines are often experiencing classic symptoms that are associated with fear and anxiety. We will show how windfarm opponents have set out to foment worry and concern about wind turbines in some communities and how, if 'wind turbine syndrome' means anything, it is best seen as a potentially contagious syndrome that can be communicated to people who are likely to be receptive to the disturbing claims being made.

---

102 Commonwealth of Australia 2015e.

5

The psychogenics of wind turbine complaints

In this chapter, we turn to the data for clues as to why some residents report symptoms of 'wind turbine syndrome' while others do not. We examine temporal and geographical patterns of symptom reporting, the social context in which symptoms are reported, and the individual and personality differences that set apart those who do and do not report symptoms. We also describe experimental research that has tested the possible role of psychological expectations in triggering health complaints.

We consider how environmental health risks tend to be assessed and what factors can predict community outrage about perceived risks. We explore how windfarm health issues have been portrayed in the media, and how that narrative has shaped perceptions of health risks in some communities.

We then explore whether heightened risk perceptions can help to explain the emergence of health complaints in windfarm communities. Evidence shows that concerns about an environmental agent can lead people to report symptoms during exposure to that agent, even when the exposure is completely benign. When people are worried about exposure and expect to experience adverse health effects, they are more likely to notice and misinterpret common symptoms, including symptoms that may be caused by anxiety. This power of negative expectations to trigger symptom reporting in response to innocuous environmental agents, also known as the nocebo effect, has been seen throughout history.

In the case of windfarms, health complaints have tended to cluster in geographical areas where there has been targeted negative publicity about wind turbines, or where people are accessing negative health information about windfarms. This indicates that these clustered outbreaks are 'contagious', spreading via communication.

Finally, we summarise experimental research that tests whether socially transmitted negative expectations may be providing a pathway for symptom reporting in windfarm communities. The practical implications of these findings are considered in light of a case study demonstrating that, in a rural community in which a windfarm was being planned, the actions of anti-windfarm advocates generated negative media stories about the alleged health risks of windfarms, which in turn provoked fear in residents.

Outrage factors

As we discussed in Chapter 2, windfarms operated for many years before complaints about health effects emerged, with aesthetic objections being the dominant reason given for opposing windfarms in their early years. The environmental health scientists Loren Knopper and Christopher Ollson had attended numerous public consultation meetings about proposed windfarm developments in Canada when they noticed in 2011 that fears about health risks had started to become the primary focus of opposition at many of these meetings.[1] As we saw earlier, these fears are often expressed in frightened, outraged language. To understand how unwarranted and disproportionate health concerns can take hold in a community, it is useful to consider how people assess risk. In general, public perception about the relative harm posed by exposure to environmental agents has little to do with actual toxicological evidence.[2] Research in the area of risk perception and communication indicates that people are more likely to assess environmental health risks by the strength of community 'outrage' associated with the purported threat rather than in terms of objective risk of harm.[3] Outrage can be predicted by the presence or absence of various factors, which in Table 5.1 we have applied to the case of

1 Knopper and Ollson 2011.
2 Leslie 2000.
3 Covello and Sandman 2001.

windfarms.[4] Peter Sandman[5] has produced matrices of factors that have been often found to be associated with increased levels of community 'outrage' about putative environmental threats to health. Sandman distinguishes 'primary' from 'additional' factors, with primary factors being those that have been shown to be more strongly associated with increased levels of community concern.[6]

Perceptions of the risks posed by environmental agents, particularly those not yet directly experienced by people, tend to be informed by information provided through the media. Given the public does not generally have direct access to scientific reports, which are often hidden behind paywalls in research journals, the media have, in effect, become the public's proxy science interpreter, translating the current state of scientific knowledge for a lay audience.[7] However, content analyses of media reporting about environmental health risks, such as those posed by new technologies, have consistently shown that the media often misrepresent the current state of scientific evidence and overstate the potential for harm.[8]

Relevantly, acoustician Geoff Leventhall has considered historical media reporting about infrasound.[9] Although continuous exposure to sub-audible environmental infrasound is a normal part of everyday life, there continue to be pervasive misapprehensions about the nature of infrasound.[10] Misperceptions are likely to have evolved from mid-20th century misrepresentations about infrasound in popular science journals and books.[11] In the 1960s and 1970s, various sensational claims were made about infrasound, ranging from the completely absurd (e.g. that infrasound 'vibrations' mashed a technician's internal organs into an amorphous jelly, leading to his spontaneous death) to the patently misinformed (e.g. that testing of infrasonic generators had broken all the windows within a half mile of the test site).[12] The mischaracterisation of infrasound as a silent killer led to media

---

4 Sandman 1989.

5 Sandman 1991.

6 I applied these to a case study of mobile phone tower complaints in the 1990s. See Chapman and Wutzke 1997.

7 McCluskey, Kalaitzandonakes and Swinnen 2016.

8 Eldridge-Thomas and Rubin 2013; Leslie 2000.

9 Leventhall 2006; Leventhall 2007; Leventhall 2013.

10 Leventhall 2006.

11 Leventhall 2007.

12 Leventhall 2006.

Outrage higher if:	Outrage lower if:
Primary factors	
exposure is coerced (e.g. among those not electing to house turbines on their land)**	exposure is voluntary (e.g. among those electing to house turbines on their land)**
agent is industrial**	agent is natural
agent is exotic**	agent is familiar (e.g. higher outrage for newly built windfarms, less for long-running more familiar farms)
agent is memorable**	agent is forgettable
consequences are dreaded (e.g. cancer, birth defects)	consequences are not dreaded*
consequences are catastrophic (e.g. many people suddenly and badly affected)	consequences are chronic*
true hazard is unknowable (because of many confounders)*	true hazard is knowable (e.g. broad scientific consensus about effects)
hazard is controlled by others**	hazard is individually controlled
exposure is unfair (e.g. not all citizens exposed equally)**	exposure is fair
sources are seen as untrustworthy (e.g. wind companies)*	sources are seen as trustworthy
process is unresponsive (e.g. demands for action not quickly met)**	process is responsive
Additional factors	
affects vulnerable populations*	affects general population
health effects are delayed*	effects are immediate*
poses substantial risk to future populations	poses no threat to future populations*
victims are identifiable (e.g. named complainants)**	victims are statistical
not preventable	preventable*
few benefits	many benefits**

Outrage higher if:	Outrage lower if:
substantial media attention**	little media attention
opportunity for collective action**	no opportunity for collective action

Table 5.1 Primary and additional components predicting community outrage about putative environmental risks to health: the case of wind turbines. (** = applies strongly to wind turbines; * = likely to apply less strongly)

speculation that infrasound exposure was responsible for a variety of maladies and calamities from brain tumours and sudden infant deaths to road accidents.[13] A selection of UK press headlines from the period captures the mood:[14]

> The silent sound menaces drivers (*Daily Mirror*, 19 October 1969)
>
> Does infrasound make drivers drunk? (*New Scientist*, 16 March 1972)
>
> Brain tumours 'caused by noise' (*Times*, 29 September 1973)
>
> Crowd control by light and sound (*Guardian*, 3 October 1973)
>
> Danger in unheard car sounds (*Observer*, 21 April 1974)
>
> 'The silent killer all around us' (*Evening News*, 25 May 1974)
>
> 'Noise is the invisible danger (*Care on the road*, Royal Society for the Prevention of Accidents, August 1974)

Over the past decade, allegations that windfarm sound, particularly infrasound, causes health effects have proliferated through the media. Such claims have persisted despite consistent evidence, outlined earlier in this book, that there is nothing unusual about the levels of infrasound produced by windfarms and that infrasound generated by

13 Leventhall 2013.
14 Leventhall 2013.

wind turbines does not significantly contribute to background levels of infrasound in the environment.[15]

Historically, unfounded media health scares were propagated through traditional broadcast and print media and so have generally had a limited lifespan, with public concern dying away when the media have finished covering the story (as the adage goes, 'Today's news is tomorrow's fish-and-chip paper'). However, the advent of the internet has meant that media health warnings about windfarm sound have been perpetuated well past their date of initial publication or broadcast. The internet has also become a major conduit for the dissemination of misinformation about windfarm health effects by anti-windfarm activists. In particular, there has been a significant use of social media to propagate anti-windfarm messages.[16] Those seeking information about windfarms by employing simple internet searches can very easily land on sites dedicated to disseminating anti-windfarm messages. Evidence also suggests that, after repeated exposure to the deceptive claim that exposure to windfarm sound poses health risks, there will be a default tendency to believe the information is correct, a phenomenon known as the illusory truth effect.[17] In the face of such illusory truth, particularly if it is based on information from multiple sources, people may even abandon their prior belief or knowledge that such fears are unwarranted.[18]

The following exemplify news articles currently available on the internet:

> Wind turbines cause heart problems, headaches and nausea, claims doctor … Wind turbines can cause heart problems, tinnitus, nausea, panic attacks and headaches among people living nearby, according to a US doctor who has studied their effects for five years. (*Telegraph*, 3 August 2009)[19]

> Wind turbines are either making people sick or driving them crazy … For sufferers of 'wind-turbine syndrome', renewable energy is the stuff of nightmares. (*Salon*, 16 September 2013)[20]

15 Evans, Cooper and Lenchine 2013.
16 Leventhall 2013; Munk 2014.
17 Dechene, Stahl, Hansen and Wanke 2010.
18 Leventhall 2017.
19 Johnston 2009.

> Wind turbine infrasound' may be making thousands sick in UK, US ... If it is directed at you, you can feel your brain or your body vibrating. (*Daily Caller*, 11 August 2014)[21]

> An ill wind blows as the surge of turbines stirs fears of silent danger to our health ... Tens of thousands of Scots may be suffering from a hidden sickness epidemic caused by wind farms, campaigners have warned. (*Express*, 10 August 2014)[22]

Risk perceptions are also heightened when there is an impression that the scientific community does not fully understand the nature of a risk.[23] As scientific understanding is rarely, if ever, complete this factor provides fertile ground for public anxiety. A media tendency to give equal weight to both sides of a story, even when the science overwhelmingly favours only one side, can result in what has come to be called 'balance as bias'.[24] Despite overwhelming empirical evidence confirming that wind turbine infrasound is not causing health effects, news stories often 'balance' the current state of the science with the counter-narrative by citing Pierpont, Laurie, or others. In some cases, the science is egregiously misrepresented. This is seen in an article published in the (UK) *Telegraph* in 2015 with the headline 'Wind turbines may trigger danger response in brain' and the strapline 'The low frequency noises from turbine blades can be picked up and can trigger a part of the brain linked to emotions, scientists have found', which misreported the science and the study it purported to summarise.[25] The headline and strapline remain misleadingly intact online, despite the correction found at the foot of the article, which reads:

> CORRECTION:
> The University of Munich research mentioned in this article did not examine 'noise levels similar to living near wind farms', as reported

20 Abrams 2013.
21 Bastasch 2014.
22 Murray 2014.
23 MacGregor and Fleming 1996.
24 Boykoff and Boykoff 2015.
25 Knapton 2015.

> in an earlier version, nor did it find that these 'could lead to severe hearing damage or even deafness'.

Further, some anti-windfarm websites publish stories intended to create fear and undermine public trust. For instance, a story headlined 'Is big wind the new big tobacco?' on one such website conveys a disturbing picture of an attempted cover-up. It is a story designed to create suspicion that the public is being lied to.[26] Such a story is bound to create unease, if not anger and fear, in some readers. Content analyses of media stories published in geographical areas where health fears are prominent have revealed a media tendency to publish negative stories likely to amplify health concerns. For instance, in Canada, where concern about the health effects of windfarms has led to a huge publicly funded epidemiological study, evidence indicates that media reports about windfarms contain factors likely to induce anxiety and concern about health risks posed by turbine sound.[27] Further, the trend for newspapers to portray windfarms negatively has been shown to be even more evident in community newspapers covering local windfarm issues.[28] This finding may explain regional differences in health-risk perception seen in Ontario, where opposition to windfarms has been stronger in smaller regional communities than in the population at large. In Australia, mainstream media reporting about windfarms has also been criticised for misreporting the scientific evidence about alleged health effects; in a recent case of misreporting, one national newspaper made the flagrantly erroneous statement that a 'ground-breaking' study had concluded that people living near windfarms faced a greater risk of suffering health issues caused by exposure to turbine-generated low frequency noise.[29] Overall, there is currently a propensity, in the countries where concern about windfarms is highest, for some mainstream media to misreport the physiological effects of infrasound exposure, and to suggest that infrasound causes adverse health effects in residents living in proximity to wind turbines. Studies indicate that, as the issue receives more prominent treatment by the media, anticipatory fear of health effects become more evident in communities faced with the prospect of windfarm development.[30] This

26 Devlin 2014.
27 Deignan, Harvey and Hoffman-Goetz 2013.
28 Deignan and Hoffman-Goetz 2015.
29 Australian Broadcasting Corporation 2015.

is highlighted by reports from residents of West Lincoln in Ontario of stress-related health effects related to the idea of the construction of a proposed windfarm. Consider the statements made by some residents when interviewed by a community newspaper, *Niagara This Week*:

> 'We are already affected by the turbines. Our stress is already high.'
> 'I've been to the doctor. They told me to move. My stress level has skyrocketed. My physician told me my stress will kill me before the wind turbines.'[31]

Wind turbines can apparently make some people sick before they are even built.

Health concerns inform negative expectations

Groups opposed to wind turbines have galvanised opposition to proposed windfarms by calling public meetings and disseminating negative information designed to stimulate health concerns. Such fear mongering is designed to heighten anxiety and create specific concerns about potential symptoms. This was epitomised in a full-page advertisement in placed by the anti-windfarm group the Western Plains Landscape Guardians in the *Pyrenees Advocate* in Waubra in 2009, warning residents that they could expect to experience sleep disturbance, vertigo, irritability, nausea and a range of other symptoms if they lived within five kilometres of a turbine.

The question that logically follows is whether heightened concern can explain the appearance of health complaints in communities near windfarms.

Field research indicates that the more worried individuals are about the health effects of an environmental exposure, the more likely they are to report symptoms, even when no health risk is posed. As discussed in Chapter 4, a field study conducted in Germany revealed that residents' *concern* about the health effects of proximity to mobile phone base stations adversely affected their sleep quality, while

30 Baxter, Morzaria and Hirsch 2013; Mroczek, Banas, Machowska-Szewczyk and Kurpas 2015.

31 Moore 2013.

exposure to electromagnetic fields itself had no such negative impact.[32] In another study, Keith Petrie and his colleagues investigated symptom reporting during a suburban insecticide spraying program.[33] Worries about the health risks posed by aspects of modern life, such as environmental pollution, appeared to prime some residents to expect symptoms, so that they started to monitor their bodies for adverse health impacts. As a result, common symptoms and sensations were noticed and misattributed to exposure to the insecticide.

Our bodies are constantly subject to vague, diffuse, and fluctuating physiological sensations that generally go unnoticed.[34] When we are worried about our health, particularly if we suspect we have been exposed to a pathogen or toxin, we are more likely to attend to and monitor our bodies to evaluate whether we are becoming ill. Normal bodily sensations that have previously passed undetected are then easily misinterpreted as a new and worrying reaction to a noxious agent. Experiencing physical symptoms is also common. A recent population survey conducted in New Zealand found that, on average, respondents experienced five different symptoms during the previous week. In fact, almost 90 percent of respondents experienced at least one symptom, and 23 percent reported ten or more symptoms.[35] It is understandable that individuals would misattribute such symptoms to an innocuous environmental agent if they already have health concerns about exposure to that agent. In addition, increased anxiety about perceived toxic environmental exposure is in itself likely to cause an increase in symptoms such as dry mouth and rapid heartbeat.[36] Evidence suggests that people may misinterpret symptoms of anxiety as signs of illness, particularly if the symptoms experienced are consistent with pre-existing health concerns.[37] When symptoms stem from negative expectations, rather than from pathogenic exposure, this is a manifestation of the nocebo phenomenon, whereby 'expectations of sickness and the affective states associated with such expectations cause sickness in the expectant'.[38]

---

32 Danker-Hopfe, Dorn, Bornkessel and Sauter 2010.
33 Petrie et al. 2005.
34 Pennebaker and Skelton 1981.
35 Petrie, Faasse, Crichton and Grey 2014.
36 Pennebaker 1994.
37 Moss-Morris and Petrie 1999.
38 Hahn 1997.

Placebo and nocebo effects: an illustration from drug trials and pain studies

While people are often aware of the placebo effect (also called the 'positive expectation' effect),[39] many are less familiar with the concept of the nocebo effect (or the 'negative expectation' effect).[40] A good understanding of placebo and nocebo effects can be found by considering data from randomised controlled drug trials.

Participants in drug trials are generally randomly assigned to receive either the drug being tested or an inactive placebo, such as a sugar pill, to determine whether the active drug has any efficacy over and above an inert treatment. The participants are not told whether they are receiving the active drug or the placebo. Analyses of the results of drug trials have consistently shown that participants who receive a placebo often experience clinical improvements that can substantially enhance their treatment outcomes.[41] A review of randomised placebo-controlled drug trials found that approximately one in five participants who received an inert placebo spontaneously reported experiencing side effects.[42] Another study found that these side effects often mirror the side effects of the active treatment, and that between 4 and 26 percent of patients in placebo control groups discontinued use of the placebo because of the perceived side effects.[43]

Evidence indicates that participants in drug trials often have both positive and negative expectations: they anticipate improvements, and worry about the possible side effects of the drug being tested (because participants must give informed consent, they must be made aware of possible side effects).[44] It is because expectations formed from informed consent processes provide an idea of the symptoms to look for that reported side effects in the placebo arms of drug trials often reflect the type of symptoms associated with active treatment. The powerful influence of such expectations has been nicely demonstrated

39 Benedetti, Durando and Vighetti 2014.

40 Benedetti, Lanotte, Lopiano and Colloca 2007. A useful and entertaining explanation of the nocebo effect is available on YouTube, and had nearly 5.7 million views as of May 2017: http://bit.ly/2ciSTSc.

41 Enck, Bingel, Schedlowski and Rief 2013.

42 Rosenzweig, Brohier and Zipfel 1993

43 Rief, Avorn and Barsky 2006.

44 Wells and Kaptchuk 2012.

in experimental pain studies using neuroimaging techniques. In one study, the effect of positive and negative expectations on experimentally induced visceral pain was investigated using functional magnetic resonance imaging (fMRI).[45] Participants received an inert substance intravenously, accompanied by either positive instructions that they should expect to experience pain relief, or negative instructions that their pain would increase. The participants' reported experience and their neural processing of visceral pain as measured by fMRI were both consistent with the instructions they had been given, confirming that their reports were not the result of 'response bias' (the tendency to give an expected or socially desirable answer) but reflected their authentic experiences.

Nocebo effects may arise as an adverse effect of placebo therapy, but they have also been shown to occur more widely. There are numerous examples of people reporting symptoms that are unrelated to any biological or pathogenic cause but which are triggered by expectations of adverse health effects.[46] This has been seen throughout history; as Francis Bacon (1561–1626) famously noted, 'infections … if you fear them, you call them upon you'.[47] The common expression that someone is 'worried sick' goes to the heart of this phenomenon. When people mistakenly believe they have been exposed to an ongoing environmental health threat, negative expectations and symptomatic experiences may persist for years, particularly if the concern has been amplified by media attention.[48] In one example, residents of a small Memphis town exhibited a dramatic escalation in symptom reporting following a health scare fuelled by media reports that they were living near an old toxic waste dump.[49] Residents were not reassured by soil toxicity tests which showed that no hazard existed, and increased symptom reporting continued. It was only when it came to light that authorities had been mistaken as to the location of the dump site, which had in fact been situated many miles from the town, that symptom reporting began to subside. However, even this information was not convincing to some residents, who continued to believe they were experiencing adverse health effects from the phantom dump site.

---

45 Schmid et al. 2013.
46 Maugh 1982.
47 Page et al. 2006.
48 Bacon [1597] 2005.
49 David and Wessely 1995.

Nocebo responses have also been implicated in health scares involving other modern technologies. As we saw in the Introduction, the advent of new technologies has consistently been associated with complaints involving a constellation of symptoms akin to those attributed to windfarms.[50] In recent years a number of people have expressed health concerns about technologies that emit weak electromagnetic fields, such as mobile phones, and have attributed a range of symptoms to exposure to these technologies.[51] However, evidence from a number of double blind provocation studies suggests that negative health effects are caused not by exposure to electromagnetic fields, but rather by worry about such exposure.[52] In a double-blind provocation study, participants are exposed both to the stimulus to which they attribute symptoms (such as low-level electromagnetic fields) and to a neutral control stimulus (such as sham or fake electromagnetic fields). During the experiment both participants and the experimenter are unaware whether the exposure is to the real or the sham stimulus. Such studies have consistently shown that sham exposure to electromagnetic fields can activate symptoms in individuals who believe that they suffer from electromagnetic hypersensitivity.[53]

It is important to reiterate that while the exposure itself might be benign, the symptoms reported are not imaginary. As noted above, neuroimaging has confirmed this. In one study, for subjects who self-identified as sensitive to electromagnetic fields, exposure to sham mobile phone radiation was accompanied by activation of brain areas involved in pain perception and the elicitation and control of sympathetic autonomic arousal.[54] When we suggest that nocebo responses may be responsible for health effects, we are not dismissing these symptoms as imaginary or 'all in the mind'. What the evidence demonstrates, however, is that, to responsibly alleviate suffering, treatment options should target sufferers' expectations, rather than having sufferers simply avoid the technologies they believe are causing their problems.

---

50 Petrie and Wessely 2002; Spurgeon 2002.

51 Rubin, Cleare and Wessely 2008.

52 Rubin, Nieto-Hernandez and Wessely 2010.

53 Rubin et al. 2010.

54 Landgrebe et al. 2008.

In the case of windfarms, the type of health complaints attributed to wind turbines, as well as the timing and location of these complaints and who is making them, all suggest that negative expectations may explain the appearance of symptoms in windfarm communities.

The symptoms attributed to windfarms

Many of the symptoms said to arise from exposure to windfarms, such as headaches, tinnitus, fatigue, concentration difficulties, insomnia, gastrointestinal problems, and musculoskeletal pain, are commonly experienced by healthy individuals living in all communities, regardless of whether they are near a windfarm or not. Further, some health complaints attributed to windfarms, such as vestibular symptoms of dizziness and nausea, are symptoms commonly experienced when a person is anxious or distressed.[55] As previously discussed, such symptoms are easily misinterpreted as being directly caused by an environmental agent, rather than a result of stress exacerbated by ongoing concern about perceived toxic exposure.

It is true that symptoms such as tinnitus and sleep disturbance can also be indicative of harmful sound exposure. However, the idea that people living in the vicinity of windfarms can expect to experience these symptoms has been widely promoted in the media, and by windfarm opponents increasingly using the portentous-sounding diagnosis of 'wind turbine syndrome'. As we saw from the evidence from drug trials, such negative expectations are powerful: they will guide people to notice these symptoms and to attribute them to windfarms. An analysis of symptom reporting by people living near wind turbines in Canada found that the reported symptoms were no more prevalent in windfarm communities than in the general population, suggesting that people were misattributing their common symptoms to wind turbines, rather than becoming more symptomatic.[56]

It is interesting that in households where health complaints are reported, adverse effects often extend to every family member in residence, although the effects may take different forms.[57] In one family,

55 Moss-Morris and Petrie 1999.

56 Hamilton 2014.

57 Thorne 2011.

exposure to windfarm sound was said to have caused allergies in a child, social withdrawal in a teenager, symptoms of tinnitus in the mother, and a constant discomforting sensation in the chest of the father.[58] This suggests a process whereby all health complaints are attributed to the household's proximity to windfarms, rather than to other, more likely, causes.

Retrospective symptom reporting: subjectivity and recall bias

Windfarm opponents sometimes counter the suggestion that symptoms could arise from negative expectations by arguing that this 'cannot account for those who were pro-turbine prior to commissioning only to experience adverse health effects post-commissioning'.[59] However, there are a number of reasons why a person's expectations may change. Social context can play a role, such as exposure to intra-community conflict about windfarms. Negative expectations may develop because of exposure to anti-windfarm rhetoric and warnings about the purported health effects of turbine sound. Being told that there is a health risk associated with something you previously supported can be enough to elevate concern and create negative expectations. Once these expectations are formed it is easy to retrospectively misattribute the ordinary experience of symptoms or illness to wind turbines.

Retrospective reports of symptoms are also likely to suffer from recall bias, where there is a tendency to overestimate the incidence and intensity of past symptoms.[60] Research consistently shows that when people are remembering past symptoms they are likely to rate the symptoms as being more frequent and more severe than at the time they were actually experienced. Interestingly, this bias may occur immediately after the symptom episode.[61] In the case of windfarms we see this in research comparing objective and subjective measures of sleep disturbance, discussed in Chapter 4.[62] In this instance, participants were studied before and after the installation of wind

58 Phillips 2011.
59 Commonwealth of Australia 2015c.
60 Houtveen and Oei 2007.
61 Walentynowicz, Bogaerts, Van Diest, Raes and Van den Bergh 2015.
62 Jalali et al. 2016.

turbines in their community. Objective data collected using polysomnography to measure physiologic signals showed that there were no significant changes in the sleep of participants when they were exposed to wind turbine sound. However, subjective data collected using sleep diaries revealed a deterioration in reported sleep quality over time. The issue was apparently one of biased recall. Without the benefit of objective measurement it would have erroneously appeared as though wind turbines had adversely affected residents' sleep.

It is notable that diseases such as diabetes, duodenal ulcers, skin cancer, herpes and stroke, have been ascribed to exposure to windfarm sound.[63] This strongly suggests the involvement of negative expectations, given there is no evidence that windfarms could be responsible for any of these diseases. Over recent decades people have become more inclined to believe that ill health is a by-product of exposure to a toxic environment, and to look for environmental explanations for illness.[64] This is illustrated by research indicating a tendency among survivors of the ten most common cancers to believe that environmental factors play a much more significant role in carcinogenesis than is indicated by the scientific evidence.[65] Negative expectations arising from health concerns about environmental agents can lead sufferers to misattribute their illness to environmental exposure, rather than to more likely influences such as aging, genetic predisposition or lifestyle.[66]

The social transmission of symptoms

As we have seen, while windfarms have been operating in many countries for over 25 years, health concerns about them are much more recent. The vast majority of health complaints arose after the self-publication of Pierpont's *Wind turbine syndrome* in 2009 (see Chapter 2). There is also evidence of a clustering effect, whereby symptoms tend to arise in geographical locations where there has been targeted negative publicity about wind turbines, or where people are accessing negative health information about windfarms. Thus, there are clear

63 Chapman 2014b.
64 Page et al. 2006.
65 Ferrucci et al. 2011.
66 Petrie and Wessely 2002.

indications that exposure to information about purported health risks might be playing a determinative role.

There is consistent evidence from both experimental and field research that media warnings and information circulated via social discourse may create negative expectations and prompt complaints of symptoms, even when the environmental exposure is completely benign.[67] Merely watching a television report promoting a link between exposure to wi-fi and adverse health effects has been shown to increase the likelihood of experiencing symptoms following exposure to a sham wi-fi signal, and to increase the risk of developing an apparent sensitivity to electromagnetic fields.[68] In the Netherlands, exposure to media reports about a fireworks explosion was associated with increased reporting of medically unexplained symptoms, not only by victims directly impacted by the disaster but also by people not directly affected.[69]

The social contagion effect

As already noted, of the small proportion of people worldwide who have reported symptoms ascribed to windfarms, many live in households where multiple occupants report adverse health effects. This suggests a process of social transmission whereby negative expectations and symptoms are discussed within the family, or through wider social networks. Research shows that simply hearing someone talking about their symptoms or observing someone exhibit symptomatic behaviour, such as wincing in pain, can result in the observer manifesting the same symptom.[70] Symptoms such as dizziness, nausea and headaches have been shown to be particularly susceptible to social transmission in both experimental and real-world settings.[71]

In one innovative study, the experience of headache was elicited in a subset of a group of students visiting a research facility at an altitude of 3500 metres.[72] All the students who experienced headaches

---

67 Winters et al. 2003.

68 Witthoft and Rubin 2013.

69 ten Veen, Morren and Yzermans 2009.

70 Faasse, Grey, Jordan, Garland and Petrie 2015.

71 Broderick, Kaplan-Liss and Bass 2011.

had heard rumours about the risk of headaches at high altitude from a single study participant. This participant, known as the 'trigger', had been randomly chosen by the experimenters to receive information, prior to the trip, about the possible occurrence of severe headache at high altitudes. Results showed a significant increase in headaches in those who were vicariously exposed to this information through the naïve trigger, but not in the remaining students who remained unaware of the rumour. Further, the headaches were not a result of reporting bias. Tests indicated that the headaches were accompanied by biochemical changes – increased salivary prostaglandins and thromboxane – that caused the pain to worsen. Administration of a placebo 'analgesic' was shown to reduce this effect, by inhibiting the nocebo component of pain and prostaglandins synthesis. This study highlights that socially transmitted expectations can influence both symptom reporting and biochemical pain pathways.

The power of observation and modelling has also been investigated in experimental studies considering factors involved in mass psychogenic illness – that is, the collective manifestation of physical symptoms in the absence of an identifiable pathogenic cause.[73] In one study participants were asked to inhale a suspected environmental toxin (actually plain ambient air). They were told the agent was known to provoke headache, nausea, itchy skin and drowsiness.[74] The researchers had also enlisted actors (known in psychology as 'confederates') to pretend to be study participants. The genuine participants reported significantly more symptoms if they saw a confederate inhale the suspected toxin and feign the expected symptoms. Observing someone else modelling the expected ill effects amplified their own symptoms.

Evidence also indicates that medically unexplained pain and health complaints in children can sometimes be influenced by a parent modelling similar symptoms, which could explain why some children in windfarm communities have reported symptoms.[75] Both experimental and clinical evidence therefore supports the likely role of social contagion in the transmission of symptoms attributed to windfarms.

---

72 Benedetti et al. 2014.

73 Lorber, Mazzoni and Kirsch 2007.

74 Mazzoni, Foan, Hyland and Kirsch 2010.

75 Osborne, Hatcher and Richtsmeier 1989; Wolff et al. 2010.

Individual differences

Of course, not everyone who is exposed to negative health misinformation about windfarms will experience a nocebo response. This will depend on whether individuals are likely to accept, and be worried by, the narrative that windfarms cause health effects. The evidence from field research shows us that there are personality and attitudinal differences between those who do and do not report symptoms, and that these differences support the thesis that symptoms are triggered by negative expectations.

Most of us have experienced 'negative' people in our families, friendship networks and workplaces. Negative people cause discreet eye-rolling in others when they launch into their predictable whinging about all manner of things. Psychologists have studied this phenomenon and have developed various measurement scales and questionnaires to evaluate where people fall on the negative–positive personality spectrum. There are a number of negative-oriented personality traits. Neuroticism is a stable tendency to respond to threat, frustration or loss with negative emotions such as anxiety, worry, hostility or sadness.[76] Negative affectivity reflects a propensity to experience elevated levels of distress over time and in diverse circumstances.[77] Frustration intolerance is a tendency to be unable to cope with negative emotions, thoughts and events.[78]

People who report symptoms and attribute them to windfarms are more likely to view life through a negative lens and to experience more negative emotions over time. This was highlighted when an English research group investigated whether having a generally negative mindset was associated with negative feelings about ten small and micro wind turbines near two English cities.[79] A relationship between perceived wind turbine noise and medically unexplained non-specific symptoms was only found in people who scored highly when assessed for negative-orientated personality traits (neuroticism, negative affectivity and frustration intolerance).

Effectively, the people attributing symptoms to windfarms are the same people who are likely to complain in other situations. There is

76 Goldberg et al. 2006; Taylor et al. 2013.

77 Watson and Pennebaker 1989.

78 Harrington 2005.

79 Taylor et al. 2013.

consistent evidence that people who exhibit negative-oriented personality traits are more inclined to believe negative narratives about health, to notice and report symptoms consistent with perceived health threats, and to be more susceptible to illness by suggestion.[80] Importantly, increased symptom reporting in this group is generally unrelated to objective markers of ill health.[81]

Negative attitudes to wind turbines and noise annoyance

Negative attitudes to wind turbines are associated with increased symptom reporting. In a recent study, residents living in the vicinity of wind turbines reported poorer sleep quality if they had a negative attitude to wind turbines, if they had concerns about property devaluation, and if they could see wind turbines from their property.[82]

As discussed in Chapter 4, there are also inter-relationships between reported annoyance with the noise produced by windfarms, psychological distress, and reports of stress-related symptoms such as dizziness.[83] While noise annoyance is not closely related to any neurophysiological sensitivity to noise, it is consistently related to *perceived* noise sensitivity, which is a personality trait reflecting a predisposition to attend to and negatively evaluate noise.[84] If annoyance were purely a reflection of the character of windfarm sound, or of the noise sensitivity of residents, we would not expect to see substantial variations in the proportion of people reporting noise annoyance across geographical locations. However, there is considerable variability in noise annoyance reported in field studies. An investigation conducted by Health Canada in relation to two Canadian provinces with equivalent residential noise exposure showed that 6.3 percent of Prince Edward Island respondents were highly annoyed by wind turbine noise, compared with 16.5 percent of respondents from Ontario.[85] This indicates that situational and contextual variables are influencing annoyance reactions.

---

80 Petrie, Moss-Morris, Grey and Shaw 2004; Put et al. 2004.
81 Pennebaker 1994.
82 Jalali et al. 2016.
83 Michaud et al. 2016b.
84 Schutte, Marks, Wenning and Griefahn 2007.
85 Michaud 2015.

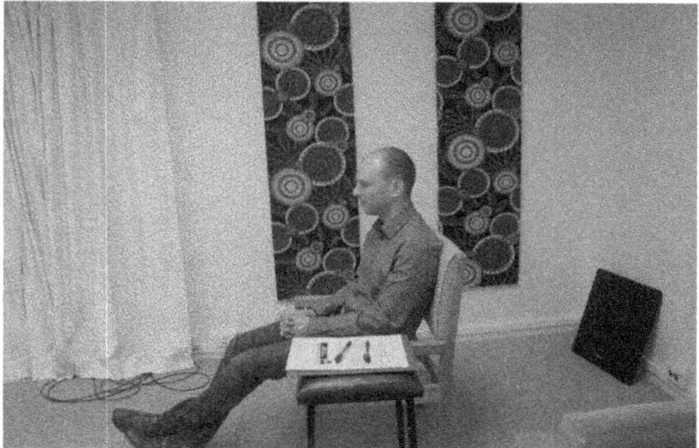

Figure 5.1 Subject being contemporaneously exposed to infrasound and audible windfarm sound in the Acoustic Research Centre listening room.

There is also evidence that noise annoyance is more strongly related to negative attitudes about wind turbines than to the actual level of noise exposure.[86] Noise annoyance is associated with concerns about the health effects of windfarms, aesthetic objections to wind turbines, and simply knowing that the sound is caused by turbines.[87] Increased noise annoyance is also associated with negative publicity about windfarm health effects, indicating that negative expectations play a role.[88] The provincial differences seen between Prince Edward Island and Ontario may, at least in part, be explained by a propensity for media in Ontario to favour negative health stories about windfarms.[89]

Positive context

Finally, residents who have received economic benefit from a windfarm are likely to have more positive attitudes about windfarms and,

86 Pedersen and Waye 2004.

87 Magari, Smith, Schiff and Rohr 2014; Pedersen, van den Berg, Bakker and Bouma 2009; Van Renterghem, Bockstael, De Weirt and Botteldooren 2013.

88 Crichton, Chapman, Cundy and Petrie 2014.

89 Deignan and Hoffman-Goetz 2015.

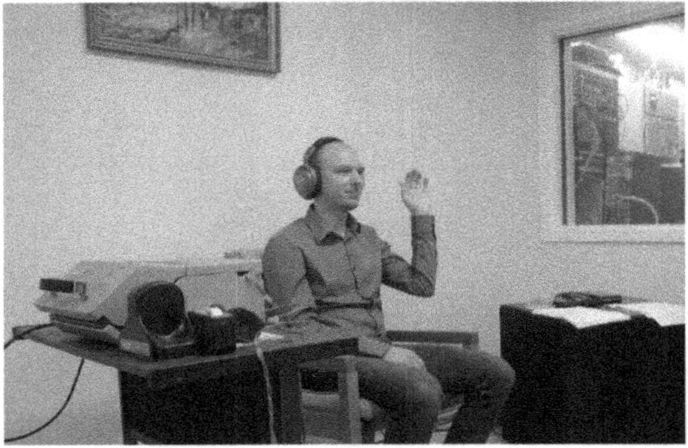

Figure 5.2 Subject undergoing hearing screening test in the listening room with view into the sound control room.

correspondingly, are unlikely to be noise annoyed or to report symptoms, even at relatively high sound exposure. In fact in the recent large scale Health Canada study participants who did not receive personal benefits had 12 times higher odds of being annoyed by wind turbine noise.[90] As we noted in Chapter 3, evidence suggests payment may be one protective factor against anti-windfarm rhetoric, and so an effective antidote to wind turbine syndrome.

A series of experimental studies

To test the broad hypothesis that increased annoyance and health complaints can be explained by negative expectations, we conducted a number of experimental studies. The experiments were performed at the Acoustic Research Centre at the University of Auckland, in a listening room built to international standards for experiments assessing subjective responses to sound (IEC268-13). Over the course of the studies, 246 people, ranging in age between 17 and 70 years old, took part in experimental procedures. We recruited healthy volunteers on the basis that when describing the onset of symptoms, complainants

90 Health Canada 2015.

generally self-identify as previously healthy members of the community. Take for example the acute health effects described below:

> Within twenty minutes ... we each experienced unpleasant symptoms of motion sickness, including ear pressure, headache, nausea, dizziness, vertigo, especially when moving about ...[91]

Over the course of the experiments participants were exposed to infrasound, or to infrasound overlaid with audible windfarm sound, and were asked to report on their current symptoms, mood, and annoyance reactions during two exposure sessions. During the sessions where infrasound was combined with audible windfarm sound, the infrasound at 9 Hz was transmitted at 50.4 dB, to replicate as closely as possible the pressure level at 9 Hz measured in field studies at a distance of 350 metres from wind turbines.[92] Audible windfarm sound was transmitted at 43 dB, a level comparable to the maximum noise exposure level in New Zealand, as set by the windfarm noise standard NZS 6808:2010. The sound recording was taken from a location on a small road approximately one kilometre from the nearest turbine of a windfarm that consisted of 134 turbines (103 turbines of 660 KW and 31 turbines of 3 MW).

Sham controlled study

In the initial sham controlled double blind provocation study, 54 participants were exposed to ten minutes of infrasound and ten minutes of sham infrasound (actually silence), in counter-balanced order – that is, half the participants were exposed to genuine infrasound in their first listening session and sham infrasound in their second, and the remaining participants in the opposite order.[93] However, participants were led to believe that they would be exposed to infrasound during both listening sessions. Participants were asked to evaluate the extent to which they experienced 24 physical symptoms, such as headache, nausea, and dizziness, on a scale from 0 (not at all) to

91 Ambrose, Rand and Krogh 2012.

92 Turnbull et al. 2012.

93 Crichton, Dodd, Schmid, Gamble, Cundy and Petrie 2014.

6 (extreme), both before and during listening sessions. The participants' level of concern about the health effects of windfarm sound exposure was also assessed over the course of the experiment.

Prior to exposure, 27 participants viewed audio-visual material integrating information from the internet suggesting that people were experiencing symptoms when exposed to infrasound generated by windfarms (we will refer to this as the high expectancy group). The remaining 27 participants viewed material in which experts explained that infrasound exposure is an everyday experience and that infrasound produced by windfarms would not cause symptoms (the low expectancy group).

The high expectancy participants reported significant increases in the number and intensity of symptoms experienced during exposure to both real and sham infrasound, relative to the baseline level of symptoms they had reported before the listening sessions. This demonstrated that their symptom reports were provoked by expectations rather than as a result of infrasound exposure. Participants in the high expectancy group tended to report symptoms that had been suggested to them as typical symptoms of infrasound exposure, indicating that their symptom expectations were very specific. As predicted, this increased symptom reporting was associated with increased concern about the health effects of windfarms which developed in the high expectancy group over the course of the study. Importantly, participants in the low expectancy group exhibited no increase in symptom reporting during either listening session, further suggesting that symptom reporting in the high expectation group was a result of a nocebo response.

Building on these findings, our next experimental studies involved simultaneous exposure to sub-audible infrasound and audible windfarm sound during two discrete listening sessions.[94] In keeping with the sham study, expectations were manipulated prior to the listening sessions by exposing participants to media sourced from the internet. As we found in the initial sham study that negative expectations formed from accessing information on the internet triggered symptoms during exposure to windfarm infrasound, our first follow-up study was designed to assess whether positive expectations could produce the opposite effect, in terms of a reduction in symptoms

94 Crichton, Dodd, Schmid, Gamble and Petrie 2014; Crichton, Dodd, Schmid and Petrie 2015; Crichton a Petrie 2015a, 2015b.

and improvements in reported health (Crichton, Dodd, Schmid, Gamble, Cundy et al., 2014). In this study 60 participants were randomly assigned to receive either positive or negative expectations prior to listening sessions. Negative expectation participants watched audio-visual material incorporating television footage about health effects said to be caused by infrasound produced by wind turbines. In contrast, positive expectation participants viewed material that explained infrasound exposure was a normal, natural experience, and also outlined the possible therapeutic effects of infrasound (there are infrasound producing devices promoted on the internet as alleviating the very symptoms windfarm infrasound is said to trigger).

We discovered that, during simultaneous exposure to audible windfarm sound and infrasound, symptoms and mood were strongly influenced by the type of expectations received. Negative expectation participants experienced a significant increase in symptoms and a significant deterioration in mood, while positive expectation participants reported a significant decrease in symptoms and a significant improvement in mood (Figure 5.3). At the conclusion of the experiment 90 percent of positive expectation participants reported that, during listening sessions, they had experienced an improvement in symptoms, while 77 percent of negative expectation participants reported a worsening of symptoms.

In further experiments we found that, once formed, negative expectations could be positively changed and symptom reporting reversed. This was achieved in one experiment by providing negative expectations before the first listening session, during which participants experienced a nocebo response, and by then delivering an alternative positive narrative before the second listening session.[95] This positive narrative emphasised that infrasound was found throughout nature, had alleged health benefits, and exposure was actually a normal experience. We also found that creating positive expectations about infrasound had a buffering effect on the later delivery of negative health information about windfarms; so that, although nocebo responses in response to negative information occurred, they were blunted and less severe. Importantly, we also discovered that, after the initial delivery of negative expectations and consequent symptom reporting during the first listening session, we could reverse symptom reports by providing, before the second session, an explanation of the nocebo effect and

95 Crichton and Petrie 2015a.

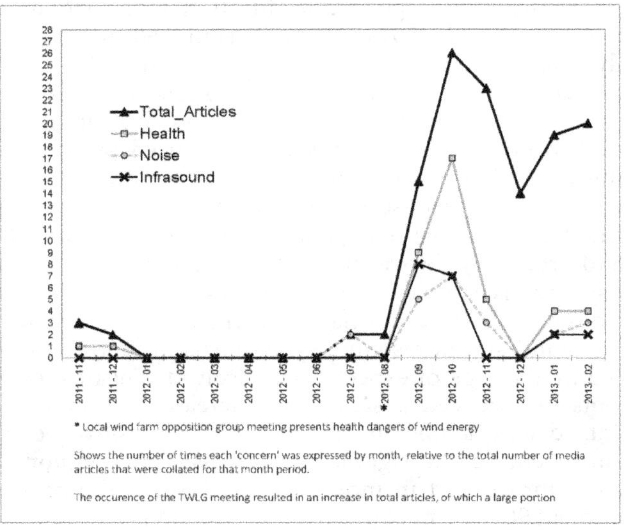

Figure 5.3 Incidence of negative news media mentions of health, noise and infrasound about the proposed Cherry Tree windfarm, Nov 2011–Feb 2013.

its likely role in the participant's symptomatic experiences.[96] These findings provide preliminary indications that disseminating a more positive narrative about windfarms may protect against and improve symptom reporting in community settings.

Overall, across all the experiments, participants who were exposed to warnings about the purported health risks posed by windfarms consistently reported an increase in their symptoms and a deterioration in mood when exposed to windfarm sound. In fact, when participants were given only negative information about windfarm sound, without any counter-narrative, their symptom reporting increased over time, suggesting that their experiences were reinforcing their negative expectations, leading to further anxiety and heightened symptomatic responses. Importantly, however, their symptoms were reduced and their mood improved when infrasound was framed as simply sub-

96 Crichton and Petrie 2015b.

audible sound created by natural phenomena such as waves crashing on the shore or wind blowing through trees, with purported health benefits.

In light of evidence showing interrelationships between noise annoyance, distress, and stress related symptom reporting, reducing noise annoyance is an important strategy to optimise overall health benefits associated with windfarms.[97] To this end we also examined whether negative expectations could be exacerbating annoyance reactions, and whether creating more positive expectations could help to reduce noise annoyance during exposure to wind turbine sound. Given that, as previously discussed, perceived noise sensitivity is said to constitute an underlying vulnerability to annoyance reactions, we also assessed the relationship between perceived noise sensitivity and noise annoyance, and whether expectations influenced that relationship. In keeping with studies of noise annoyance in windfarm communities[98] participants evaluated their own noise sensitivity on a scale from not at all sensitive to extremely noise sensitive, before experimental procedures began. Again, positive and negative expectations were delivered prior to listening sessions using audio-visual presentations incorporating existing internet material.

We found that participants exposed to negative expectations were significantly more annoyed by windfarm sound than participants exposed to positive expectations, illustrating the potential for media and social narratives to influence noise annoyance in windfarm communities. Somewhat surprisingly, while perceived noise sensitivity predicted annoyance, this was only true for the negative expectation group. In other words, individuals in the negative expectation group experienced higher levels of noise annoyance if they were noise sensitive – while positive expectation participants were not annoyed by the sound, even if they were noise sensitive.

Tellingly, in each group, noise sensitivity was related to the participants' experience of negative mood during sound exposure, but the influence ran in opposite directions. In the negative expectations group, participants who considered themselves more sensitive to noise experienced a more negative mood, including more worry, anxiety and distress. However, in the positive expectation group, noise-sensitive participants reported lower levels of worry, anxiety and distress. This

97 Michaud et al. 2016b.

98 Pedersen and Persson Waye 2007.

suggested that these participants experienced significant relief from an underlying tendency to be anxious about the negative effects of sound exposure. This supports the view that perceived noise sensitivity reflects attitudinal and evaluative responses to sound, rather than sensory aspects of auditory processing.[99] These findings are in keeping with other evidence that the context of environmental sound exposure can determine whether perceived noise sensitivity predicts annoyance reactions.[100]

Implications for windfarms

These results have important implications, as anti-windfarm campaigners often cite noise sensitivity as an intractable vulnerability to the negative effects of windfarm sound, and argue that this requires precautionary changes to the regulations governing the location of windfarms. Instead, our research suggests that the answer does not lie in regulatory change, as the vulnerability is not to the acoustic characteristics of windfarm sound. Rather, noise-sensitive individuals are more susceptible to negative suggestions about sound exposure, and, as a result, are more at risk of negative reactions triggered by the dissemination of misinformation about the health risk posed by windfarms. Importantly, our results suggest that creating more positive expectations about windfarm sound exposure should reduce annoyance reactions, even in noise-sensitive residents. This is also indicated by field evidence revealing that where people adopt positive attitudes to windfarms, this operates as a protective factor against annoyance, even if residents are noise-sensitive.[101]

Critically, we discovered that it is possible to reverse negative expectations after they are formed, and thereby alleviate annoyance and symptom complaints during exposure to windfarm sound. This is important if we are to address health complaints in the community. Results showed that nocebo responses were reversed when participants were provided with an alternative, positive narrative about the health effects of windfarm sound, whereby infrasound was depicted as a

99 Ellermeier, Eigenstetter and Zimmer 2001.
100 Oiamo, Baxter, Grgicak-Mannion, Xu and Luginaah 2015.
101 Pedersen et al. 2009.

normal component of environmental sound and reference was made to the use of infrasound in therapeutic contexts.[102]

We also found that nocebo responses could be reversed by explaining to participants that their symptomatic experiences were prompted by negative expectations formed from viewing internet material suggesting that windfarms posed health risks.[103] The way in which the nocebo effect was explained to participants was designed to normalise the nocebo response, eliminate blame, and ensure that their experience of symptoms was validated. Evidence demonstrates that if people feel they are not being believed or not taken seriously, they may become resistant to psychological explanations for their symptoms, and will therefore be more likely to persist with the belief that their symptoms have a biological cause.[104]

As we have previously discussed, brain imaging studies reveal that symptoms experienced as a result of nocebo responses are authentic experiences. Therefore, reversing negative expectations about windfarms is likely to be a vital strategy to address genuine suffering in windfarm communities. This highlights the need for responsible and careful framing of messages about windfarms: the aim should be to minimise anxiety and avoid creating unfounded negative expectations. Importantly, our experimental findings suggest that creating more positive expectations about windfarm sound may ameliorate health complaints and reduce annoyance in affected communities.

The first report of Australia's National Wind Farm Commission,[105] released in 2017 and discussed in Chapter 6, revealed that, in its first year of operation, all of the 46 complaints the commission received about operational windfarms related to just nine of the 76 existing farms in Australia. Further, there were only 42 complaints regarding 19 proposed windfarms. These are very small numbers relative to the numbers of residents living near windfarms across Australia. Field evidence indicates that generally, over time, residents develop more positive attitudes to windfarms in their community.[106] However, in communities where anti-windfarm advocates are actively attempting

102 Crichton and Petrie 2015a.
103 Crichton and Petrie 2015b.
104 Liden, Bjork-Bramberg and Svensson 2015.
105 Office of the National Wind Commissioner 2017.
106 Wilson and Dyke 2009.

to provoke anticipatory anxiety, there is a real risk that negative expectations will produce annoyance and symptoms.

Case study in fomenting anxiety

To understand how anti-windfarm advocates foment anxiety in communities, it is useful to consider a case study from rural Victoria.[107] In 2011, Infigen Energy applied to construct and operate a 16-turbine windfarm known as Cherry Tree, near the top of a 550-metre ridge. Australian census data show that the three settlements nearest to the proposed windfarm had the following populations: Trawool (376 dwellings with 789 people), Whitehead's Creek (9.5 kilometres away from the site, with 159 private dwellings and 373 people) and Seymour (12.7 kilometres away; 2923 dwellings with 6370 people).[108]

On 28 August 2012, a newly proclaimed local anti-windfarm group, the Trawool Valley Landscape Guardians (TWLG), organised a public meeting at Trawool, the small settlement nearest the proposed site. There was an estimated attendance of 100. The meeting was addressed by two residents (Donald Thomas and Noel Dean) who have property near the already operational Waubra windfarm, 230 kilometres by road from Trawool; Max Rheese, a member of the Australian Environment Foundation, an activist group sceptical about global warming and opposed to wind energy; and Steve Campbell, then chief of staff to Senator John Madigan, who at the time was minor party politician outspoken in his opposition to windfarms. A video produced by the Waubra Foundation was shown at the meeting, and a then-director of the foundation, Kathy Russell, was in attendance. Notes taken at the public meeting by an attendee were provided to us, and two news reports highlighted points made by speakers.

In 2013, the Victorian Civil and Administrative Tribunal (VCAT) conducted a hearing to consider objections to the proposed windfarm. In the months prior to this hearing, we documented examples of negative information disseminated through the news media, online, and through other channels.

---

107 This account is based on a paper first published in 2014 and co-authored with my colleagues Ketan Joshi and Luke Fry: Chapman et al. 2014.

108 This short video shows views from the planned site for the 16-turbine, 50 megawatt windfarm: http://youtu.be/JpxNcTCWXIQ

We obtained all media coverage of the proposed windfarm from a commercial media monitoring company (iSentia) for the period between 9 November 2011 and 28 February 2013. This covered the period from the public announcement of the proposal until soon after the commencement of the VCAT hearings. We also searched Google News for the same period, using combinations of the search terms 'Cherry Tree', Cherry Tree, Infigen (the wind company), and 'windfarm'. The records retrieved included news, letters and editorials from local, state and national newspapers, but not local radio or state-wide television. We examined this material for any negative content about noise and/or health issues, which we then grouped into free broad categories, namely expressions of concern or direct assertions that:

- the windfarm would have a direct impact on human health ('Health')
- the windfarm would generate audible noise that would cause annoyance or affect residents' quality of life ('Noise')
- the windfarm would have a direct impact on human health through inaudible noise in the infrasonic range ('Infrasound').

As we have discussed, the internet provides ready access to an abundance of claims about diseases and symptoms said to occur in humans and animals exposed to wind turbines (see Appendix 1). On 21 August 2014, we conducted a Google search using five different search strings likely to be used by anyone seeking broad information about windfarms and health. Jessica Lee has analysed search engine data and shown, among other things, that the first page of Google results account for 33 percent of all reader click-throughs. We weighted the results of our searches using Lee's click-through data,[109] and calculated the probabilistic click-through rankings of the top ten sites returned by each of the five searches. (For more details, see our open-access paper.[110])

We also searched submissions made to VCAT, which are public documents. We examined 75 opposing submissions for any mention of health concerns, and recorded other concerns. Multiple concerns were recorded separately and the postcodes of the writers were recorded. We provide illustrative examples of these concerns in Table 5.2 below.

109 Lee 2013.
110 Chapman et al. 2014.

Quote	Source
'After attending the urgent community meeting regarding the Cherry Tree windfarm proposal, we are now more than ever gravely concerned members of the community'	Letter from four residents. *Seymour Telegraph*, 12 September 2012.
'The major concern of the audience was health including sleep deprivation, increased blood pressure, heart racing, nosebleeds and constant headaches derived from the noise, vibration and infrasound produced from the 160m turbines'	*Seymour Nagambie Advertiser*, 4 September 2012.
'Headaches, wanting to vomit all the time, pains in the chest, blood pressure, can't sleep, sleeping tablets do nothing for you'	Resident featured in a Waubra Foundation video screened at the Trawool meeting.
'Really bad chest pains in the night, and a lot of blood noses, I'd be asleep and then wake up, and my nose would be bleeding. It's just pretty scary stuff'	Resident featured in a Waubra Foundation video screened at the Trawool meeting.
'Symptoms have been consistently reported in Australia, up to 10 kilometres from homes. Most symptoms disappear when people leave the area, or when the turbines are switched off	Waubra Foundation video screened at the Trawool meeting.
'[There's] not a single credible research paper in the peer reviewed literature stating that chronic wind turbine noise is harmless to human health but there is now over a dozen peer reviewed papers that say the opposite'	Max Rheese, climate change sceptic and windfarm opponent, at the Trawool meeting.
'It's the most bizarre thing. It just sounds so weird but you lay down and you can hear the turbines in your pillow'	Waubra resident Donald Thomas at the Trawool meeting

Table 5.2 Illustrative examples of negative statements about windfarms and health from news media and public meeting convened by opponents.

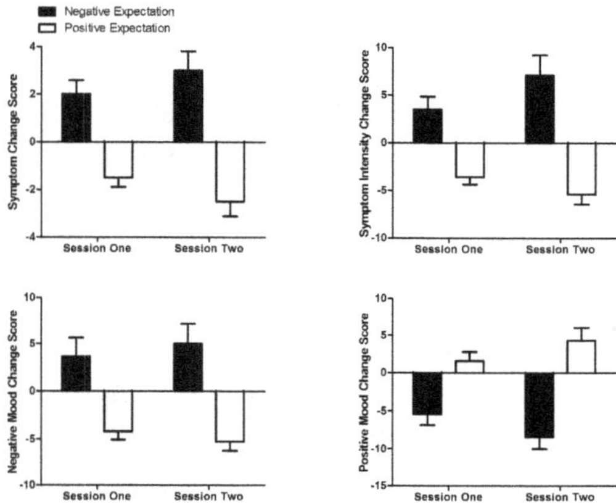

Figure 5.4 Changes from baseline in symptom number, symptom intensity, and mood scores. Source: Crichton, Dodd et al. 2014.

Dissemination of negative information in the local community

Of 126 media articles retrieved, 41 (33 percent) contained concerns about the health impacts of the proposed windfarm. Ninety-five percent of these were published after the anti-windfarm meeting organised by TWLG in August 2012. Figure 5.4 shows the number of times each concern was expressed in the collated media content, along with the total number of articles, and a marker showing the timing of the TWLG meeting.

Negative information from the internet

Using our five different search strings, 27 different sites were retrieved in the top ten hits thus returned. Of these, eight (30 percent) were stories or pages that described the alleged negative health impacts of windfarms, and two were ranked in the top ten weighted click-ranked sites.

Submissions to VCAT

There were 75 submissions made to VCAT from 53 households (several households sent separate submissions by different family members). Of these 53 households, 14 were in Trawool households (representing 3.7 percent of Trawool residences), 16 from Whitehead's Creek (10.1 percent of residences) and 13 from Seymour (0.4 percent of residences). Three were sent from Melbourne addresses (110 kilometres away) and two from known anti-windfarm activists in other states. The remaining five were from hamlets at direct distances ranging from 4.6 to 26.4 kilometres from the proposed site.

All but one submission mentioned health concerns, with reduced visual amenity and bird deaths also being commonly mentioned. Thirty-three (44 percent) of submissions together named 28 different symptoms or health concerns, with the most common being sleep problems (17 mentions), headache/migraine (11), anxiety (9), stress (8), tinnitus (6), and memory loss, nausea and hypertension (5 each). (Table 5.3)

Across the 75 submissions, there were many examples of people expressing concern after having been exposed to alarming, negative claims and testimonies from victims, scientists and doctors. These were often sourced from the anti-windfarm movement, particularly the Waubra Foundation, and from the TVLG public meeting.

For example, from a chiropractor:

> After reading and hearing many accounts of anecdotal evidence given by people living within the vicinity of the wind turbines we are concerned that the turbines may impact on our health. Although we were unable to find any published research on the health problems associated with wind turbines we feel that it better not to take the risk until appropriate research is carried out. Innumerable letters and reports have been written by general practitioners who have witnessed first-hand the negative effects of wind turbines on the health of patients in their community. The results are alarming to say the least.

Many submission writers mentioned that they had met people who claimed to have been made ill by turbines: 'seeing how sick people have become horrifies us'. Many also referred to 'research conducted by the

Concerns expressed	N (% of submissions)
Health related	
General concern about health impacts	74 (99)
Concern that sound or noise will cause health impacts	58 (77)
Specific symptoms, illnesses named	33 (44)
Anticipated abandonment of home	17 (23)
More research needed on health impacts	17 (23)
Blade glint/ shadow flicker	14 (19)
Concerns pre-existing illness will worsen	11 (15)
Electromagnetic interference	10 (13)
Comparisons with tobacco, asbestos or lead as previously benign re health	4 (5)
Economic impact	
Visual amenity marred	57 (76)
Fire risk	47 (63)
Traffic and access problems	37 (49)
Loss of tourism	21 (28)
Decline in local business	15 (20)
Other	
Fauna deaths (esp. birds)	64 (85)
Flora destruction	37 (49)
Community divisiveness	16 (21)
Concern over wind company's multi-national status	15 (20)
Belief windfarms are uneconomic	12 (16)

Table 5.3 Concerns expressed in 75 submissions opposing the windfarm development.

Waubra Foundation', despite the organisation having recently declared that they do not conduct medical research:

> From research from the conducted Waubra Foundation [sic] and international acoustic technicians, we know that the following medical conditions have been identified in people living, working or visiting within 10km of operating wind turbines.

No submissions showed awareness that nobody involved with the Waubra Foundation has conducted any research authorised by a human ethics review committee, nor published any research on the area in an indexed peer-reviewed journal.

As we saw in Chapter 3, windfarm opponents have circulated the factoid that 'over 40' Australian families have abandoned their homes.[111] 'Walking off farms' was mentioned in 17 submissions (23 percent): 'This is evidenced by the fact people are walking off their farms and leaving their houses as a result of the health effects' and 'I believe at this stage that there is too much evidence of people becoming sick and even having to walk off of their land in other areas because of the negative effects of the turbines'. Those leaving were said to include turbines hosts: 'People who have permitted to have put wind turbines on their property, have had to leave their homes because of illness, problems sleeping and noise.' One submission threatened abandonment before any adverse effects were experienced: 'I won't wait to become sick, I would leave'.

The spectre of a distant and venal transnational corporation putting profits over local residents' health was raised in 20 percent of submissions. The company concerned, Infigen, operates windfarms in Australia and the USA.

> One must ask the question of what is more important – that a multinational corporation generates higher profits or that the mental and potentially physical health of the local community is compromised by allowing the wind farm to operate in this location.

(Significantly, Australia's only community-owned windfarm at Leonards Hill, also in Victoria, was not spared opposition despite its ownership structure.)

Three quarters of submissions expressed concern that existing health problems would be exacerbated:

111 Chapman 2014b.

> My eldest son and mother-in-law suffer from severe migraine headaches, often brought on by changes in air pressure, always exacerbated by any loud or ongoing noise. The noise from the wind turbines would make their condition unbearable.

One submission referred directly to claims made by the two Waubra residents who had addressed the meeting: 'One man got sick and he sold his farm because the wind turbines made him sick. The other man could hear the wind turbine noise in his pillow'.

Our results described the dramatic increase in expressed concerns about health and other issues published in local news media immediately following a public meeting organised and addressed by dedicated opponents of windfarms from outside the area. The meeting exposed the small proportion of local residents in attendance to a powerful mixture of sometimes emotional testimony from two complainants from another community, and to contributions from the Waubra Foundation presumably intended to provoke health concerns in those attending and their social networks. Our data also show that anyone searching the internet in Australia for information on health and windfarms will readily find negative material published by opponents.

Confirmation bias is a well-documented cognitive heuristic whereby people search for, interpret, and prioritise information in ways that confirm their beliefs.[112] If individuals have been primed by exposure to events like the Trawool meeting to understand that windfarms threaten health, subsequent searches for information may see confirmation bias operate and lead them to select information that is consonant with their existing negative beliefs.

Victim testimony can be a powerful ingredient in fomenting anxiety in those exposed to their claims. As was noted in a study of Dutch media coverage, 'Scientists, technicians and experts get significantly less space, than laypeople, government, industry and interest groups, in media coverage of EMF health impacts'. In reporting on the proposed windfarm, local news media highlighted the testimony of purported victims:

> Mr Dean said he suffered balance-related problems which he believed were caused by low frequency sound waves generated

112 Klayman 1995.

> turbulence created by wind coming into the turbines. He had suffered head pains, tinnitus and muscle spasms. He had sold most of his land 'and got the hell out of there' telling the audience 'I hope other people don't have to go through what we've gone through.'[113]

During the meeting, an audience member thanked the speakers and said, 'I think it's been extremely informative. A lot of the health issues have come out that we probably weren't aware of.' The meeting provided attendees no exposure to the many who live near windfarms who have no noise or health complaints. A selection of such people from the Waubra area can be seen in a video produced by Vic Wind,[114] featuring landowners talking about their experiences of hosting turbines. Instead, the Trawool public meeting provided a concentrated and memorable set of highly negative claims. This was followed by a surge in local media reporting, although only one third of this raised concerns about noise or health. In total, only 53 of the 3458 residences (or 1.5 percent) in Trawool, Whitehead's Creek and Seymour submitted objections to VCAT.

In the submissions that were submitted, there was considerable evidence of shared or identical wording. Six contained an identical paragraph disputing the wind company's statement that the noise of wind turbines would be comparable to background noise at a beach. These similarities suggested there had been networking between opponents.

VCAT allowed the windfarm to proceed. Of the health considerations raised by opponents, VCAT rejected the hypotheses that wind turbines directly cause adverse health outcomes, implying instead that psychogenic factors were relevant to understanding such experiences:

> The Tribunal has no doubt that some people who live close to a wind turbine experience adverse health effects, including sleep disturbance. The current state of scientific opinion is that there is no causal link of a physiological nature between these effects and the turbine … The totality of material before the Tribunal suggests, but does not conclusively prove, that these effects are suffered by only a small proportion of the population surrounding a wind farm …

113 Sonti 2012.

114 See http://www.windalliance.org.au/waubra-videos.

> The position now, as then, stated by the NHMRC in summary, is that there is no evidence that wind turbines cause adverse health effects.[115]

Every Australian planning case to date considering the issue of 'wind turbine syndrome' has found the evidence offered by proponents of the disease to be insufficient.[116]

Finally, it is interesting to compare the Cherry Tree windfarm development with the Coonooer Bridge windfarm, developed and approved at approximately the same time in Victoria. The latter utilised a community sharing model to distribute income equitably among neighbours. A scientist from the CSIRO noted of the difference between the two projects: 'When we dug a little deeper, we often found their opposition was based more on concerns about process'.[117] Although our research shows the clear impact of the activities of anti-windfarm groups on the expression of health concerns, further research may shed light on what inspires both acceptance rather than resentment.

115 Bergin 2014.
116 Barnard 2014.
117 Green 2013.

6
Opponents of windfarms in Australia

In this chapter, we will take a close look at some of the leading opponents of windfarms in Australtia. We will first consider the two main interest groups (the Waubra Foundation and the various whack-a-mole 'branches' of the Landscape Guardians) that have most often led the small chorus against windfarm development. We will also touch briefly on several other groups that have had a mainly local focus on particular windfarm projects, and on the anonymous, openly defamatory website Stop These Things. We will then profile some of the most prominent Australian individuals who do whatever they can to demonise windfarms, including Sarah Laurie, the indefatigable public voice of the Waubra Foundation.

How widespread is opposition to windfarms in Australia?

The organised anti-windfarm movement in Australia is very, very small. There is no de facto register of the individuals involved but browsing through the lists of public submissions to various government inquiries or calls for comments, anti-wind blogs, and media monitoring records, it is hard to avoid the same few names appearing repeatedly.

In our 2013 study of windfarm complaints across all (at that time) 51 Australian windfarms, we found records of only 129 individuals across Australia who had *ever* complained. Even if all of these individuals lived within five kilometres of a windfarm, this figure would equate to just one complaint for every 254 residents living in the vicinity of wind turbines. In fact 94 of the complainants (or 73 percent of them) lived near one of six particular windfarms targeted by anti-windfarm groups. There were no complaints from either Western Australia or Tasmania.[1]

The main outcome of the 2015 Australian Senate Committee on Wind Turbines report was the establishment of a National Wind Farm Commissioner charged with investigating complaints about windfarms. In March 2017, the commissioner, Andrew Dyer, released his much anticipated first report.[2] In its first 14 months of operation until 31 December 2016, the commission received:

- 46 complaints relating to nine operating windfarms (there were 76 operational windfarms in Australian in 2015)
- 42 complaints relating to 19 proposed windfarms
- two complaints that did not specify a windfarm.

Of the 90 total complaints about operational or planned windfarms, 40 came from Victoria, and 23 each from South Australia and New South Wales. Just two complaints were received from Queensland about planned farms.

As of 31 December 2016, 67 of the 90 complaints had been classified as closed, with the remaining 23 matters still in process. Of the 67 closed complaints, 31 were closed because the complainant decided not to progress the complaint. Another 32 were closed after the complainant was sent relevant information. This left only four in need of any sort of 'negotiated' resolution. According to the report, two of these were settled after negotiations between the parties; the other two were classified as 'other'. Some of the 23 complaints still in process may require similar negotiation, but the numbers remain small.

These desultory figures are frankly devastating to the case that was pushed by the Senate committee. We now have a complaint-investigating mechanism that will cost taxpayers undisclosed millions of dollars, to deal with a problem Madigan and his group swore was widespread, urgent and unacceptable. But the hordes of complainants who apparently needed such a mechanism have mysteriously now gone all shy.

1 Chapman et al. 2013.
2 Office of the National Wind Commissioner 2017.

Shooting themselves in the foot

The anti-windfarm movement's jubilation over the establishment of an independent investigative commissioner was a classic example of the need to be careful in what you wish for.

What has happened has put egg all over Stop These Things' anonymous visage. Simon Holmes à Court, who chaired the community-owned Hepburn Community Wind Project in Victoria, told us:

> Windfarm companies like Infigen can spend hundreds of thousands in legal fees on a single case like the Cherry Tree windfarm VCAT hearings, where the antis used the VCAT process as an expensive taxpayer-funded form of therapy. They've done the same at countless planning panels and senate inquiries. And that's just in the planning process.
>
> I've spent months of my life cutting through the absolute bullshit of the anti-wind brigade in order to have sensible conversations with the people in our community who had genuine interest or concerns.
>
> Now every complainant has a direct conduit to the Wind Commissioner. For those with genuine concerns or grievances, he's in a position to mediate, but looking at the commissioner's complaints-handling policy I doubt the activists are getting much traction: there's a clause that says the Office of the Commissioner won't tolerate abuse and is prepared to refer people to the authorities if they engage in threatening behaviour.
>
> No developer could get away with requiring objectors to be civil! Most wind company staff working in the field have been subjected to obscene behaviour, about which they can do nothing but turn the other cheek and then later read defamatory material about how evil they are on Stop These Things – though everyone I know in the sector stopped reading the site after their failed rally in 2013!
>
> From a purely economic point of view, I believe the commissioner is having much more success for a much lower cost than was being achieved by the (sometimes valiant and sometimes wrong-footed) wind sector. While the taxpayer is covering the costs of the Commissioner, it's a lot cheaper for everyone than endless planning panels, appeals and senate inquiries.

The senators and ex-senators who were so enthusiastic about getting the commission established may today be reflecting that they might have kicked a massive own goal. The commission has the authority to investigate complaints and require complainants to furnish corroborative information, such as medical records and utility bills (which would allow claims about abandoned houses to be checked). If complainants refuse to co-operate, the commission can decline to investigate the complaint.

These men must be embarrassed by the small number of complaints received so far. It will be extremely hard for anti-wind advocates to get any further parliamentary indulgence for their cause. The low numbers, however, should come as no surprise. A 2007 UK report based on 100 percent returns from all local government authorities found that of 133 windfarms in the United Kingdom, only 27 had ever received a noise complaint since the first farm commenced operation in 1991. The complaints that had been received came from just 81 households across the entire country.[3]

A 2012 CSIRO study of community attitudes to windfarms found there was 'strong community support for the development of windfarms, including support from rural residents who do not seek media attention or political engagement to express their views.'[4] Public opinion over the last decade has also showed consistently high levels of community support for renewable energy. In September 2016, 65 percent of Australians thought the nation should take a global leadership position in the roll-out of renewables, and 77 percent agreed that climate change is happening.[5] Australia has the world's highest rate of household uptake of solar energy, with 15 percent of houses having installed solar panels by 2015.[6] Against such a backdrop, it would be surprising if anti-windfarm sentiment were anything but a fringe phenomenon.

3 Moorhouse, Hayes, von Hünerbein, Piper and Adams 2007.
4 Hall, Ashworth and Shaw 2012.
5 Whitmore 2016.
6 Sawa 2015.

A failed rally

A 2013 event organised by Stop These Things (STT) illustrates this perfectly. In the early months of 2013, the people behind STT began organising a protest rally for 18 June on the lawns of Parliament House in Canberra. The master of ceremonies would be the prominent Sydney-based radio announcer Alan Jones. Jones and the STT website relentlessly promoted the rally in the months leading up to it, with those behind STT clearly very close to the planning for the big day.

Brave, anonymous bluster like this was published for weeks on the STT website:

> STT thinks that the wind industry is well and truly on the ropes, but our 'never say die until it's dead and buried' attitude means we won't be happy until there is a garlic-coated crucifix driven through the heart of this rort-ridden scam of the century. Turn up, be loud and take our country back. Let 18 June 2013 be a day the Coalition won't forget.[7]

(The Liberal–National Coalition was then in opposition, but heading towards an election victory in September 2013.)

In the end, the day was certainly one STT would have liked to forget. It was an embarrassing fizzer. I was sent the photograph in Figure 6.1 by an observer in attendance. He suggested that there were probably as many journalists and security staff there as anti-windfarm protestors. The *Australian*, known for its anti-wind stance, put the attendance of the rally at 'only about 100' and reported that a counter pro-wind rally on the other side of Canberra attracted more than 1000 attendees.[8] Even STT's own photographers could not put lipstick on the pig. A series of photographs of the 'throngs' in attendance is a sad spectacle.[9] It is unlikely Jones had ever acted as master of ceremonies to a smaller gathering. Not surprisingly, no other rallies have been attempted since.

7 Taylor 2013.
8 Australian Associated Press 2013.
9 Stop These Things 2013g.

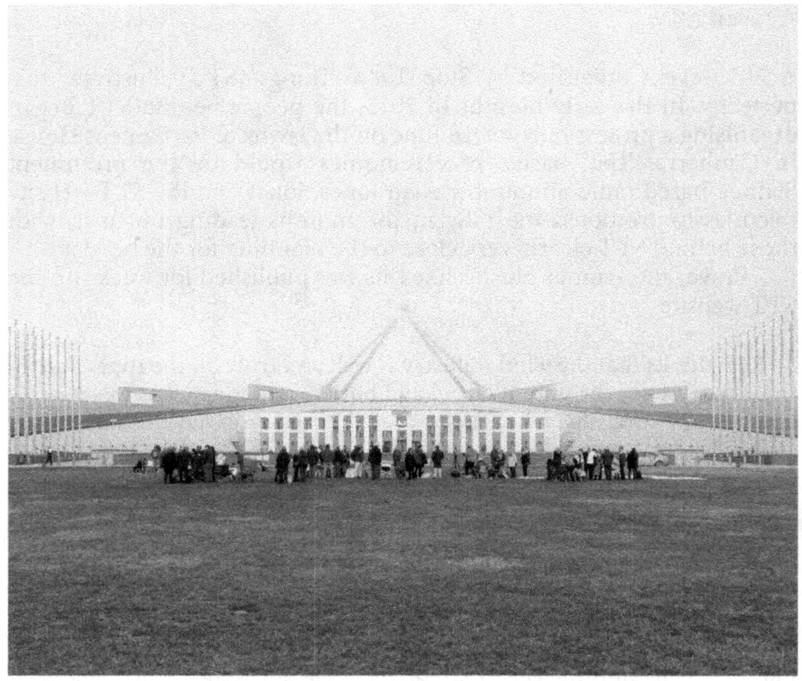

Figure 6.1 A desultory anti-windfarm rally organised by Stop These Things, Canberra, 18 June 2013. Photograph by Leigh Ewbank.

The Landscape Guardians

The very earliest objections to windfarms in Australia were voiced by spokespeople for 'branches' of the Landscape Guardians (for example Prom Coast, Spa Country,[10] Grampians-GlenThompson,[11] Western Plains, Daylesford and District, Leonards Hill). A 2010 report in the *Ballarat Courier* stated that there might have been some 70 branches of the organisation in Australia at the time.[12] Key figures in the Landscape

10 van Tiggelen 2004.
11 Parliament of Victoria 2009.
12 Gullifer 2010.

Guardians have had links with the nuclear energy, mining and fossil-fuel industries.[13] Predictably, the Landscape Guardians have never tried to guard our landscape from open-cut coal, coal-seam gas mining or even residential developers. Such developments involve incomparably more destruction and ongoing pollution of the areas in which they are located than do windfarms. Yet these virtuous people seem only concerned to protect communities from windfarms.

The Landscape Guardians Association Inc. was registered in 2007 by Andrew Miskelly, possibly in preparation for legal proceedings.[14] The Taralga Landscape Guardians failed in a court action in 2007 in which they sought to stop the construction of a windfarm near the NSW southern tablelands town of Taralga. The windfarm was eventually constructed from 2013.[15]

A 2006 *Sydney Morning Herald* report noted that:

> a loose association of anti-windfarm groups that goes by the names of Landscape Guardians or Coastal Guardians relies heavily for its information and campaign tactics on overseas groups that have been linked to the nuclear power industry.
>
> The forerunner of the anti-windfarm pressure group was Britain's Country Guardians, established by Sir Bernard Ingham, a spin doctor for the former British prime minister Margaret Thatcher. He is a director of Supporters of Nuclear Energy. He was also a paid consultant to the British nuclear group BNF.[16]

The Landscape Guardians are something of a peripatetic organisation, announcing and re-announcing themselves to the world, often with many months or sometimes years between appearances, with the same individuals bobbing up as representatives of different branches. Journalist Sandi Keane described how Kathy Russell, a registered director of the Waubra Foundation, was:

> Vice President of the Australian Landscape Guardians, Vice President of the Victorian Landscape Guardians, spokeswoman for

13 Keane 2011.
14 SourceWatch n.d.
15 Preston 2007.
16 Frew 2006.

> the Western Plains Landscape Guardians, Mt Pollock Landscape Guardians and the Barrabool Hills Landscape Guardians.[17]

It has been claimed, and seemingly with justification, that the various Landscape Guardians groups have more officials than ordinary members. Russell opposed the Mount Pollock windfarm near her property (now renamed the Winchelsea Project). Those opposed argued that 'the development would restrict views, create a traffic bottleneck on Mount Pollock Road, devalue neighbouring properties and detrimentally impact on flora and fauna in the area'. She has written a detailed critique of renewable energy for *Quadrant*.[18]

The Waubra Foundation

The Waubra Foundation has been Australia's most prominent anti-windfarm group. Since late 2015, its public activities have been greatly diminished – Google Alerts now produces only rare notices of any media or website activity. At one point it was posting several news articles a week on its website, but at the time of writing it had posted just six articles in 12 months.

The foundation was set up in March 2010 by Peter Mitchell, a Victorian mining, oil and gas investor, who chaired it until January 2015, then spent some 14 months as its patron. He ended his office-bearing involvement in March 2016. Mitchell's antagonism to windfarms sprang from a proposal by Origin Energy to build a windfarm near his country estate:

> As owner of the historic property Mawallock, he successfully objected to the number of turbines proposed for the Stockyard Hill wind farm near Beaufort, Victoria. He also managed to have them removed from the ridge overlooked by his property.[19]

Mitchell wrote at least one submission to parliament for the Landscape Guardians using the South Melbourne post office box of Lowell Capital

---

17 Keane 2011.
18 Russell 2010.
19 Keane 2011.

post office box address, the same address later used by the Waubra Foundation. Sarah Laurie from the Waubra Foundation explained this arrangement, writing on 22 September 2011:

> The Waubra Foundation is not a front for the Landscape Guardians … Peter Mitchell … has kindly made his mailbox available for the use of the Foundation, as we have extremely limited financial resources.[20]

Things must have been tough for the foundation: a post office box at that time cost about 50 cents a day. Perhaps stung by public exposure of this intriguing interconnectedness, the Waubra post box was changed in 2013 to one in Banyule, near the home of the foundation's honorary secretary.

The Waubra Foundation's first patron was the late Alby Schultz, federal member of parliament for the seat of Hume in New South Wales from October 1998 until August 2013. Schultz was an implacable opponent of windfarms, but his electorate hosted a number of them. On 27 July 2011, the *Daily Telegraph* reported Schultz as saying that after surgery to have a pacemaker fitted, his doctor advised him to avoid turbines. 'The thinking is the electromagnetic field generated by windfarms could shut down my system,' he said.[21] Neither Schultz's doctor nor any doctor in Australia came forward to support this bizarre statement. In the whole of Europe, where the concentration of global windfarms in greater than in any other region, and where tens of thousands of residents would have pacemakers, there has never been such a report.

As of 27 September 2017, the Waubra Foundation's website listed four board members: Sarah Laurie (chief executive officer), Charlie Arnott, Michael Crawford, and Tony Edney.[22] Past members have included the founder and chairman Peter Mitchell, Kathy Russell, Michael Wooldridge and Tony Hodgson. As of 30 June 2016 the foundation had net assets of just $8050, no employees, and five volunteers.[23]

20 Walker 2011.
21 Rehn 2011.
22 Waubra Foundation n.d.
23 Australian Charities and Not-for-profits Commission 2016.

Name	Residence (postcode)	Distance from Waubra (km)
Peter Mitchell	Portarlington (3223)	122
Sarah Laurie	Crystal Brook (5523)	668
Tony Hodgson	Mosman (2088)	793
Kathy Russell	Barwon Heads (3227)	127
Michael Wooldridge	Surrey Hills (3127)	141
Clive Tadgell	Malvern (3144)	135

Table 6.1 Distance from Waubra to homes of Waubra Foundation founding directors.

However, as of 25 September 2017, the Australian Securities and Investment Commission (ASIC, the corporate register), showed that Tony Edney had not yet been registered and five of the six founding directors (Peter Mitchell, Robert Tadgell, Kathy Russell, Michael Wooldridge, and Tony Hodgson), as well as Alexandra Nicol (a former staffer for Western Australian Liberal senator Chris Back) and Michael Crawford were still recorded as directors. As mentioned earlier, Michael Wooldridge, a former federal minister for health, was a director until he was barred from serving as such by the corporate regulator.[24] This decision was overturned by the federal court on 1 November 2017.

None of the Waubra Foundation's founding board lived in the Waubra district (see Table 6.1), a fact that has caused widespread anger among local residents who see their town's name being used to advance a wider agenda.

The foundation is registered with the Australian Charities and Not-for-profits Commission (ACNC) and once held Deductible Gift Recipient (DGR) status, meaning that donations were tax deductible. However the foundation's DGR status was revoked on 11 December 2014 after ACNC received a letter from Senator Richard Di Natale of the Australian Greens party challenging the legitimacy of its

24 Janda, Frazer and Caldwell 2014.

classification as a 'health promotion charity'.[25] The foundation has since exhausted all internal ACNC appeals processes and in 2016 subjected the Australian taxpayer to a 12-day hearing with the Administrative Affairs Tribunal. At the time of writing the decision was still pending.

If ACNC's decision to revoke the foundation's tax-deductible status is upheld, $83,790 of donations made to the foundation will have to be distributed to one or more organisations with DGR status and similar objectives. This will be an interesting one to watch.

Activities

One of the Waubra Foundation's governing principles, enshrined in its constitution, is 'At all times to establish and maintain complete independence from government, industry and advocacy groups for or against wind turbines.' The foundation may be 'independent' of other opposition groups, but their relationships are often close, as we saw with the case of Peter Mitchell.

The foundation runs a website and its principal spokesperson, Sarah Laurie, has done a vast number of radio and TV interviews, submission writing, letters to editors and politicians, appearing in support of anti-wind organisations at planning hearings, and speaking at meetings.

On 29 June 2011, the Waubra Foundation moved its aggression needle up several notches by sending a melodramatic 'Explicit Cautionary Notice to those responsible for wind turbine siting decisions' to Australia's wind energy companies, citing a list of health problems that wind turbines might cause.[26] It put the companies on notice that they could be held liable for damages. Predictably, this theatrical bluster has come to nothing over seven years later.

The notice listed a range of very prevalent health problems that collectively are experienced by millions of Australians (sleep deprivation, hypertension, heart attacks, diabetes, migraine, depression, tinnitus, post-traumatic stress, irreversible memory deterioration). The notice stated that all of these conditions 'correspond directly with the operation of wind farms' and that the foundation had conducted its 'own field research'. In the foundation's 2016 report to

---

25 Sturmer 2014.

26 Waubra Foundation 2011b.

the ACNC, it claimed to be 'facilitating multidisciplinary acoustic field research by independent researchers'.

Another publicity stunt by the foundation in 2012 saw a notice on its website call for volunteers to offer respite accommodation for windfarm 'refugees', whom we considered in Chapter 3. Had the stunt met any demand it is hard to imagine the foundation not milking the publicity this would have provided. Unsurprisingly, the notice was quietly removed from the website.

Stop These Things

As we have seen throughout this book, the anonymously authored anti-windfarm website Stop These Things (STT) has become a mecca for a rag-bag of Australian and international climate-change denialists and frothing conspiracy theorists. The great majority of its obsessed correspondents write bravely behind pseudonyms. Its website domain is registered in the USA, but the registrants are inaccessible, cloaked behind a paid anonymity service.

STT began publishing in December 2012. Since then various attempts have been made to sleuth the names of those responsible, both to expose them and to pursue them for defamation. These attempts have involved using analytical software to compare passages of text published on the STT website with public writings of those suspected of being involved. This has often resulted in matches of unusual and characteristic turns of phrase, with three individuals strongly suspected of being involved.

The STT operator or operators appeared to have a very close relationship with the office of Senator John Madigan before he lost his seat in 2016. Madigan's speeches would appear rapidly on the STT website. Brendan Gullifer, who was chief of staff in Madigan's office for several years, is a former journalist who between 2010 and 2012 wrote for the *Ballarat Courier*. He often covered the windfarm issue in a way that excited wind opponents. In 2011, Nina Pierpont's partner, Calvin Luther Martin, awarded Gullifer 'journalist of the year' for his reports on windfarms.[27]

27 Martin 2011.

Gullifer told me by email in 2013 that he had allowed edited excerpts from an abandoned book he had been writing on windfarms to be published on the STT website but was adamant he did not control the site. The excerpts were not published under his byline. He clearly knew how to contact those operating the page.

The decision by STT's 'management' to hide behind anonymity is a double-edged sword for them. On the plus side, they get to exercise the bravery of the anonymous coward by spraying defamatory abuse. But that's about where it ends, because anonymity means no one connected with the site can ever publicly defend it or use its content to take their arguments into other media. No politician would ever stoop to acknowledging support for the site, nor to quoting it in parliament. Its content can never be cited by any authoritative report or investigation. Even a cursory browse through its pages shows fanatical hatred of renewable energy and language that would alert anyone other than those sharing the same values that this is clearly a lunatic fringe at work.

Other opponent groups

Beyond the Landscape Guardians and the Waubra Foundation, other groups that have enjoyed a few moments in the limelight include the Friends of Collector (based in New South Wales near Canberra) and the Flyers Creek Wind Turbine Awareness Group (led by Patina Schneider and opposing the Flyers Creek windfarm development between Orange and Blayney in central western New South Wales). The Noise Watch website, set up in 2014, appears inactive, with no new postings since June 2015.[28] The Waterloo windfarm in South Australia has seen one resident, Mary Morris, who lives some 17 kilometres from the turbines, become prominent in activism against the farm speaking for the Waterloo Concerned Citizens Group.[29]

---

28 See http://www.noisewatchaus.org.au.

29 See http://ramblingsdc.net/Australia/WPowerLies.html.

Prominent individual windfarm opponents

With few exceptions, those who have been prominent in anti-windfarm activism in Australia fall into one of several camps. There is considerable spill-over between these, and they are certainly not mutually exclusive, with some individuals fitting into more than one category.

First, there are those whose hostility to wind power is driven by their contempt for green values and politics. As we wrote in the Introduction, an ideological recoil from climate science, and from wind turbines as totemic reminders of green values, underscores the passion of many objectors. Green politics has polled badly in most rural areas of Australia (with the exception of opposition to coal-seam gas), and for those sceptical or hostile to climate change, wind turbines symbolise values that they reject.

A subset of the anti-green ideologues consists of those with commercial interests in fossil fuels. The journalist Sandi Keane explored this in her 2011 examination of the various Landscape Guardian groups in Australia.[30] Their interest in denigrating renewable energy is obvious, as is their willingness to harness health scares in service of that wider objective.

Next, there are NIMBYs (not in my back yarders) – those who may or may not have any antipathy to renewable energy, but whose main objection is that they just don't want wind turbines anywhere near their properties. Their main objections are usually aesthetic, with other arguments, including health, being pulled in as extra ordinance in their battles with local and state governments. NIMBYism can be expressed by people of any social class or background, but many have remarked on the prominence of a handful of wealthy or well-connected individuals with rural properties who have objected to Australian windfarms.

These include:

Peter Mitchell, now in his 80s, has a long history in mining investment. He has been involved in the Landscape Guardians and the Waubra Foundation, which he founded in March 2010. A submission sent in February 2011 to the Senate inquiry into windfarms, authored by Mitchell on behalf of the Australian Landscape Guardians, is addressed from PO Box 1136, South Melbourne, Victoria 3205, the

30 Keane 2011.

same address as Mitchell's Lowell Resources Funds Management Limited, a mining investment company.[31] Its portfolio represents 'a range of commodities including gold, iron ore, coal, oil, gas, uranium, rare earths and strategic minerals, copper and other base metals'.[32] Mitchell owns a country estate with an acclaimed garden not far from the proposed Stockyard Hill windfarm, which, after many delays, will proceed to construction in 2018.

Maurice Newman chaired then Prime Minister Tony Abbott's Business Advisory Council, as well as the Australian Broadcasting Corporation and the Australian Stock Exchange. Newman and his wife hosted a meeting of the Crookwell and District Landscape Guardians at their country house, the minutes of which were leaked; they included a discussion among those attending of how best to oppose windfarm developments.[33] Newman wrote in the right-wing *Spectator*:

> Even before they threatened my property, I was opposed to windfarms. They fail on all counts. They are grossly inefficient, extremely expensive, socially inequitable, a danger to human health, environmentally harmful, divisive for communities, a blot on the landscape, and don't even achieve the purpose for which they were designed, namely the reliable generation of electricity and the reduction of CO_2 emissions.[34]

Charlie Arnott, a cattle and sheep farmer from Boorowa in New South Wales (and great-great-great-grandson of the Arnott's biscuits founder), has been spokesman for the Boorowa District Landscape Guardians and, since 2013, a board member of the Waubra Foundation.

Tony Hodgson, with Rodd Pahl (see below), co-founded the Friends of Collector opposition group.[35] Hodgson was joint founding and managing partner of Australia's leading corporate and insolvency firm, Ferrier Hodgson. In 2013, he threatened to sue any neighbours who put wind turbines on their properties near his cattle farm.[36]

31 Mitchell 2011.
32 Lowell Capital Ltd 2011.
33 Taylor 2013.
34 Newman 2012.
35 Boland-Rudder 2013.
36 Francis 2013.

Rodd Pahl is the managing director of Bluegrass, a PR consulting firm that has helped to promote opposition to windfarms. Bluegrass' website once advised: 'We have developed a set of online tools to augment more traditional advocacy techniques and help you build grassroots movements that result in real action.'[37] Echoing the core lesson promulgated by the 'merchants of doubt',[38] it continued 'Look to create political uncertainty, strong voices on opposing views leads to hesitation'.

In November 2013, Pahl established the Association for Research of Renewable Energy in Australia Limited (ARREA). Its Australian Securities and Investment registration shows its business address is at Bluegrass' office in Sydney, with Pahl listed as one of three directors. ARREA commissioned a report that was summarised in a submission to the 2015 Senate inquiry. Its main conclusion was that:

> Wind power duplicates electricity production, distorts market signals, especially compared to other renewable energy sources, and leads to inappropriate public perceptions about the value of wind power to the long-term sustainability of our nation.[39]

During the Senate inquiry, Senator Urquhart asked another ARREA director, Douglas Bucknell, how many members ARREA had. He responded, 'Seven'. Senator Urquhart then asked, 'I understand that spokespeople for your organisation are Tony Hodgson and Rod Pahl – is that correct? And are they also spokespeople for an opponent wind group called Friends of Collector – is that right?' Bucknell answered elliptically, 'I understand that to be right.'[40]

Michael Wooldridge, former health minister in the Howard Coalition government (1996–2001), was a board member of the Waubra Foundation but resigned in 2014 following an adverse finding (subsequently overturned) by the Federal Court about his role as a director of a retirement village company.[41] Wooldridge had opposed the proposed Bald Hills windfarm, which bordered his family's farming interests in Gippsland, Victoria. The Bald Hills project (now

---

37 Chapman 2011.
38 Michaels and Monforton 2005.
39 Association for Research of Renewable Energy in Australia 2015.
40 Commonwealth of Australia 2015a.
41 Janda, Frazer and Caldwell 2014.

operational) was almost scuttled by the Landscape Guardians' heartfelt concern for the safety of the orange-bellied parrot (see Chapter 1).

Two *BRW* 'rich list' multi-millionaires, **Bill James** and **Michael Crouch**, helped to support legal action against a large windfarm planned for Tasmania's King Island, although neither personally lived there.[42] According to *BRW*, Bill James is one of three founders of the travel giant Flight Centre and is worth $855 million. His family is believed to own land on King Island, but according to locals he does not live there. Crouch, the other major donor, is worth $310 million after founding Zip Industries, says *Crikey*.[43] He owns Waverley Station, a cattle farm on King Island, but also does not live there.

Gillon McLachlan, the CEO of the Australian Football League, commenced legal action in 2016 to stop an approved windfarm on the doorstep of his family's historic Rosebank property, near Mount Pleasant and Adelaide. The Mount Lofty Landscape Guardians are also involved in the action. McLachlan withdrew his participation in the action in March 2017.[44]

Ted Baillieu, as Liberal premier of Victoria (2010–13), introduced a range of planning measures designed to shut down wind development, including the establishment of a series of 'no-go zones' for windfarm construction zones across Victoria. The only non-coastal no-go zone was in the McHarg Ranges (an area unknown to most Victorians), where Lady Marigold Southey – former Victorian lieutenant-governor and Baillieu's second cousin – owned an 800-hectare farm and vineyard near the hamlet of Tooborac. Southey had been an active opponent of a proposal for an 80-turbine windfarm in the area.[45]

Upstairs–downstairs: the sociology of opposition

There is a fascinating sociological side to the prominence in the anti-windfarm movement of well-to-do individuals. When wind energy companies scout potential locations for windfarms, land exposed to high winds understandably has high priority. Accessible land on

42 Anon. 2014.
43 Whyte 2014.
44 Booth 2017.
45 Millar and Morton 2012.

mountain ridges has premium attractiveness. Herein we find an interesting dimension to what is often a class-based opposition to windfarms.

Mountainous and hilly land is generally worth far less that flat land. Flat land can be used for cropping and grazing stock, while hilly land and the ridges of mountains are far less economically useful to farmers.

Because of this basic difference, flat land is more expensive to buy than hilly land, with the result that those with properties suitable for cropping and grazing tend to be more well-to-do than those who have only been able to afford hilly scrubland. In rural areas, it is common for there to be old established family holdings of landed gentry who have enjoyed local privileges of wealth and status, as well as more recently arrived city folk who have bought prestigious old country properties and hobby farms and often move between these and their city addresses.

Such landowners may have little interest in earning extra income from wind turbines as for them the property is a lifestyle asset, a 'bolt-hole' to escape the city on weekends. By contrast, far less well-off landowners who own less valuable land may see windfarms as manna from heaven: as an opportunity to turn non-arable or grazing land destined to be perpetually marginal into a cash cow. More than that, the guaranteed income they earn from turbines adds to their property value and 'drought proofs' their income in dry seasons when their agricultural earnings may be way down.

These differences foment interesting frictions between less well-off local landowners who stand to earn an ongoing windfall of cash from turbine hosting and implacably opposed wealthier 'upstairs' landowners who see the good fortune of their 'downstairs' neighbours as an affront to the natural social order of things. The landed gentry and weekend 'Pitt Street/Collins Street' farmers are outraged that their bucolic vistas might be spoilt by the sight of wind turbines and care little for the good fortune of local farmers who stand to benefit greatly from hosting them.

Members of the wind sector have explained to us that almost every organised opposition group is funded by a wealthy landowner with a country estate. Draw a pair of circles at a distance of one and three hours' drive around each capital city and the vast majority of opposition to windfarms has taken place between these circles, with very little in the rural areas far from capital cities. (A former staffer of the NSW Office of the Environment and Heritage once remarked off the record that of the six members of one lobby group who attended a meeting, five had their primary residences in the well-to-do Sydney suburbs of Mosman and Balmain.)

Not often appreciated is the inevitable tension between the two socio-economic groups – those who come to the area on weekends for the pastoral scenery and who pine for the charm of 1950s country Australia, and those who live full-time in the community and rely on its economic health not only for their own livelihoods but also for their children's future prospects in the area.

At the time of writing in mid-2017, the success of prominent anti-windfarm NIMBYs in thwarting windfarms in their districts looks decidedly disappointing for them (Table 6.2).

Perennial victims and professional objectors

In Australia, a small number of individuals and families have long been the public face of anti-windfarm victimhood. They often appear in media reports, and are feted by radio hosts and the few politicians who are opposed to renewable energy. They are invited to tell their stories to public meetings organised by opponent networks, and have been given the limelight at Senate inquiries and administrative affairs tribunals. They get to meet 'important people'. I have been told more than once by residents who support windfarms that these people appear to 'like getting their pictures in the paper', or that opposition to the windfarm has 'given purpose to an otherwise unremarkable life'. Such attention can be intoxicating and can be hard to walk away from.

Rejected or ineligible windfarm hosts

When a wind energy company announces plans to develop a windfarm in an area, they will already have undertaken extensive land, wind and electricity network surveys before settling on a prospective location. In small rural communities, word spreads quickly that a company is scouting the area, and with potentially lucrative land rentals on offer, some landowners inevitably see dollar signs.

Windfarm developers work through a very complex process to put in place the lease agreements. These include negotiations with landowners on commercial terms and the layout for an optimal

Objector	Organisational affiliation	Windfarm	Status
Peter Mitchell	Waubra Foundation, Landscape Guardians	Stockyard Hill (Vic)	530 MW (largest in Australia) in development (Vorrath and Parkinson 2017).
Tony Hodgson	Waubra Foundation	Collector (NSW)	55 turbines received final approval. Awaiting construction.*
Sarah Laurie	Waubra Foundation	Crystal Brook Energy Park (SA)	250 MW Land agreements signed December 2016.**
Kathy Russell	Waubra Foundation, Landscape Guardians	Winchelsea/ Mt Pollock (Vic)	Winchelsea farm (44 turbines, 132 MW) being built (Fowles 2016).
Michael Wooldridge	Waubra Foundation	Bald Hills (Vic)	52 turbines operational since 2015 (Parkinson 2015).
Maurice Newman	Crookwell and District Landscape Guardians	Crookwell (NSW)	91 MW, 28 turbine construction begins in 2017 (Burgess 2016).
Angus Taylor MP	Liberal Party	Boco Rock (NSW)	Received development approval from the NSW government in 2010 for up to 122 turbines.***
Charlie Arnott	Boorowa District Landscape Guardians	Boorowa (NSW)	Boorowa did not proceed but nearby Rye Park development recommended for approval (Coote 2017).

Table 6.2 Status of windfarm developments opposed by prominent Australians. *http://ratchaustralia.com/collector/about_collector.html **http://crystalbrookenergypark.com.au/history/ ***https://www.bocorockwindfarm.com.au

windfarm. The developer is optimising the number and size of turbines, the wind resource in the turbine locations (it can vary significantly around the local topography), access to turbine sites (construction roads are a major cost for a windfarm), electricity grid connection costs, planning system constraints, and the developer's access to capital through its financing.

Throughout this process, which can take many months or even years, the proposed windfarm layout can change many times, with the ultimate result only knowable at the end. Some landowners who believed they were assured of a lucrative annuity may end up with nothing – upon investigation their property may not have been as suitable as expected, a neighbour might have thrown a spanner in the works, their property may never have been in consideration in the first place, planning regulations might have changed, or, all too commonly, the developer may determine that the entire project is not viable and abandon the project.

It is a rollercoaster ride for all those involved and, as with all development, there are plenty of examples of bad behaviour on both sides of the table. In the early days of the sector in Australia there was plenty of money to be made in signing up a number of landowners, securing a planning permit and on-selling the project. Unfortunately, some opportunists ruffled feathers in more than a few communities. Many a developer also inadvertently stirred up long-festering family feuds, which can be caused by big issues such as disputes over inheritance or small issues such as a poorly maintained fence or night-time noise from an irrigation pump.

Savvy wind developers nowadays are careful to engage as often as possible with the community, employ staff in the local area from day one, ensure that all landowners receive equal financial terms, develop benefit-sharing schemes, and, in some cases, offer payments to landowners nearby who miss out. In the past some developers had landowners sign confidentiality agreements, but as the industry has developed it has become generally accepted that such agreements only serve to foment suspicion and jealousy.

Even when there is a contractual agreement that rental payments should remain confidential, rumours of the often large sums involved tend to leak and circulate among local residents. While there are some who might regard the income going to the hosts as simply their good luck, it is understandable that others may deeply resent the apparent unfairness of some residents getting paid while others miss out, especially when community engagement has not been handled well, benefits haven't been shared, and there is a sense that an outsider has arbitrarily created 'winners' and 'losers'. We take up this issue in Chapter 8, where we look at ways in which this resentment might be reduced.

Before I attended a National and Medical Research Council meeting on windfarms and health in Canberra on 7 June 2011, I had never met any of those involved in the wind industry or those supporting or opposing windfarms. All of these interest groups were present at the meeting. The 'antis' kept well clear of me, probably because I had by then already written an article for the *Croakey* blog that would have greatly displeased them.[46]

At the lunch break I met several of those representing the wind industry. One of them pointed out one of the 'antis'. The wind company representative said words to the effect of:

> When we were first assessing the suitability of various farms for hosting, one local approached us hoping that we would put as many on his property as we could. Unfortunately for him, his land was unsuitable because of its topography. It wouldn't have been commercially viable for us. From the moment we told him that, he turned from a strong supporter into a sworn enemy who is now making things as hard as he possibly can.

He added that he had kept various correspondence written by the farmer and was looking forward to it finding its way into the public domain, should the farmer's efforts continue.

In another account I was given, a family not being considered for turbine hosting nonetheless approached the wind company representatives, seeking a deal. The family wanted the company to have their entire house lifted onto a truck and moved to a picturesque lake at the back of their property. The family proposed that the company would pay all costs and erect a jetty so that a boat could be moored near the house. The family threatened to make things difficult for the company if their demands were not satisfied.

This is an extreme example, but tales of families requesting extensive renovations, ostensibly in order to 'sound-insulate' their houses, are more common. The proposed renovations are often

---

46 Chapman 2010.

extravagant and include works that could not be considered noise mitigation. When they are agreed to, word spreads and others join the queue to see what they can get. Local narratives develop about cashed-up multinationals who will bend to such demands given what is at stake. It becomes part of the cost of doing business. But truly extravagant demands are often refused, and long-term acrimony can then set in.

'Professional' opponents

Various anti-windfarm websites around the world proudly list the names of 78 'professionals' who, according to the European Platform Against Wind Farms,[47] which assembled the list, have 'investigated or voiced concern for the health and well-being of wind turbine neighbors'. Fourteen of the paltry global 78 are from Australia: Steven Cooper (acoustician), Con Doolan (engineer), Colin Hansen (engineer), Les Huson (acoustician), David Iser (GP), Sarah Laurie (former rural GP), Peter Mitchell (engineer), Andja Mitric Andjic (rural GP), George Papadopoulos (pharmacist), Wayne Spring (physician), Scott Taylor (rural GP), Bob Thorne (psychoacoustician) and Carcoar husband and wife Alan Watts (rural GP), and Colleen Watts ('scientist'). 'Professional' here is of course code for anyone with a tertiary qualification in any field who concludes that wind turbines cause health problems.

It's important to put these numbers in perspective. There were 102,804 registered medical practitioners in Australian in 2015. Given Sarah Laurie is unregistered to practise medicine (see below), that leaves just five registered medical practitioners in Australia who have expressed concerns about windfarms in Australia, according to the anti-wind groups. That's just one in 20,561 registered doctors whom windfarm opponents claim as theirs, an almost homeopathic concentration of concern.

In the following pages, we profile several prominent Australian windfarm opponents to give a sense of the some of their more interesting beliefs. We also considered David Mortimer in Chapter 3.

47 European Platform Against Wind Farms n.d.

Sarah Laurie

The high priestess of windfarm opposition in Australia is undoubtedly Sarah Laurie. She has been the public face of the Waubra Foundation, although in recent years she has been much less prominent. Google alerts for her name since about mid 2015 have rarely flagged any news coverage.

Laurie lives a short distance from the site of a windfarm once proposed for Crystal Brook in South Australia in 2010. The project did not proceed at the time, but has recently been picked up by another developer and is again progressing. Laurie's concerns about windfarms seem to date from around that period. She has been a prolific writer, although mainly confines her efforts to submissions to windfarm enquiries, lengthy letters to politicians, bureaucrats and journalists, the web pages of the Waubra Foundation and other international anti-windfarm websites. She seldom, if ever, writes for scientific journals. On 8 May 2017 PubMed returned no results from the advanced search author=Laurie S, and all fields=wind.

Laurie is a medical graduate who obtained her bachelor degrees in medicine from Flinders Medical School in Adelaide in 1995. She practised medicine for seven years before ceasing practice in April 2002. She let her registration lapse some two and half years later. Since graduating she has to date therefore spent more than twice as long not practising (15 years) as she did practising (seven years). She was awarded a fellowship with the Royal Australian College of General Practitioners in 1999, and a fellowship with the Australian College of Remote and Rural Medicine in March 2000, although she relinquished her membership of the latter in 2004. Laurie has explained that her decision to stop medical practice was because of personal health and family reasons.

When the Waubra Foundation formed in 2010, its website described Laurie as its 'medical director'. This later changed to 'chief executive officer'.[48] She is unaffiliated with any accredited research institution. Therefore, if the Waubra Foundation under her direction was conducting 'field research' involving human subjects, this would not have been approved by any institutional ethics committee. She would have been unable to publish any papers arising from that

48 See http://waubrafoundation.org.au/about/people.

research in any reputable medical journal where formal ethics clearance is mandatory whenever human subjects are involved.

In 2013 Laurie gave evidence about her views on wind turbine health impacts to the Ontario Environmental Review Tribunal. The tribunal noted that she 'has not conducted formal structured research. She states that she conducts an ongoing survey, where, to date, she has spoken with approximately 130 people in Australia who live in the vicinity of industrial wind turbine projects.' This semantic distinction between her 'field research' and 'formal structured research' would make a fascinating case study in human research ethics.

The December 2013 judgment of the Ontario tribunal includes some 12 pages discussing whether Laurie's qualifications and experience entitled her to be considered an expert witness in the tribunal's deliberations, and the evidence she gave. On the matter of her use of the title 'Doctor' in association with her Waubra Foundation activities, the judgment states:

> As a result of a complaint filed with the AHPRA [Australian Health Practitioner Regulation Agency] in 2013 that her current activities (discussed below) constituted practice as a physician, she voluntarily agreed not to use the title/honorific 'Doctor' or 'Dr'. She states that she has done so, in order to avoid any potential misunderstanding by members of the public regarding her status as a practicing physician. Documentary evidence respecting the complaint was adduced in evidence and marked confidential, i.e., it is not included in the public record in this proceeding. Ms Laurie was cross-examined on this evidence. The Tribunal finds that this evidence supports Ms Laurie's assertion that the AHPRA did not make any finding in respect of the complaint made against her.[49]

Two years later, the transcript of Laurie's evidence to the 2015 Senate committee on wind turbines describes her as 'Ms Laurie', but those who signed off the final majority report still allowed her to be described in the report as 'Dr' on seven occasions. Stop These Things and other anti-windfarm websites have no doubt that she should still be called 'Dr'.

Laurie has sometimes had a hard time in courts and tribunals when she has sought to be or been called as an expert witness in wind turbine cases.

---

49 Environmental Review Tribunal of Ontario 2013.

The South Australian Environment, Resources and Development Court, in its judgment of *Paltridge & Ors vs District*, was satisfied that public health would not be put at risk by a proposed windfarm development. Commenting on Laurie's evidence to the court and comparing it to that provided by Professor Gary Wittert from the University of Adelaide, the bench wrote:

> With regard to the interviews [of those said to be suffering from wind turbine exposure] conducted by Dr Laurie, we accept the criticisms of this evidence made by counsel for Acciona [the windfarm developer], namely, that they suffer from the following defects:
>
> 1. The absence of a formal medical history having been taken from the subjects of her interviews;
> 2. The absence of a formal diagnosis of alleged symptoms from these subjects; and
> 3. The absence of any enquiry, as to the prevalence of the symptoms reported by these subjects, when compared to any other population or a control population.[50]

The court also noted:

> After reviewing the evidence of Dr Laurie, Professor Wittert concluded that: 'There is no credible evidence of a causal link, between the physical outputs of a turbine (or sets of turbines), at the levels that are described … and adverse effects on health'.

The judgment concluded: 'We accept his [Wittert's] conclusions and, where his evidence differs from that of Dr Laurie, prefer the evidence of Professor Wittert.'

Wittert examined Laurie's 'research' data, which she claimed showed an association between the morning blood pressure of three individuals living near the Waubra windfarm and the power output of the turbines. Wittert concluded (as anyone with even basic ability to interpret graphic associations can see immediately by looking at the data): 'These data are inconsistent with any assertion that the output from wind turbines has an adverse effect on blood pressure.'[51]

---

50 Environment, Resources and Development Court of South Australia 2011.

51 Wittert 2011.

The same 2013 Ontario Environmental Review Tribunal judgment states:

> In terms of her other professional training and experience, Ms Laurie acknowledges that she has no training or experience in conducting medical or scientific research. She further acknowledges that she also does not have any training or experience in research methodology and design, other than some undergraduate exposure when obtaining her medical degree, and does not have postgraduate experience in this area. She acknowledges that she is not a qualified acoustician, and she has no experience or training in acoustics generally, or, in particular, pertaining to noise generated by industrial wind turbines, although she has reviewed publications in the subject area of acoustics, and has consulted with acousticians.[52]

A South Australian court made a similar observation in 2014:

> Dr Laurie is not an expert in assessing whether there is a causal link between windfarm noise and health impacts. She has no relevant qualifications or experience in this kind of research. However, in case we are wrong in rejecting Dr Laurie's as an expert, we will consider her evidence.

The judgment noted that:

> Dr Laurie rejects all of the studies, including the EPA studies, which are not consistent with her theories. She admits that evidence showing a causal connection between contemporary windfarms and health effects does not exist, and she seeks to have more research done in the hope that such evidence will be generated in the future.[53]

The 2013 Ontario judgment determined that while Laurie could give evidence, deficiencies in her training and expertise and current status as an unregistered doctor meant that:

52 Environmental Review Tribunal of Ontario 2013.
53 Environment, Resources and Development Court of South Australia 2014.

The Tribunal accepts that it is appropriate for Ms Laurie to consider existing published research or other literature in formulating her opinions. However, the Tribunal has already found that Ms Laurie cannot be qualified to give opinion evidence based on formal medical or scientific research, or research design and methodology. The Tribunal has also found that she cannot be qualified to give opinion evidence requiring diagnostic opinions, or the application of diagnostic interpretation to formulate conclusions on the potential health impacts of exposure to operating 'industrial wind turbines. This raises the question whether she can be qualified to give her proposed opinion evidence on the basis of the experience she has obtained through self-study of the published research and other literature. The Tribunal accepts that the time Ms Laurie has devoted to this aspect of her work experience is not insignificant. However, Ms Laurie's evidence does not indicate that she has conducted a comprehensive review of all literature, nor that she has the expertise to assess the sufficiency of the research methodology in individual research studies. Consequently, the Tribunal finds that her self-study of the published literature, as described in her witness statement, even if considered in conjunction with her survey of self-identified participants, is not sufficient to meet the basic threshold of reliability necessary to assist the Tribunal in making a sound decision.

[456] In summary, the Tribunal has found that the Appellant, Mr Sanford, has not established a basis on which Ms Laurie can be qualified to give her proposed opinion evidence in this proceeding.

[457] The above finding, however, does not preclude Ms Laurie from giving evidence.

It noted that while her status as a medical graduate who was now unregistered did not permit her to make medical diagnoses of persons she interviewed, this is in fact what she was doing when providing her opinion about those whose health she described:

[449] … the Tribunal has found that most of the opinions expressed by Ms Laurie do require the making of a diagnosis, or the application of diagnostic interpretation. Therefore, the Tribunal finds that it cannot ascribe sufficient reliability to these opinions, in contradictory circumstances where diagnostic opinion is being

> proffered by the witness, while, at the same time, the witness stipulates that she cannot provide such diagnostic opinion.
>
> [450] The above analysis and findings address the opinions in Ms Laurie's witness statement which require the making of a diagnosis and/or the application of diagnostic interpretation as described above.

Laurie was allowed to testify in a 2014 hearing for the Bull Creek Wind Project in Alberta, Canada. However, the commission gave its opinion on her skills and training and testimony, stating:

> Dr Laurie's written evidence also included her interpretation and discussion of numerous published and unpublished epidemiological and acoustical reports and studies. In the Commission's view, Dr Laurie lacks the necessary skills, experience and training to comment on the interpretation of epidemiologic studies or the interpretation of acoustical studies and reports. The Commission gave little weight to this aspect of Dr Laurie's evidence.[54]

Laurie sometimes goes out of her way to explain that she and the Waubra Foundation are not opposed to windfarms, but rather that they are an organisation focused on publicising and ameliorating the health effects of noise and infrasound regardless of its source. The Ontario Environmental Review Tribunal summed up this distinction:

> Ms Laurie explained that the Waubra Foundation is solely concerned with the human health consequences of exposure to operating 'industrial wind turbines and other sources of infrasound and low frequency noise'. She states that she does not oppose industrial wind projects per se, but is concerned about the current practice of siting wind turbines in locations where, in her view, they are likely, on the basis of current knowledge, to cause harm to human health.[55]

This is hard to reconcile with the overwhelming focus of Laurie's attention on windfarms. Any Google search for her statements and writings provides a deluge of evidence that her primary target is

54 Alberta Utilities Commission 2014.

55 Environmental Review Tribunal of Ontario 2012.

windfarms, with only occasional passing mentions of noise problems from other industries.

Laurie has spoken often at public meetings organised by the Waubra Foundation and local opposition groups. In early October 2010, residents of Leonards Hill in central Victoria were encouraged to attend a presentation in nearby Evansford, given by Laurie. In the same week, the Australian Environment Foundation, a climate change denialist group, arranged a protest meeting at the opening ceremony for the beginning of works on a two-turbine, 2000-shareholder community-owned windfarm at Leonards Hill, near Daylesford. Banners with 'Windfarms make me sick' were prepared and some 50 people (almost all of them out-of-towners) attended the protest, which was reported in the local press.

In November 2010, Laurie was reported in the local newspaper, the *Advocate*, as saying, 'If I were living right there I would be very concerned. I would be beside myself.' She highlighted acute hypertensive crisis as a potential effect and said it warranted 'immediate attention'. Scary stuff. In early December 2010, the 'president' of the Daylesford Landscape Guardians (since deceased) told the *Australian*, 'I've been on medication for the last five years just fighting this.'[56] The windfarm had not even opened but the president was already worried sick.

On 22 June 2011, one of the two wind turbines at Leonards Hill began operating at 25 percent capacity. The president was interviewed by ABC News less than 48 hours later and said, 'I've heard the turbines the last three nights and I'm finding that it feels inside the house like it's being pressurised. And so I've not been sleeping until later on.' In mid-August 2011, the *Ballarat Courier* reported that Leonards Hill received its first health complaint from a 57-year-old woman with sleep problems. She described the sound of the two turbines, half a kilometre away, as at times 'like a jet engine'. The next day, the Landscape Guardians president went public as the second health complainant about the windfarm.

Laurie has made some quite extraordinary statements in her public pronouncements. She claims she has 'heard from [unnamed] ex-employees that if they have disclosed their health problems [caused by wind turbines] their employment has been terminated – in their words, they have been dropped like "hot cakes".'[57] We are unaware of

56 Akerman 2010.

any former employees in Australia ever taking legal action over a dismissal, going public in the media to describe their experiences, or making a submission to a parliamentary inquiry.

In 2012, Laurie wrote to the NSW planning minister, Brad Hazzard, and others advising them that alleged rapid fluctuations in barometric pressure around windfarms could sometimes 'perceptibly rock stationary cars even further than a kilometre away from the nearest wind turbine.'[58] This is a claim that would have made a fascinating story for a *Mythbusters* investigation.

Laurie may be a country and western fan, channelling the Patsy Kline and Kitty Wells duet 'Talk back trembling lips' (in which they sing 'shaky legs, don't just stand there') when she told the South Australian court in 2011 that wind turbines can make people's lips vibrate 'from a distance of ten kilometres away'.[59] That's about the distance from downtown Sydney to the northern suburb of Chatswood. Indeed, these vibrations are 'sufficient to knock them off their feet or bring some men to their knees when out working in their paddock', she added elsewhere.[60]

These fascinating claims could of course easily be subjected to tests under blinded experimental conditions. Windfarm operators would willingly co-operate in the experiment by powering turbines on and off unbeknown to the experimental subjects, whose lip trembling, ability to stand in paddocks, and claims to hear the turbines from massive distances could all be tested. We would encourage budding experimental psychology students to consider approaching the Waubra Foundation and inviting them to co-operate in such a study. They could collaborate in setting out the experimental protocols and testing procedures, and could name in advance any confounders they might be likely to raise in the event of the study showing that none of these effects could be demonstrated.

Finally, a South Australian court at which Laurie appeared as a witness apparently couldn't resist this priceless comment in its judgment:

57 Laurie 2011a.
58 Laurie 2012a.
59 Barnard 2012.
60 Laurie n.d.

> Dr Laurie wishes to have investigated the theory that some people are 'so exquisitely sensitised to certain frequencies that their perception of very, very low frequency is right off the shape of the bell curve', such that they can, for example, from Australia, perceive an earthquake in Chile.[61]

Chile is a mere 11,365 kilometres from Australia's east coast.

Noel Dean

Noel Dean and his wife have owned a property in the Waubra area since 1970. They had lived there since early November 1974, but left their home on 25 May 2009 because they were experiencing extremely bad headaches and felt unwell. Dean wrote in a Senate submission that:

> It took three months to identify why we were experiencing these severe adverse health effects. In that time I had done very little work, [and] spent many hours in bed during the day not knowing what was wrong.[62]

Construction of the Waubra windfarm began in December 2007 and was completed in June 2009. The first turbines began generating green power in February 2009 and the entire site was fully operational by July 2009.

Dean told the ABC *Four Corners* program, in an episode broadcast in July 2011:

> The first time that I got affected was just after they started up. I woke with headaches of a morning. I had to have Panadol [paracetamol]. It hadn't happened before. It happened two mornings in a row and then because we had a property up north, I went up there for the night. I woke up without headaches and then when I come back I did get headaches again.[63]

---

61 Environment, Resources and Development Court of South Australia 2014.
62 Dean 2011b.
63 Fowler 2011.

He repeated this to the 2011 Senate inquiry in March that year, stating that his family had to move very soon (perhaps only one night) after the Waubra wind turbines started up: 'My family was fairly affected because we had to move straight away; we could not stay another night because my head felt as if it was going to burst.'[64]

Dean has appeared at public meetings organised by opponents in other areas, where he gives emotional accounts of his health and his belief that the Waubra windfarm is responsible for his situation. In his 2011 Senate submission he described his belief that the 'frequencies produced by the turbines are the same as those that operate the brain, the interference of frequencies of the brain by those that are produced by the turbines is why the lower parts of our bodies went cold.'[65]

However, in his Senate submission he also stated: 'I have been in brain training care and rehabilitation for about ten years because of an unfortunate, unrelated incident.'[66] Dean would thus appear to have been in rehabilitation for a pre-existing health problem for some eight years prior to his exposure to the Waubra windfarm and still required 'brain training and rehabilitation' during the period in which he attributed various adverse health conditions to his exposure to the turbines near his property. Dean also advised the Senate that he was a polio survivor who had to 'rub liniment into my legs during the night, thankfully now only once during the night'.[67] Yet he appeared to attribute this nocturnal problem, and others, to the wind turbines.

In the 2011 anti-windfarm film *Pandora's pinwheels*, Dean stated: 'If I'm not careful it will take me out. I suffer from … they say sleep apnoea'.[68] Dean does not say in the film how long he has suffered from sleep apnoea, and whether this preceded his exposure to the wind turbines (an exposure that, according to his account, may have lasted for as little as one night).

Dean once told an anti-windfarm meeting at Baringhup in Victoria on 19 March 2013 that wind turbines started charging his mobile phone without it being plugged in. 'I've had my … mobile phone go into charge mode in the middle of the paddock, away from everywhere.'[69] This extraordinary claim would certainly be of great

64 Commonwealth of Australia 2011.

65 Dean 2011b.

66 Dean 2011b.

67 Dean 2011a.

68 PR Resources Inc. 2011, at 1 hour, 8 minutes.

interest to manufacturers of mobile phones, who to date have apparently not been advised that this remarkable charging ability is something all phone users should be aware of.

Ann and Gus Gardner

Ann (often referred to as Annie) and Andrew 'Gus' Gardner are two of Australia's most determined windfarm opponents. They live near the AGL-operated Macarthur windfarm in Victoria, which is the largest in Australia. It commenced construction in October 2010 and the first turbines were connected to the electricity grid in September 2012. The Gardners live on a farm there, where they keep sheep with fine wool. They appeared on an ABCTV *7.30 Report* report on 12 October 2011.[70] Ann Gardner explained about wind turbines that 'The ultra-fine sheep are highly strung. They are highly vulnerable if they are stressed,' while her husband worried that the windfarm would harm their income: 'My hard-earned capital [would be] threatened by this monster'.

Two other fine-wool growers interviewed on the program, Noel and Lyn Hartwich, who have a property near the Callicum Hills windfarm, said:

> I don't think that ever happens … That's just a myth … Well, why can we grow fine wool and we haven't had any problems? And I don't know whether to say this, but our sheep have won prizes. Last year, they won the Victorian ewe of the year.

Both Ann and Andrew Gardner are on record as saying they are still affected even when the turbines are off. In Chapter 3, we described how those claiming to suffer from acute effects of wind turbine exposure say that they get immediate relief when the wind stops turning the turbines or when they move away from their residences. But on 7 February 2015, Ann and Andrew Gardner wrote a letter to the local newspaper, in which they claimed:

---

69 Chapman 2015f.
70 Hoy 2011.

> Around the Macarthur wind farm, residents suffer from infrasound emitted by the turbines, even when they're not operating … Even when the turbines are turned off, we feel the same 'sensation', being headaches, ear pressure, nose pressure, heart palpitations, nausea, dizziness etc., and still cannot sleep at night.[71]

How is it that while many complainants argue that their symptoms stop when the turbines are not turning, the Gardners claim that their symptoms continue?

Andrew Gardner sent the email below to 189 recipients, including politicians and journalists, on 26 April 2015 (he did not bother to 'bcc' their addresses). The politician who forwarded it to me commented about the irritating frequency with which he received these unsolicited multi-addressed emails from the Gardners. Gardner's email read:

> Dear All,
> The 'torture' continues … every night I find my sleep is severely disturbed, due to infrasound emitted by turbines at Macarthur Wind Farm. I suffer from neck pain/headaches and 'bolts' of pressure during the night which means I wake up feeling just exhausted, as if I haven't been to bed.
>
> During the day, whilst trying to work on our farm, in the paddocks, I'm hammered with infrasound from the forest of turbines surrounding our property. The impact of the infrasound is getting worse as time goes by and I find it quite impossible to work on some days, let alone have to put up with the danger of tiredness whilst driving machinery and vehicles.
>
> The 'sensation' from which I suffer would register close to the maximum level of 5, according to Steven Cooper's Cape Bridgewater community health survey.
>
> AGL turn the turbines off at night *so we can sleep in our own homes* [our emphasis]. Every week we are forced to leave our home and farm for at least two nights, which means three days with travelling, and trying to look after animals part-time is impossible. This just should not be allowed to happen in Australia, but the money is just too good for all those involved, no doubt.
>
> I require a receipt number for this complaint.
>
> Andrew Gardner

71 Gardner 2015b.

Note that elsewhere the Gardners have said that even non-operating turbines disturb them, yet here they say the turbines are turned off so that they can sleep. So which is it?

Les Huson

Victorian acoustician Les Huson is one of 14 Australian 'professionals' named on a list of people promoted by anti-windfarm groups who have 'investigated or voiced concern for the health and well-being of wind turbine neighbours'.[72]

In 2015 Huson presented a poster at a conference on windfarm noise in Glasgow that impressed Ann Gardner, prompting her to advise the 2015 Senate committee that 'It is now accepted that infrasound DOES come from wind turbines that are not operating.'[73] Gardner provided no evidence for such 'acceptance'. Huson's paper described his measurements of infrasound inside dwellings when the turbines were not running compared to when they were operational.[74] He concluded that:

> Upwind indoor measurements at the Macarthur wind farm during an unplanned shutdown from full power and subsequent start-up to 30 percent load has shown that stationary turbines subject to high winds emit infrasound pressure below 8 Hz at levels similar to the infrasound emissions at blade pass frequencies and harmonics.
>
> The stationary V112 turbine infrasound emissions are caused primarily by blade and tower resonances excited by the wind.

There was a rather important problem with Huson's conclusion. His declaration that the infrasound he recorded was from the high wind interacting with the stationary blades and towers takes no account of whether it might have in fact been infrasound in the wind itself, or perhaps from sources like refrigerators or fans within the houses in which he did the recording. He undertook no pre-construction recordings of infrasound in the same locations to see what the infrasound readings were in when the same 'high winds' were blowing.

72 European Platform Against Wind Farms n.d.
73 Gardner 2015.
74 Huson 2015.

This obvious problem may explain why his paper seems never to have been published in any research journal.

Huson notes in his paper that he was 'not affiliated with any pro- or anti-wind organisation.' Perhaps. But he has a track record as being a 'go-to' acoustician whose work is lauded by anti-windfarm groups.

George Papadopoulos

Some anti-windfarm advocates appear to have almost superhuman auditory capacity. General Electric has compared the diminishing dB of a wind turbine over distance with the volume of other common noise sources. For example, at a distance of 400 metres, the audible noise from a turbine is comparable to to that emitted by a household refrigerator.[75]

George Papadopoulos, a pharmacist, may be peerless in his auditory acuity. He lives near the town of Yass in New South Wales and is an avid writer about windfarms online, to inquiries, and to anyone who might listen. He has often emailed me oddly worded letters, often commencing with the baroque 'My dearest Professor'. He is apparently possessed of extraordinary aural abilities, almost as if he has bionic ears. Here are some examples.

In May 2011, he wrote on a homeopathy website about visiting a windfarm with two others:

> Almost immediately, pressure sensations in the head abruptly started – plus blocked ears that could not be relieved by swallowing or yawning. We couldn't hear any loud deafening noises, but the constant whooshing noise was phenomenal – enough to drive you mad. We were ultimately compelled to leave the site due to severe nausea in all three of us. Perhaps it wasn't a good idea to get so close to the turbines. Eventually it was only at 5 kilometres away that we finally felt totally relieved and normal – we had finally escaped this whirlpool of disaster.[76]

But by March 2012, Papadopoulos was writing that he could now hear turbines 35 kilometres away – a seven-fold increase in less than a year!

75 For a useful diagram illustrating the loudness of wind turbine noise at different distances, see http://invent.ge/2y8dAv2; Kellner 2014.

76 Papadopoulos 2011.

> Should anyone wonder why I am so against wind turbines, it is because the recent installation of 40 of them 35km away at times has turned the quiet rural area of the northern hills of Yass into a rumbling mess.[77]

His amazing abilities then increased further and by October 2012, he reported:

> There have been two reports from Warrnambool, Victoria, which include details very similar to what I describe above. The closest turbines appear to be about 35–50 km away with many more about 70 km away … Where does the problem stop? This is a difficult question to answer. On two occasions when the ILFN [infrasound and low frequency noise] nuisance was at its worst, I travelled out west. On one occasion, I discovered that it appeared to have dissipated at Wee Jasper, 70 km away from the closest turbines. On another occasion, and by far the worst of all days, the problem had dissipated when arriving at Young about 100 km from the closest turbines … Truly these figures appear subjective, outrageous, and for most, impossible to believe. However, I am reporting my findings that have taken hours and days to determine. I'm not just plucking figures out of the air.[78]

As the crow flies, 100 kilometres is about the distance from the central business district of Sydney to the town of Lithgow on the other side of the Blue Mountains. Papadopoulos has been confronted with his '100 kilometre' statement several times and has never taken a backward step from it.

George and the world of woo

For a time after he began agitating against windfarms, Papadopoulos linked up with an entity called Geovital Academy as an 'assessor'.[79] Thanks to the Wayback Machine, we can still read his

77 Papadopoulos 2012a.

78 Papadopoulos 2012b.

79 See http://web.archive.org/web/20130419232329/http://geovital.com.au/geovital_assessors.html.

deleted particulars, which have since been removed from the Geovital site:

> An in-depth knowledge of health
> George is a pharmacist with many years' experience. He is now expanding his skills to include natural and holistic health approaches and has a longstanding interest in how electromagnetic radiation affects human health. George travels between Sydney, Canberra and Yass NSW on a regular basis and is available to communities and people around and between these areas. George became a member of Geovital Academy in 2013.

Geovital's website is quite something. It sells blankets, shields, paints and pillows to protect gullible people from the evils of electromagnetic radiation invading their houses. From at least 8 May 2012 until 31 May 2013, the Wayback Machine shows, the website included a statement from 'Noble [sic] Prize winner Ivan Engler Dr.med.univ., PhD':

> With almost all of my (roughly 300 patients) with a cancerous disease, their bed was placed for years on an energetically unfavorable place in a Geopathic Zone.[80]

No one named Ivan Engler ever won a Nobel Prize in any category. He may have won a Noble prize, whatever that might be.

It gets worse. In 2013, the Cancer Council Victoria had its attention drawn to a section of Geovital's website inviting people to participate in 'a blind study about the occurrence of cancer in geopathically disturbed areas'. The study was open to 'cancer-suffering households' in Melbourne. The study involved an examination of radiation in the houses of those with cancer. Following the assessment, the illnesses of the participants would be revealed to a 'geobiologist' to be compared with the measurements taken during the assessment. Participants were required to pay $45 toward travel expenses and a fee of $95 per room assessed.

The Cancer Council wrote to the Australian Competition and Consumer Commission on 20 August 2013, complaining in detail about the study. It argued:

---

80 https://web.archive.org/web/20130501000000*/http://www.geovital.com.au/geopathicstressshielding.html.

> no authoritative studies have shown a causal link between 'geopathic stress' and adverse health effects … we believe that Geovital's conduct may mislead people affected by cancer and their families as to the causes and appropriate treatments for cancer. This could have serious implications for the health of people with cancer.
>
> Additionally, we are concerned about the study's financial cost to people with cancer, many of whom are already facing significant financial burdens associated with cancer diagnosis and treatment. [these people] are likely to be encouraged … to purchase 'shielding' devices sold by Geovital in order to reduce the 'health burdens' suggested by Geovital to cause cancer.

The application of 'shielding paint' promoted on Geovital's website was said to have been followed by '76 percent of 250 chronically ill people recovered to good health within 3 months of having Geovital shielding solutions put into place'.

The ACCC contacted Geovital and all mentions of the study were quickly removed from its website. Papadopoulos has ended his association with Geovital, but his judgment in being associated with them in the first place is notable. In spite of this, Papadopoulos is listed on anti-windfarm websites as a 'professional' who has raised concerns about windfarms.[81]

Bruce Rapley

Bruce Rapley is a New Zealander who made a submission to the 2015 Australian Senate inquiry. Senator Madigan and his committee were apparently impressed with his expertise and invited him to give oral evidence to the committee.

Like Noel Dean, Rapley appeared in the 2011 amateur movie *Pandora's wheels*.[82] At different times in the film he describes himself as 'a biologist', 'a scientist' and 'a philosopher of science'. At the time the film was made, Rapley had no PhD (his degree was awarded in 2015 by Massey University in New Zealand). In the film he refers to 'our research [on windfarms] over the last three years', that is, from 2009 onward, and talks about 'our records'. So where is this research and these records? A PubMed search conducted on 9 May 2017 found

---

81 European Platform Against Wind Farms n.d.

82 PR Resources Inc. 2011.

five papers published by Rapley between 1995 and 2007 on bioelectromagnetics, but nothing on windfarms, acoustics or the philosophy of science. Massey University advised me in 2016 that his 2015 PhD thesis, on sound in the military environment, was publicly unavailable as it was under restriction for unstated reasons, a ruling that is apparently ongoing. His research is thus not available to anyone for review.

Rapley's spoken evidence to the 2015 Senate committee was something to behold. A supremely self-confident person, his testimony is highly recommended for enthusiasts of bluster.

His opening oral statement worked up to a final farrago of outrage:

> In the future, I believe that the adverse health effects of wind turbines will eclipse the asbestos problem in the annals of history. In my opinion, the greed and scientific half-truths from the wind industry will be seen by history as one of the worst corporate and government abuses of democracy in the 21st century.

Rapley spent much of his allocated time blasting research on the nocebo phenomenon as it has been applied to research on wind turbines. He started with:

> The nocebo principle cannot be applied to a palpable phenomenon by definition. To continue to fly this particular flag is to insult the intelligence of genuinely impacted people and to bring the scientific method and science into disrepute. It is a staggering misuse of the scientific method and does nothing to advance the understanding of this complex problem.

Asked to expand on this by Senator Back, Rapley waded in:

> Firstly, quite bluntly, on first scientific principles it is the wrong terminology. It is a piece of very poor academic science to even invoke the term. The definition of nocebo, in medicine, is – from the Latin 'I shall harm' – an inert substance or form of therapy that creates harmful effects in a patient. Therefore, the nocebo effect is the adverse reaction experienced by a patient who receives such a therapy. Wind turbines are not a therapy. Sound is not an inert substance devoid of biological perception or effect. Nocebo is the wrong word. It is very simply a bastardisation of a term invented

> for nefarious purposes to attempt to invoke some sort of pseudoscientific authenticity. The term that should be used is psychogenic or psychosomatic. It just stuns me that people continue to use this. It is the wrong term to begin with and it does not explain the effects that we see. It is simply a ruse. It is a red herring that is put out and promoted by certain academics and the industry to explain a phenomenon.

Rapley continued displaying his limited understanding of how nocebo effects can occur:

> It [the nocebo hypothesis] fails on first principles ... because it cannot account for those who were pro-turbine prior to commissioning only to experience adverse health effects post-commissioning that they were later able to relate back to turbine emissions.[83]

As we discussed in Chapter 5, this objection is easily countered by pointing to the way that complainants are often exposed to new negative information after a period of never having heard or considered that wind turbines may be harmful.

He finished by arguing that since 'we have animals affected by this' and that 'animals are not really susceptible to media hype', the nocebo hypothesis had to be bunkum. Appendix 1 documents many claims about animals that we highlighted in Chapter 2. None of them has ever moved beyond evidence-free assertion.

Some might care to weigh the value of Rapley's opinions about nocebo research and windfarms against those of Sir Simon Wessely, recent president of the Royal College of Psychiatrists, who has published on the subject.[84]

In 1995, the New Zealand Skeptics Society reported that:

> Rapley is a leader of something called Resonance Research, a non-profit organisation involved in 'furthering the understanding of phenomena occurring at the margins of traditional knowledge'. RR offers 'a variety of inspirational seminars and workshops', and

83 Rubin, Burns and Wessely 2014.
84 Rubin, Burns and Wessely 2014.

networks in the areas of Bio-Energy, Counselling, Geopathic Stress, Homeopathy, Radionics/Radiesthesia, and Vibrational Memory.

In particular, Mr Rapley has recently been energetically arranging a visit to New Zealand by Viera Scheibner, PhD, who warns against vaccinations. In particular Dr Scheibner finds 'obvious' the connection between 'vaccine injections and cot death'.[85]

Politicians

Several federal politicians in the Liberal and National parties and on the crossbench have been stalwart critics of windfarms.

These have included former prime minister Tony Abbott,[86] former treasurer Joe Hockey,[87] the current minister for resources Senator Matt Canavan (Queensland), Senator Chris Back (Western Australia),[88] the late Alby Schultz (MP for Hume in New South Wales) and his successor Angus Taylor,[89] ex-senators John Madigan (Democratic Labour Party), Bob Day,[90] Steve Fielding (Family First) and Nick Xenophon (independent), and current senators Jacquie Lambie (independent)[91] and David Leyonhjelm (Liberal Democratic Party).

Madigan, Back and Taylor, along with Senator Ron Boswell (National Party, Queensland, since retired) and MP Craig Kelly (Liberal Party, New South Wales) spoke at the 2016 Stop These Things rally, so were clearly comfortable assisting the group in its mission.[92] As of 8 May 2017, a collection of 12 videos of the rally published on YouTube in July 2013 had been viewed on average just 211 times each.[93]

A few of these politicians are worthy of special attention.

John Madigan arguably made little impact on the Australian political landscape during his six-year tenure in the Senate, despite expending superhuman effort to oppose windfarm development.

85 Dutton 1995.
86 Cox and Arup 2015.
87 Bourke 2014.
88 Back 2012.
89 Ewbank 2014.
90 Day 2015.
91 Lambie 2015.
92 Stop These Things 2013e.
93 Stop These Things 2013e.

Madigan introduced, along with co-sponsor Nick Xenophon, the Excessive Noise from Wind Farms Bill 2012, which was ultimately rejected by parliament. He chaired the Senate Select Committee on Wind Turbines, whose recommendation to set up a Wind Farm Commissioner was ultimately an own goal (see earlier in this chapter). Throughout 2012 and 2013 his staff were in the audience at community windfarm consultations in South Australia, New South Wales and Victoria and eagerly asked attempted 'gotcha' questions.

When asked who invited him to address the Stop These Things rally, Madigan claimed that he did not know. He frequently started interviews and speeches with an assurance that he was 'not against turbines', yet on his website he boasted of his 'fight' against wind energy.

Xenophon, seen by many as a moderate voice, worked closely with Madigan on a wide range of anti-wind activities, including a series of community meetings around south-eastern Australia in 2012, one of which 'activated' David Mortimer (see Chapter 3). Xenophon was slated to appear at the Stop These Things rally in 2013 – a coup that STT breathlessly boasted about prior to the rally. When the progressive GetUp! and Friends of the Earth organisations arranged a pro-renewables rally in Canberra on the same day, Xenophon attempted the politically impossible: he agreed to front both rallies. A freelance filmmaker had planned to document his appearance at the rallies and his mad dash between the two (set to the Benny Hill theme 'Yakety Sax'?). Perhaps word reached his office – Xenophon pulled out of both at the 11th hour.[94]

Several Coalition MPs have informed contacts of mine that behind the scenes no one was working harder or smarter to stop the development of wind energy in Australia than Angus Taylor, federal member for Hume. Having become engaged in the windfarm debate around 2003, Taylor spoke at many community meetings around his electorate, assuring the locals that a solution to their concerns was in train. He authored and widely distributed a report to his party room called 'A proposal to reduce the cost of electricity to Australian electricity users'. The report suggested that if Australia immediately abandoned the renewable energy target and moved instead to gas generation, Australian energy consumers would save $3.2 billion by 2020. He was ignored, as wind energy has become cheaper than gas-generated electricity by a wide margin. Taylor (nicknamed by Stop

94 See Nick Xenophon's Facebook post of 17 June 2013: http://bit.ly/2wwATHt.

These Things as 'The Enforcer') addressed the 2013 rally, an odd move for an Oxford-educated junior MP known to have an eye on the top job.

In June 2015, after describing windfarms as 'visually awful' while a review into renewable energy he'd commissioned was ongoing, Prime Minister Tony Abbott went on to say, 'Up close, they're ugly, they're noisy and they may have all sorts of other impacts.'[95] When questioned whether he'd actually visited a windfarm, he declared that he once rode a bicycle past the single small wind turbine on Rottnest Island, off Perth. If only Tony Abbott had submitted a formal complaint about this turbine, it would not only have been the first against the Rottnest turbine: it would have been the first complaint against any windfarm in Western Australia.

The media

I have done many interviews with Australian news media on windfarms and health issues since 2010. These have rarely if ever been hostile, with program researchers, journalists and on-air staff often remarking to me off-the-record that the 'other side' of this issue are often decidedly oddball.

There are only three outlets that have regularly given anti-windfarm activists a warm embrace: the *Australian* newspaper (particularly its 'environment' writer Graham Lloyd; 2GB radio announcer Alan Jones, whose program is broadcast live into many other linked stations in the Macquarie network; and the bizarre internet radio program Fair Dinkum Radio, hosted by the conspiracist Leon Pittard, who gives a platform to every conceivable type of truther and nut-job. Pittard has given several lengthy, fawning interviews to windfarm opponents.

For a while, the *Ballarat Courier*, thanks to reporter Brendan Gullifer, who went on to become Madigan's chief of staff, was a wellspring of anti-windfarm reporting, and arguably was the first Australian paper to give prominence to the theory that windfarms made people sick. When Gullifer left, anti-windfarm reporting at the paper dried up entirely.

95 Glenday 2015.

Sydney-based radio announcer Alan Jones has unquestionably provided more exposure to windfarm opponents than anyone else in Australia, and possibly in the world. Jones, who thinks global warming is 'witchcraft',[96] regularly gives extensive airtime to these opponents. In October 2016, in one of his typical bombastic preambles that lasted longer than the interview itself, he referred to 'renewable energy rubbish', claimed that there was 'harrowing evidence' that windfarms were 'buggering up people's health', and rattled off portentous references to the Japanese and Iranian studies that we critiqued in Chapter 4.

This chapter has considered the range and apparent motivations of the small number of interest groups and individuals who have been prominent in opposing windfarms in Australia. We have profiled some of the more 'interesting' people among them and statements they have made. In the next chapter, we will look at the themes and strategies that some of these opponents have used in their efforts to attack and discredit those whom they see as standing in the way of their efforts.

96 Cubby 2012.

7

How the anti-wind lobby reacts when challenged

Throughout my career in public health I have upset powerful interest groups and impassioned activists for several health-related causes. Since the late 1970s, when I worked successfully with others to have actor Paul Hogan removed from Winfield cigarette advertising because of his appeal to children,[1] I have often been attacked by those who stood to lose by having the full glare of media attention being trained on their activities, nonsense or lies. Sunlight is a powerful antiseptic and, like cockroaches that can carry disease, many exponents of mendacity and nonsense have a strong dislike for the glare of sunlight on their activities and react badly to it.

Over the years I've published research papers and books that have challenged the position of interest groups in several areas. These include the anti-vaccination movement, the gun lobby, those opposed to mandatory fences around domestic swimming pools, the tobacco and e-cigarette industries and their supporters, those arguing that mobile phone towers and wi-fi cause cancer, and, most recently, opponents of windfarms who invoke health concerns in their arguments.

In this chapter, I'll describe some of the attacks that have been made on me by opponents of windfarms: by activists, their political barrackers, and by various journalists employed by the *Australian*. As will be seen, those opposed to windfarms are determined, aggressive and sometimes unprincipled. The attacks I received can be seen in

1 Chapman 1980.

the context of the global movement to discredit concern about anthropogenic global warming and renewable energy.

My first sense that I could expect vigorous pushback from the anti-windfarm camp if its claims were ever challenged came within hours of publishing my first contribution on the issue. In February 2010, I had begun following various stories about windfarms allegedly causing health problems and decided to write a piece for the blog *Croakey*.[2]

Shortly afterwards, the comments page began brimming with responses, with 53 landing in the next three days. Many of these were from a small number of people who quickly became heated and hectoring.

The volume and intensity of the responses sent me a very strong message that this was an issue heavily pregnant with emotional intensity and pseudoscience, and was likely to become a fascinating case study of how networks can be used to promote highly dubious claims. It was an issue right up my street.

My next encounter with apoplectic windfarm opponents came at a meeting I had been invited to attend in June 2011 at the National Health and Medical Research Council (NHMRC) in Canberra. In 2010 I had been invited by the NHMRC to review a draft of its forthcoming rapid review of the evidence.[3] I wrote a few pages about the importance of any review needing to consider psychogenic factors in understanding why small numbers of people complained about some windfarms while most were indifferent. At the meeting, I joined a panel in the morning and gave a brief presentation to the meeting, summarising these considerations.

Those attending the meeting included windfarm opponents, government public and environmental health experts, and wind energy company employees. Several presentations were made, including two via video by the English acoustic scientist Geoff Leventhall (who had also reviewed the NHMRC report)[4] and Mariana Alves-Pereira,[5] a Portuguese researcher who identifies wind turbines as one cause of the unrecognised disease of 'vibroacoustic disease' (see Chapter 2).

In the afternoon we were allocated to different tables and asked to discuss future research priorities, in the unlikely chance that any

---

2 Chapman 2010.
3 National Health and Medical Research Council 2010.
4 Leventhall 2011.
5 Alves-Pereira 2011.

consensus might emerge from such wildly different interest groups. At my table there was a wind industry representative, a state government scientist, and a Waubra farmer, Donald Thomas, who opposed the local windfarm and claimed that he and his mother were badly affected by the local wind turbines. Also at my table was Peter Mitchell, the founder and then chair of the Waubra Foundation and a long-time windfarm opponent (see Chapter 6).

Thomas told me across the table that the location of his property in the Waubra district made it unsuitable to host turbines. He made the same comments when he was interviewed for an anti-windfarm film: 'We live in the valley where we were never going to get the turbines.'[6] I saw Mitchell stiffen when he heard the comment, perhaps concerned that others at the table might wonder if envy and resentment may have conditioned Thomas' negative reaction to the turbines.

Discussion was fairly civil until Mitchell, *sotto voce*, leaned forward and told me that I was a disgrace and that someone who had been as influential as I had been in the field of tobacco control should get myself informed about the real health problems arising from windfarms and join in opposition to them.

Mitchell, a company director with extensive oil, gas, and other mining interests, seemed to me to have the patrician air of a wealthy man used to getting his way with perceived underlings. If he harboured the slightest expectation that his theatrical, clenched-teeth advice would cower me into joining his cause, he was going about it in a decidedly strange way.

Ever since those early days, my participation in public discussion about windfarms has drawn the ire of those opposed to them. The attacks have concentrated on three main themes. First, as a social scientist, it was surely self-evident that I was totally unqualified to make any informed comment about any matter to do with windfarms. Second, my growing scepticism about the alleged health risks of wind turbines could only be explained because I must be a paid agent of the wind industry and, worse, had not declared this. I must therefore also be a deceitful liar whose every word should be discounted. Third, I am a coward because I have allegedly continually refused to meet with windfarm complainants, because such meetings would clearly show me that I am utterly wrong about windfarms not being a direct cause of health problems in those exposed.

---

6 PR Resources Inc. 2011.

I'll now look at each of these accusations and describe the various strategies windfarm opponents have used to undermine my and others' work.

I am by no means the only person who has been vilified by these opponents. We are aware of others who have spoken out about this issue who have been subjected to racist name-calling, or whose employers have been petitioned with threats of reputational risk. Employees of several wind energy companies have told us about vandalism to their cars and months of personal abuse. The then Victorian energy minister, Peter Batchelor, even suffered physical assault when his leg was jammed in a car door as he tried to exit a community forum in Colac in August 2009.[7]

Unqualified to contribute

On many occasions during my career, those who dislike an argument I am making have sought to discredit it by arguing that as a social scientist, despite being a professor with nearly 40 years of postgraduate teaching and research in the School of Public Health within the Faculty of Medicine at the University of Sydney, I am unqualified to be advancing the arguments I am making. The problem, apparently, is that only a narrow range of expertise can ever be relevant to advancing evidence in health matters. It doesn't matter what the evidence in question is. What is critical is what undergraduate degree was obtained by the person making the argument at the very start of their career: in my case, 45 years ago. The 2015 Senate majority report on wind turbines set out which qualifications it considered relevant:

> The committee highlights the fact that Professor Chapman is not a qualified, registered nor experienced medical practitioner, psychiatrist, psychologist, acoustician, audiologist, physicist or engineer.[8]

Apart from the awkward observation that none of the members of the Senate committee making this call had any of these qualifications either

7 Lynch and Himmelreich 2009.
8 Commonwealth of Australia 2015b.

(but nonetheless felt themselves suitably qualified to make judgments on the evidence they received), most of the witnesses they cited in their final report also had none of these qualifications. In addition, the list of 78 concerned 'professionals' around the world whose names can be found on anti-windfarm websites contains 11 people who also don't make the cut, including two sociologists (see Table 7.1).[9] For windfarm opponents, sociologists are apparently legitimate experts if they express concerns about wind turbines and health, but are to be dismissed if they do not.

In particular, the chair of the Senate committee, John Madigan (who was a blacksmith before entering parliament) appeared to be quite obsessed with my qualifications. On 15 April 2014 I gave notice of potential legal action for defamation against him, following public remarks he made about me on Alan Jones' radio program on 27 March 2014. My notice referred to a statement made by Madigan, following a remark by Jones:

> **Alan Jones:** You've got people like this fellow Chapman, calling himself a professor at Sydney University, preaching also the windfarm propaganda. They are everywhere these people.
> **Senator Madigan:** Yes and Alan, when we talk about people using the title ... using a title like professor, let us be crystal clear that most people in the community assume when you use the title professor that you are trained in the discipline of what you speak. And I ask people, look and check what is the person making these proclamations about some other people's health, what is the discipline they are trained in of which they speak. Because most people in the public assume that when you speak on an issue of health that you are trained in the discipline of which you speak and there are people making pronouncements and denigrating people who are not trained in human health.

My lawyers wrote to Senator Madigan about what he had said:

> The imputations of concern (arising as a matter of ordinary meaning and by way of true innuendo) are, among others, that Professor Chapman
> (a) is not trained in the discipline he purports to be trained in;

9 European Platform Against Wind Farms n.d.

Name	Qualifications
Members of the Senate committee's majority report	
John Madigan	blacksmith
Chris Back	veterinary science
Bob Day	science technician
David Leyonhjelm	veterinary science
Nick Xenophon	law
Witnesses cited in in the health section of the Senate committee's majority report	
Lilli-Anne Green	none stated
Bruce Rapley	'scientist'
Nine complainants	none stated
'Professionals' noted by anti-windfarm groups who have expressed concerns about wind turbine effects	
Jeffery Aramini	veterinary science
Mrs June Davis	nursing
Ms Carmen Krogh	pharmacy
Mr George Papadopoulos	pharmacy
Dr Robyn Phipps	'researcher' (architecture)
Dr Eja Pedersen	medical sociology
Prof [sic] Carl Phillips	epidemiology (no primary medical degree)
Mrs Gail Rogers	nursing
Norma Schmidt	nursing
Assoc. Prof Libby Wheatley	medical sociology

Table 7.1 Persons without the listed qualifications deemed relevant by the 2015 Senate Committee. Source: Commonwealth of Australia 2015b, European Platform against Wind Farms n.d.

(b) is dishonest;
(c) misrepresents his qualifications and expertise;
(d) denigrates people;

> (e) makes statements of opinion outside his area of expertise while misrepresenting that he is qualified in the relevant area of expertise;
> (f) is not trained in Medicine;
> (g) is not trained and/or does not have expertise in human health;
> (h) is not a Professor in health;
> (i) does not have expertise, and is not qualified to comment, about windfarms and human health.

Amazingly, Madigan replied denying that his words referred to me, but said that they were in any case true and justified. He also stated in his reply that I was a 'paid advocate of the wind industry' and that if this matter proceeded to court he would seek to expose this in court and under parliamentary privilege. My lawyers advised Madigan that I had never sought or had any paid advocacy role with any wind company nor any agent acting for them. They added:

> Our client also takes this opportunity to note that given we have now conveyed to you the matters set out above, there is no longer any basis for you to claim that our client is 'a paid advocate for the wind industry' or 'inappropriately influence[s] government departments and representative bodies', as you suggest you may do in future in Parliament. Should you, despite the matters set out above, nevertheless deliberately make such false and misleading statements to Parliament, it would constitute a contempt of Parliament and a breach of your Parliamentary privilege.

Radio station 2GB appeared to take a different view of the comments and quickly published the statement below on their website, shortly after receiving a similar letter from my lawyers:

> Correction: Professor Simon Chapman
>
> On 27 March 2014 during an interview on the Alan Jones program a reference was made to Professor Simon Chapman. Comments by the interviewee could have been interpreted by some as suggesting that he was not a qualified professor in health.
>
> 2GB accepts that Professor Chapman is a highly regarded Professor of Public Health at Sydney University who has been widely acknowledged for his work. He has been published extensively, including on the topic of windfarms and health, and been a tenured

> Professor of Public Health in the Faculty of Medicine at Sydney University since 2000.
>
> It was not intended to suggest that Professor Chapman was unqualified and we apologise if that impression was given.

Following receipt of my lawyer's letter, Madigan made a speech on 17 June 2014 to an apparently near-empty Senate chamber. Over 19 minutes, under parliamentary privilege, he made blustery accusations about my qualifications, my character, and my financial arrangements with the wind industry. The video, available online, is well worth watching.[10] Having now been defamed under the protection of parliamentary privilege, I was entitled by the rules of the Senate to have a reply published in the parliamentary Hansard record setting out responses to each of his attempted slurs.[11]

The *Australian* goes on the attack

On 20 February 2015 and again three days later, the *Australian*'s Gerard Henderson and Simon King spent a lot of ink explaining to readers that I had 'as much authority to discuss health affairs as I [Henderson] do. Namely, zip.'[12]

Their readers needed to be told this because the previous week, ABC television's *Media Watch* program had tipped a critical bucket over the *Australian*'s reportage of acoustic engineer Steven Cooper's study (see Chapter 4), which involved just three households consisting together of six long-time complainants about the Cape Bridgewater windfarm.[13]

I was one of four people quoted by *Media Watch*, and this got Henderson very excited. He wrote to the program:

> *Media Watch*'s decision to associate Professor Chapman with the words 'expert' and 'scientific' gave a clear impression that he is qualified to assess scientific research. However, Paul Barry neglected to advise *Media Watch* viewers that Simon Chapman had no

---

10 Madigan 2015.
11 Chapman 2014e.
12 Henderson 2015; King 2015.
13 Australian Broadcasting Corporation 2015.

> scientific or engineering or medical qualifications. He has a BA (Hons) from the University of New South Wales and a PhD from Sydney University. Dr Chapman's PhD is in Sociology. In other words, Simon Chapman has no qualifications to assess the research of the acoustic engineer Steven Cooper ... *Media Watch* misled its viewers last Monday by implying that Professor Simon Chapman is an 'expert' who is 'scientifically' qualified to assess the heath effect on humans of wind farms. The fact is that Simon Chapman has no formal qualifications in science or medicine or engineering.[14]

Simon King, a journalist for the *Australian*, went one better on 23 February with his discovery that I do 'not have a PhD in Medicine'. This was news to me because I do have a PhD in medicine. I do not have a PhD in sociology. My official transcript from the University of Sydney shows that I graduated in 1986 with ... wait for it ... a 'PhD in medicine'. The degree transcript states it no less than eight times, lest anyone might miss seeing it. I did my PhD, examining tobacco advertising, in the Department of Social and Preventive Medicine, in the Faculty of Medicine. A scan of the transcript can be found on the last page of my curriculum vitae.[15]

Madigan, King and Henderson appeared to know little to nothing about the nature of contemporary expertise and how nearly all complex problems in health and medicine today involve researchers from different disciplines working together. In the School of Public Health in the Faculty of Medicine where I worked, there are biostatisticians, historians, psychologists, ethicists, economists, epidemiologists, and social scientists. Only some – probably a minority – have undergraduate degrees in medicine. Of those who do, most have long not practised clinical medicine since developing careers in research. Henderson's primitive understanding of expertise apparently begins and ends with the possession of an undergraduate degree. It is rare these days for research grant applications to be submitted by people all from the same discipline. Sydney University's massive new investment in obesity and chronic disease research, the Charles Perkins Centre, epitomises the importance of contemporary trans-disciplinary research. Arguably the most renowned epidemiologist in the world, Oxford University's Sir Richard Peto, has no medical undergraduate degree. His undergraduate degree was in natural sciences.

---

14 Henderson 2015.

15 See http://bit.ly/2xvOhS8.

There are many fools other than those at *Media Watch* who have also fallen for my fake expertise about windfarms and health. They include the nincompoop editors of eight specialised international research journals (*Noise and Health*, *International Journal of Acoustics and Vibration*, *Journal of Low Frequency Noise, Vibration and Active Control*, *Environmental Research*, *Environmental Pollution*, *Journal of Psychosomatic Research* and *Energy Policy*) who asked me to review research submissions about windfarms and health for them in recent years; the editors and reviewers of the papers I published on windfarms and health listed at the end of the Introduction; the National Health and Medical Research Council, which appointed me as an expert reviewer of their 2010 rapid review of the evidence on windfarms; and the dazed incompetents running the Australian Acoustical Society, the Australasian College of Toxicology and Risk Assessment and the Clean Air Society of Australia and New Zealand, all of whom asked me to give plenary session talks to their scientific meetings of acousticians and environmental health specialists in recent years.

The duffers on the Order of Australia awards committee also seemed to believe that I contribute to health and medical research. My 2013 citation reads 'for distinguished service to medical research as an academic and author'.

The first prize for monumental ignorance about research, however, must go to the late Alby Schultz MP. Schultz told the Australian House of Representatives on 30 May 2013 that I was 'a person who is not lawfully permitted to conduct any form of medical research or study in relation to human health'.[16] This claim was faithfully parroted by Senator John Madigan in the Senate in 2014[17] and dutifully included in an article by journalist Graham Lloyd in the *Australian* on 19 August 2015.[18]

Since learning nearly four years ago that my entire research career has apparently been unlawful, I wait anxiously each day for the knock on the door from law-enforcement officers. There must also be a very long line of employees in the research grant agencies that have awarded me competitive research grants over the last three decades who are now also nervously awaiting police interrogation for awarding me research money. These include the NHMRC, the US National Cancer Institute,

16 Schultz 2013.
17 Tyrer et al. 2003.
18 Lloyd 2015d.

the Cancer Council NSW, the Heart Foundation and the Cancer Institute of NSW.

Fiona Crichton, the co-author of this book, had a related experience, which she describes in the boxed text below.

'It's not a great start for an aspiring PhD, is it?'
Fiona Crichton

Over the course of my time conducting experimental research exploring potential pathways for health complaints and annoyance reactions in windfarm communities, I had received correspondence from a number of people suspicious about my motives for conducting the research and disgruntled about my findings. In some cases, these 'concerns' were openly intimidating and apparently aimed at discouraging me from continuing my experimental work.

Although one of the accusations repeatedly levelled was that I was in the pocket of the wind industry, my research was not commercially funded. Instead I received a stipend from the University of Auckland as a doctoral scholar. I also consulted and worked with acoustic and sound experts who gave generously of their time for no monetary reward at all.

The author of the email I received, shown below, is a senior and active member of an anti-windfarm group. I had never heard of him until on 20 August 2013 he sent me an unsolicited email of a mere 3398 words after reading the first published paper (of 3015 words) in what would become a collection of papers that made up my PhD.[19] His email read like one of those later-regretted 'late-night' efforts.

Here are a few choice extracts from his efforts:

It's time to get your brain into gear, Fiona, it's time to wake up.

Do understand this: Should you and/or your colleagues continue what would seem to be your unquestioning support of windfarms as a means of achieving CO2 emissions reductions, and more particularly, should you continue to bad-mouth anyone (even subtly), who dares to question the efficacy or the impacts of this technology, then do understand that those of us who are elaborating the reality of this utterly useless technology cannot guarantee that, as the truth of the stupidity of continued support becomes obvious, you will not be subject

19 Crichton, Dodd, Schmid, Gamble and Petrie 2014.

to richly-deserved ridicule should you continue to maintain that position.

Now that you know that you have been conned by the wind industry and its academic free-loaders, don't feel too bad. To ease the pain and to help calm your nerves, could I suggest some good bed-time books?

The first is John Grant's 'Discarded Science – Ideas that seemed good at the time' … there is always Hans Christian Andersen's 'The Emperor's New Clothes'. No guesses as to who the crooked weavers are!

As I said above, we're in big school now. It's not a great start for an aspiring PhD, is it?

He copied his diatribe to a professor at my university, who was hugely amused by it, and to two professors in the UK whom I had not met and who had no knowledge of me. These professors had simply published a paper in the *Lancet* about electricity and health which I referenced in the introductory section of my first peer-reviewed article.[20] They must have been mystified.

A wind-industry stooge

> Chapman is suffering from something far more severe than 'wind turbine syndrome'. It is called 'closed mind syndrome'. It happens when promises of money and prestige, offered by the wind industry, destroys so many brain cells, that the individual can no longer function as a decent human being. They resort to spewing ignorant comments, and defending useless ideas, all for the sake of the mean green … MONEY. I hope the intelligent, moral, decent human beings in this world, are able to come up with a cure … fast!'
> *—Anonymous comment on the Stop These Things website*

Since I began writing and speaking about wind turbines and health in 2010, it has become almost standard for those who do not agree with me to say or insinuate that I am somehow being paid by the wind industry or parties acting for it. This is completely untrue and I have said this repeatedly to journalists and interviewers whenever

20 Crichton, Dodd, Schmid, Gamble and Petrie 2014.

the question has been asked. Those who continue to make this claim, particularly from the supposed protection of anonymity or parliamentary privilege, are either ignorant about my lack of competing interests or are knowingly lying.

Neither I, nor anyone acting for me, has ever sought or received any research funding, 'unrestricted educational grants', hospitality, shares or any other consideration from any wind-energy company or agent acting for them.

Madigan was clearly utterly convinced that I was deep in the wind-industry trough. When he replied to the letter from my lawyers claiming that he had defamed me on Alan Jones' radio program in 2014, he wrote that should the matter proceed to court, he would:

> be obliged to discover and produce the financial records (and other source documents) concerning payments received by him from any and all of the above [wind companies]. Your client will also be obliged to discover and produce the financial records (and other source documents) of the University of Sydney concerning any payments received by it from any and all of the above; be it from donations, research funding or research grants, for example …

Madigan could, at any time, have requested from my then employer, the University of Sydney, the details he was seeking about any funding being nefariously channelled through the university. It would have been only too happy to be fully transparent as it always is on research funding and donations. I have no knowledge that the university had any such grants or donations from wind companies. If they did, none of it ever came to me. So the reply from the university would have almost certainly been a one-sentence letter.

Expert witness in legal case

In late 2012, I was approached by lawyers acting for the wind company Infigen. Infigen was planning a windfarm, Cherry Tree Hill, on top of a large hill near Seymour in Victoria. Windfarm opponents from outside the district had been in the area and spread anxiety among residents living several kilometres away from the planned site (as we described in Chapter 2). Infigen was taking the local council to the Victorian

Civic and Administration Tribunal (VCAT) after the council opposed the development.

The Infigen lawyers asked me to provide an expert statement on the psychogenic aspects of windfarm complaints in preparation for the VCAT case. To prepare my statement, I attended a meeting in Melbourne with the law firm, visited the proposed windfarm site and spent two days writing a report during my Christmas break. I was paid $2399.90 for my time in preparing the report, including my travel costs.

I expected that windfarm opponents would henceforth attempt to argue that this reimbursement of travel costs and payment for two days of my time meant that I was now forever tainted as being 'paid' by the wind industry.

However, expert witnesses have a general duty to courts, not to any party in proceedings. This was made clear by a chief justice of the Federal Court, who wrote:

> 1.1 An expert witness has an overriding duty to assist the Court on matters relevant to the expert's area of expertise.
> 1.2 An expert witness is not an advocate for a party even when giving testimony that is necessarily evaluative rather than inferential.
> 1.3 An expert witness's paramount duty is to the Court and not to the person retaining the expert.[21]

I was well aware that windfarm opponents would try to frame my professional fees for providing expert testimony as a sign of competing interests, but accepted the commission because my research was specifically relevant to a matter of public interest and I was aware of the above guidelines on the duties of expert witnesses to courts.

In the highly unlikely event that an anti-windfarm group had invited me to provide expert advice to them on the same issue, my report would have made the same points. I claimed travel expenses and two days' writing fees because I am not in the habit of making donations to large commercial enterprises such as energy companies.

Until my retirement from the university in early 2016, I had a tenured academic personal chair in public health at the University of Sydney, where I have worked continuously since 1986. Throughout all that time, my salary was paid for entirely by the university, where I have

21 Allsop 2013.

teaching, research and research scholar supervision responsibilities. My *curriculum vitae* has a section near the end which lists every research grant I have ever received. None of these grants benefit me personally: they were principally used to employ staff and for running the projects described.

Having been an editor of an international journal for 17 years, where I handled thousands of research manuscript submissions, and head of research in my school between 2007 and 2012, I have long been extremely aware of issues to do with competing interests and the importance of declaring them. I have a long history of researching and writing about corporate influences on science. My most recent paper on the importance of declarations of competing interests was a survey of all Australian universities' practices in requiring staff to make and update declarations of competing interests.[22]

Against this background, the idea that I would secretly be accepting payments from the wind industry, and therefore publicly lying every time I said I was not in such a relationship, is ludicrous.

On 29 June 2015 I publicly offered Madigan the opportunity to inspect my banking details if he revealed the identity of the anonymous authors of the Stop These Things website.[23] No reply was ever received.

An ivory-tower academic who refuses to meet with windfarm victims

On many occasions I've read taunts that I have refused to meet windfarm complainants and that therefore I can have no understanding that they are genuinely suffering the direct impacts of wind turbines. In fact, I have never received any invitation to meet with such people, although I have quite often received hostile emails asking why I haven't.

I am aware of at least one fellow wind turbine syndrome sceptic who corresponded with two prominent long-time complainants and expressed willingness to visit their properties and, in one case, to stay overnight. He was firmly rejected both times. I have no illusions that any overtures from me would meet the same fate.

---

22 Chapman, Morrell, Forsyth, Kerridge and Stewart 2012.
23 See my tweet at http://bit.ly/2yg7itu.

Simon Holmes à Court is a Melbourne entrepreneur who has a property near Daylesford in Victoria. Being interested in renewable energy, he worked with others to set up Australia's first community-owned windfarm, the Hepburn Community Wind Farm. He chaired the windfarm's co-operative until 2012. The two-turbine farm is located at Leonards Hill near Daylesford and commenced generating power on 22 June 2011.

His role in helping to realise a community's positive wind vision made Holmes à Court a very public figure in the small world of the anti-wind movement. He was one of the first people to have his face placed on a 'hate wall' on the Stop These Things website, showing Australians who have supported wind energy.

Holmes à Court approached two windfarm complainants multiple times, asking to visit their properties so that he might try first-hand to get some perspective on the noise or vibrations being experienced. He has supplied me with copies of the two email sagas that followed. These excerpts suggest that calls by windfarm opponents for sceptics to meet with complainants are little but posturing, and that barriers are firmly put down when such meetings are attempted.

In May 2013 Holmes à Court asked a prominent complainer, Mr J, if he could visit when he was next in the area and was warmly welcomed with the response, 'Simon you are more than welcome to visit.'

As Holmes à Court attempted to firm up the logistics of a visit, Mr J began to backtrack on his invitation. Holmes à Court wrote:

> My intentions are simply to understand your position. The 'debate' has become unproductive. I'd like to understand how you see the issue and I'd like to understand what it is that you experience from the X wind farm. And perhaps, you might be interested in understanding what drives me. I would be grateful if you would please reconsider my request to meet up with you next Thursday lunchtime.

Mr J replied the same day:

> Too late for polite words. Do not even dare to enter my property looking for me or in any way disturb my peace – you are a persona non-gratis! If you fail to respect my wishes I will consider it an act of trespass.

Holmes à Court responded that he was going to be visiting a friend who lived in the area and that they'd see if he could experience the windfarm noise at such a distance themselves. Upon hearing that Holmes à Court had a friend in the area, Mr J softened his tone considerably and agreed to a meeting of the three.

However, when the third party was eventually unable to make it during the window of time when Holmes à Court would be in the area, Mr J cancelled the meeting. Simon wrote:

> I trust you are talking about noise in the audible spectrum (LFN) and not infrasound. If you are able to point me to any particular location where you find it I'll have some time Thursday afternoon and plan to drive around a bit. Don't worry – I'll respect your privacy.

Mr J replied:

> I have been quite clear in the past about the AUDIBLE nature of the problem – I do not hear INAUDIBLE noise. There is something clearly wrong with your cerebral faculties. DO NOT CONTACT ME EVER AGAIN!

Undeterred, Holmes à Court was in the region again three months later and again asked Mr J if he might show him locations where the noise was loud. Mr J replied:

> If you were here right now, it is a little uncomfortable with this horrid resonance – thanks to the wind turbines. But as far as meeting with me in person forget about it!

In a subsequent email, he wrote

> As to where to experience it? Frankly there are few place [sic] worse than my area out on the hills of [town name]. But if you are familiar with all the mockery I cop from your wind turbine co-religionists, you should be able to hear it all over the region – and of course I do on the worst nights.

If at first you don't succeed ...

Shortly after, Holmes à Court met with the outspoken anti-wind MP Craig Kelly (who would go on to chair the Coalition's Environment and Energy Committee in 2016). Kelly further encouraged Holmes à Court to spend time with the windfarm complainants he was hearing from.

Heeding this advice, on 24 August 2013 Holmes à Court wrote to a prominent opponent of a Victorian windfarm, Mrs W. He told her that he was involved in the Hepburn Community Wind Farm. He explained he was 'not formally a part of the wind industry, but in building the Hepburn Wind project I've become quite familiar with the sector and have met with people on "both sides of the debate"'. He asked Mrs W whether she would meet with him and whether she might 'even possibly allow me to stay overnight to experience a night among the turbines'.

Mrs W wrote back that night. Here are excerpts from her letter:

> Are you able to bring the media along? It would be good if you could invite as many media reporters as possible ...
>
> It would appear, from what you tell me, that you are in contact with Federal politicians. As you've been communicating with Craig Kelly and appear to have the same concerns as he, why not invite Craig to come along also, particularly as he's shown interest in visiting us for a while now ...
>
> In fact, it would be an ideal opportunity to bring some other politicians along also, as you most probably have an 'in' with them. It would be great if you could invite some of the up and coming politicians such as Angus Taylor (they say he'll win the seat of Hume no worries), Nick Xenophon would be a good one, and John Madigan shares your concern about community issues around wind farms.
>
> Ask Greg Hunt to come along too, being the Shadow Minister for the Environment, as we hear from him from time to time and he'll be able to fill you and the media in on Coalition policy for the future on the environment, whilst at the same time familiarising himself with the community concerns.

As she continued, the prospect seemed to dawn on Mrs W of something far larger than a media contingent and five national politicians including a cabinet minister. She suggested:

> The best way to do it Mr Holmes à Court, would be to get a bus load of politicians and media to visit our district. I can organise for them all to be billeted around the wind farm, as families from every direction are being impacted, depending on the wind direction.
>
> However, you must stay for a WEEK, not just a night. There's no way you'd be able to experience the true situation at all by staying for just one night, as that particular night could very well be a relatively calm one.
>
> In order for you all to experience 'life amongst the turbines' you MUST stay for at least seven nights, as surely several of those will be windy, one could be rainy and you might even experience the infrasound here. Infrasound is DEFINITELY emitted by these 140 turbines.
>
> So I look forward to hearing from you in the near future. When you're able to give me the 'heads up' on a bus load of pollies and media, then we'll start organising accommodation for you, which certainly won't be a problem.

Holmes à Court replied:

> I wouldn't be keen on being a part of a media circus. You might have seen that a handful of SA pollies and media stayed for a windy night near Waterloo this year. I don't think it was particularly useful for the local residents.
>
> I have four young kids and I run a business, so seven days away from home would be difficult, but I could try for multiple nights, especially if I can work during the day. I'd be happy to give it a go.
>
> I know it would be an imposition, but is there any chance that there's a spare room in your house or that of another affected resident at the wind farm?

Three days later Mrs W replied:

> We've already set out our conditions for a visit to our district, i.e. with a bus load comprising politicians and media spending close to a week here, to enable the real situation to be experienced. If you're really serious about finding out what it's like living next to a wind factory, we're sure you'll be able to organise this.

Holmes à Court replied:

> Thanks for your email of 28/8. As mentioned I have no interest in being a part of a media circus – that's not how understanding and trust are built. The media looks to find and sensationalise division, and few politicians behave constructively when the media is around.
>
> I am genuine in wanting to understand the experience of affected residents, but I hear you loud and clear that you are not interested in hosting me. Fair enough – you really don't know me from a bar of soap.
>
> I am wondering if you might be able to put me in contact with someone who might be open to me visiting?

Mrs W then slammed the door firmly shut, writing:

> Further to your recent email, we just do not accept that you are genuinely interested in our plight. Nobody here is interested in explaining to you their plight. We've explained our conditions, i.e. unless you're prepared to visit with many members of the new government and media, in particular Graham Lloyd of the *Australian* and Graeme Archer from *Today Tonight*, Adelaide, and stay for at least 5–6 nights, then we would appreciate if you would stop harassing us.

This exchange reveals either Mrs W's profound naïvety (as if a busload of the nation's most senior politicians and media would be able to take a week out of their schedules as she demanded – global summits on climate change like that held in 2015 in Paris saw politicians typically spend a couple of days there), or it suggests that she set such conditions knowing that they would never be met, thus allowing her to be able to claim that Holmes à Court refused to meet the conditions set.

Similar stories can be told by those who have reached out to vocal opponents of another Victorian windfarm. I have no doubt that were I to accept any such invitation that might be issued to me, there would have been complaints to my university that I was engaging in research without ethics committee approval (see below), harassing sick and vulnerable people, and so on. Yet if I don't visit, the rhetoric that I am 'refusing to visit those affected' allows windfarm opponents to frame sceptics like me as 'ivory-towered' and indifferent to real people's suffering. But there is a more fundamental reason why I have had no interest in visiting complainants. Any such meetings could do little to confirm or refute hypotheses about whether or not their claims have substance. Quite obviously, there are millions of people globally who have lived and worked for years near wind turbines and do not complain or suffer any health effects.

On 22 July 2015, following my written submission and oral evidence to the 2015 Senate committee on windfarms, Senator Madigan sent me 62 written questions on notice. He wanted answers within four working days.[24] One question went directly to this issue. Here is part of the answer I provided.

> Question 12: Have you ever visited the home of anyone claiming to be adversely effected [sic] by proximity to wind turbines and if not, why not?
> My response: No, I have not visited any such homes. Here is why. There are many people who passionately believe in things that I do not believe in. For example, every week many thousands use lottery number selection systems in the firm belief that this will increase their chances of winning the lottery; 51% of Britons believe in aliens; a majority of the population believe in the supernatural and life after death; and whole religions believe in reincarnation.
>
> Some people earnestly believe that aircraft chemtrails are chemical sprays used by governments to 'control' populations, and that mobile phones and towers and Wi-Fi are deadly. I do not need to talk personally to any of these people or visit their homes in order to corroborate the information that I can obtain from a variety of sources which tells me clearly that these beliefs are irrational, and in fact either nonsense or faith-based beliefs.

I have no doubt that visiting the homes of complainants would allow me to confirm that such people were both distressed by turbines and convinced that they were being harmed by them. But having been 'up close' to turbines often in Australia, New Zealand, France, Spain and Portugal, and taken note of the many thousands of people living adjacent to those windfarms who could also hear them but do not complain, I would be confirmed in my view that psychogenic factors explain noise complaining and that this is a phenomenon that can be 'spread' through communities, as we detailed in Chapter 5.

24 My full response to the questions can be read in Chapman 2015c.

Tactics used by anti-wind interests

We have considered some of the common discrediting themes that windfarm opponents use in attacking their opponents. We turn now to some of the tactics they have used.

Defamatory emails to politicians

Having worked in public health for nearly 40 years, I have often developed good working relationships with politicians and their staff who have sought advice. I often provide them with briefings and information and they generally reciprocate.

In July 2014, a serial agitator against windfarms, Jackie Rovensky, who is a very frequent commentator on posts on the Stop These Things website, sent an email to a large number of federal politicians, one of whom forwarded it to me minutes after having received it. The email showed the full list of politicians who had been sent the email. Typical of the many communications to politicians from anti-windfarm advocates I have seen, this one rambled on for many pages. But it contained the defamatory statement that I was 'incapable of utilising ethical unbiased standards'.

At 11.55 am on the day I received it, I emailed its author:

> I have been forwarded a copy of your recent email sent to federal politicians. In your cover note you wrote that I am 'incapable of utilising ethical unbiased standards'. This is a defamatory remark. I would strongly advise you to immediately write to all those to whom you sent this remark, retract it and apologise to me.

At 12.41 pm Rovensky emailed all the recipients and apologised. I took no further action.

However, two months later, she seemed unable to help herself and was at it again. This time she had written to 13 senior officers of Australian public health and medical associations making false and defamatory allegations that I had conducted research without Human Ethics Committee approval when researching my paper examining Sarah Laurie's public statement that 'more than 40' Australian families had abandoned their homes because of wind turbine noise.[25] She had written, 'It has subsequently emerged from inquiries made by Senator Madigan's staff, that at the time Professor Chapman conducted his inquiries, he did not have in place prior ethics committee approvals from the Sydney University Ethics Committee.' I look in more detail at this accusation below.

This time, I engaged specialist defamation lawyers to demand a retraction, which she duly issued. She also paid my legal expenses in full.

These incidents revealed both the intransigence of this person's conviction that I was an unethical researcher, her lack of elementary diligence in fact checking, and her naïvety in imagining that she could spray around such malicious accusations without me being quickly alerted to it. Presumably, her decision to distribute this material rested on her faith that the information was reliable; she stated it had been obtained from Senator Madigan's staff.

I wonder if those staff assisted her in paying her legal expenses?

Complaints to my university

Several anti-windfarm activists took to writing lengthy, often verbally incontinent letters of complaint about me to various authorities at my university. Having worked at the University of Sydney for two extended periods totalling 32 years, having a high media profile, and having served as a staff representative on the university's governing Senate for four years, I know many staff at all levels in the university.

Recipients of these complaints included the chancellor, the vice-chancellor, all members of the academic board and the Senate, the dean of the Faculty of Medicine and my departmental head. Rarely were these complaints ever copied to me by their authors, and none ever tried to make contact with me to discuss their complaints before firing them off. I would have been delighted if they had done so. They were instead clear efforts to try and have me disciplined from on high.

However, I got to read many of these complaints because those receiving them would often send them to me, as is normal practice anywhere. Several asked me to draft replies for them (also very normal) and various support staff to senior staff would pat me on the back good naturedly, saying that the work I was generating for them would surely guarantee them overtime pay.

The complaints I saw were profoundly ignorant about and, again, naïve to the nature of university research and enquiry. They assumed

---

25 Chapman 2014b.

that anything an academic said must reflect the university's 'position' on an issue. So what I might have written or said in the news media was tantamount to the university also having said it.

I repeatedly read that I had been invited to visit families who were being affected by wind turbines in their homes. As I have explained, I had never received such invitations.

Allegations of unethical research

As described above, Jackie Rovensky alleged that my research into 'abandoned' homes had not been given clearance by my university's human ethics committee. At least two parties made the same allegation directly to university authorities. The university provided me with a copy of its reply to one serial complainant, but was reluctant to reveal the identity of the other. Body language in response to queries made to various people at the university made it obvious that it was a complaint from an anti-windfarm federal politician. Whoever it was, it was someone very ignorant about research practices and human ethics oversight.

As I described in Chapter 3, my research involved using six sources to try and corroborate the statement that 'over 40 homes' had been abandoned. Three of these sources were public records (parliamentary submissions; the Stop These Things, and media reports). No human ethics committee approval is required to report on information obtained from such already public sources.

I also used three other sources:

- I invited three senators who had made public statements about 'abandoned homes' to provide me with any information they might have;
- I emailed known anti-windfarm activists and asked them for any such information;
- I asked colleagues and associates also interested in windfarms and health if they had any relevant information about home abandonment claims.

Moreover, I submitted to the university's human ethics committee, which was obliged to respond to the complaint. In my submission to the ethics committee, I argued that my research for the paper in question was not 'human research' as described in the Australian Vice Chancellors' Committee/Australian Research Council/National Health and Medical Research Council National Statement on Ethical Conduct in Human Research 2007.[26] Namely, it:

- did not involve any approaches to individuals claiming to be adversely affected by wind turbine noise; and it
- involved no risks to any person.

The National Statement on Ethical Conduct in Human Research lists the types of research it applies to. It says:

> Human participation in research is therefore to be understood broadly, to include the involvement of human beings through:
>
> - taking part in surveys, interviews or focus groups;
> - undergoing psychological, physiological or medical testing or treatment;
> - being observed by researchers;
> - researchers having access to their personal documents or other materials;
> - the collection and use of their body organs, tissues or fluids (e.g. skin, blood, urine, saliva, hair, bones, tumour and other biopsy specimens) or their exhaled breath;
> - access to their information (in individually identifiable, re-identifiable or non-identifiable form) as part of an existing published or unpublished source or database.

I argued, and the human ethics research committee agreed, that my research for this paper did not involve any of these things and so did not require prior approval from the committee. The complaint about my 'unethical' research was formally rejected by the university.

Threats of intimidation

On the morning of 15 June 2015, my attention was drawn to a publicly accessible post published late on the previous evening by Helen Dale on her personal Facebook wall. At the time, her Facebook page identified her as 'Senior Advisor to Senator David Leyonhjelm, Liberal Democrat Senator for NSW at [the] Australian Parliament.' Leyonhjelm was a

26 Cook, Ecker and Lewandowsky 2015.

member of the 2015 Senate committee on wind turbines, to which I had made a submission.[27]

Helen Dale is the latest name used by a woman born as Helen Darville, who for some time also used the pen name Helen Demidenko. As Demidenko, in 1995 she won the prestigious Miles Franklin Literary Award in highly controversial circumstances.

Her Facebook post read:

> Okay, this is a message for those skeptics friends of mine in Australia who are into Public Health.
>
> You need to pull the likes of Simon Chapman and Nathan Lee into line. First, you need to teach both of them to stop with the ad hominem. Then you need to teach the former statistics and how to read them. Then you need to teach both of them how to argue and clarify their thoughts.
>
> David and I can turn both of them into mince on Twitter – yes Twitter – without much effort. This should not happen. I'm a lawyer with a finance major and David's a vet with an MBA.
>
> Now while it's very nice to win arguments all the time, that's not the same as being right. And I'd rather be right than feel smug about my own argumentative aptitude.
>
> My suspicion is – like many people on the left – they live in a bubble and get neither their arguments nor their evidence tested severely or regularly (the very opposite of this Facebook page, for starters).
>
> I'm relying on you to fix this. And if it isn't fixed, I will take great pleasure in ensuring the individuals in question aren't just minced on Twitter.
>
> Getting minced by a Senate Committee is a lot less fun, I assure you.

Dale would have known that I might be called as a witness to the Senate committee. On 16 June 2015 I wrote to Senator Madigan in his capacity as chair of the committee, stating that I believed Dale's post was in contempt of the Senate. I wrote:

> Ms Dale's Facebook post makes no reference to wind farms and health, nor to any subject area. However, as you are aware, I have

27 Crichton and Petrie 2015b.

made a written submission to your wind farms enquiry. I have made no submissions to any other current Senate enquiry. She refers to 'a Senate Committee' which I believe the ordinary person could only take to mean the Committee you chair. There is no Senate enquiry on tobacco harm reduction, to which she refers in several of her comments below her initial post.

Ms Dale's words that 'David and I can turn each of them to mince on Twitter' and 'I will take great pleasure in ensuring the individuals in question aren't just minced on Twitter. Getting minced by a Senate Committee is a lot less fun, I can assure you' are intimidatory to me as a potential witness to your enquiry. 'Minced' is an unambiguously aggressive expression which is entirely antithetical to the spirit of any fair, open-minded and courteous consideration of Senate witnessing.

The Senate's standing orders on matters constituting contempt state in clause 10:

> *Interference with witnesses*
> (10) A person shall not, by fraud, intimidation, force or threat of any kind, by the offer or promise of any inducement or benefit of any kind, or by other improper means, influence another person in respect of any evidence given or to be given before the Senate or a committee, or induce another person to refrain from giving such evidence.[28]

I believe Ms Dale's public statement above constitutes a clear case of contempt of the Senate. She is urging others to 'pull me into line' presumably in relation to matters relevant to my evidence and then threatens to take steps 'without much effort' to ensure that I am 'minced' publicly on Twitter and then before a Senate Committee, which everything points to being the Committee you chair.

It is utterly disgraceful that a senior staff member of a Senator of your Committee should publicly make such statements.

I look forward to learning of your proposed actions in this matter, and reserve my right to subsequently refer the matter to the Senate Privileges Committee should I conclude that you have not treated this matter with the seriousness it deserves.

28 Lewandowsky, Ecker, Seifert, Schwarz and Cook 2012.

On 29 June 2015 I appeared before the Senate committee as a witness, to speak to my submission and answer questions. Leyonhjelm sat mute throughout my evidence and did not ask any questions.

On 3 August 2015 Senator Madigan wrote to me on behalf of the committee, confirming that threatening witnesses was in contempt of the Senate and that Dale has been asked to explain her Facebook post. He stated:

> The committee has written to Ms Dale to seek an explanation of her social media statement. Ms Dale has responded to the committee advising that the social media statement was not related to the work of the Select Committee on Wind Turbines and that the statement was not intended to intimidate, threaten or attempt to influence you in your role as a witness before this committee.
>
> The committee notes that you accepted the committee's invitation to appear as a witness at the committee's public hearing in Sydney on 29 June 2015. The committee further notes that questions were put to you in an orderly manner and that you were given an opportunity to make corrections to the transcript and provide additional supplementary material to the committee after the hearing.
>
> In light of Ms Dale's assurance that her social media statement is not related to the work of this committee and was not intended to influence your appearance as a witness before this committee, the committee does not propose to take any further action in respect of this matter.

I had expected no more from this group. As I had explained in my letter to Madigan, I had made no submissions to any other Senate committee other than to the wind turbine committee. So Dale's words on Facebook – 'Getting minced by a Senate Committee is a lot less fun, I can assure you' – could only have referred to the wind committee.

I therefore regarded their dismissal as a travesty of parliamentary process and appealed to the president of the Senate to refer the matter to the Parliamentary Privileges Committee. In the meantime, the wind turbines committee had been dissolved with the publication of its report, so apparently nothing more could be done. Dale stopped working in Leyonhjelm's office during the 2016 election campaign.

Defamation proceedings

I have twice received letters from lawyers claiming defamation in regard to windfarm matters.

As noted in Chapter 4, in 2015 I received a threat for defamation from lawyers acting for Steven Cooper, an acoustician who has long been championed by anti-windfarm activists. Cooper complained that my public comments about one of his reports on ABC TV's *Media Watch*,[29] and in the comments section of an article in *The Conversation*, were defamatory about his contracted research for Pacific Hydro, a windfarm operator that ran the Cape Bridgewater windfarm in Victoria. His lawyer set out a long laundry list of all the ways his client claimed to have been damaged by my comments. They sought $15,000 plus costs and an apology.

I wrote back denying most of the claims, and agreeing with some that concerned criticisms I had made about aspects of Cooper's report. I explained that:

> The methodological problems with Mr Cooper's study are frankly elementary. As Hoepner and Grant say, 'It's a study that wouldn't have done very well if … submitted for assessment in an undergraduate science degree.' Other comments by others on *The Conversation* are equally if not more scathing.
>
> *The Conversation* is a publication completely funded by Australian universities and open only to writers with university affiliations. It often reports on recently published research, sometimes highly critically. Mr Cooper may not appreciate that it is normal and expected in research communities that any criticism is expressed, even if this criticism may harm the reputation of the researcher. This is encouraged via follow-up publications, editorials, letters to the editor, rapid on-line responses and sometimes post publication seminars …
>
> Nearly every published researcher has experienced criticism of their published work. If researchers whose work was thus criticized were to seek legal action against their critics on each occasion of criticism, they would be widely ridiculed.
>
> I will be very pleased to expand on the many obvious and serious problems with Mr Cooper's study in court should he be foolish

29 Office of the National Wind Commissioner 2017.

> enough to want to expose it to further detailed public criticism. Such exposure would have the potential to greatly amplify public and professional awareness of the major problems with his work. I have close professional associations with many national and international experts in study design, and study bias, although the methodological problems with this study could be affirmed by anyone with even rudimentary knowledge of these matters.
>
> In any court hearing I would also encourage my legal team to question Mr Cooper on why his research involving human subjects was conducted without any approval from a recognised human research ethics committee. I would also encourage my legal team to invite Mr Cooper to explain why for some time he used the email drnoise@acoustics.com.au and why his company's website home page formerly referred to him as 'Dr Cooper' when he has no PhD nor medical undergraduate degree.
>
> We would also cross-examine him on statements on his website that describe him 'Australia's leading acoustical engineer', 'the industry guru' with a 'level of experience not seen in anyone else in the country'. I am aware that there are leaders in the Australian acoustics field who do not share Mr Cooper's assessments of himself.
>
> I have no intention whatsoever of settling this matter by paying Mr Cooper anything nor writing or signing any correction apology or retraction.

I never heard back from them.

When I gave evidence to the 2015 Senate enquiry at a hearing held at the New South Wales Parliament on 29 June 2015,[30] Senator Nick Xenophon concluded his questions to me by asking:

> **Senator Xenophon:** Finally, I know that this is a vexed and heated issue, but previously you have said or published about Dr Sarah Laurie from the Waubra Foundation that she is a deregistered doctor. Do you acknowledge that that is inaccurate?
>
> **Prof. Chapman:** I have never said she is a deregistered doctor. I have said she is an unregistered doctor.
>
> **Senator Xenophon:** Right, but you did republish a tweet that referred to her as a deregistered doctor, I think, in March last year.

30 Bowen, Zwi, Sainsbury and Whitehead 2009.

Prof. Chapman: I am not aware that I did that. I would like to see that tweet.
Senator Xenophon: Okay. If I am wrong, I will apologise; but, if you are wrong, you would be happy to apologise to Dr Laurie for that?
Prof. Chapman: Of course I would, yes.

On 13 July, some two weeks later, I received a letter, not from Senator Nick Xenophon, but from Nick Xenophon & Co. Solicitors. The letter alleged that by retweeting a tweet that falsely stated that Sarah Laurie was a 'deregistered' doctor, I had defamed her. She sought $50,000 in damages and a public apology (the text of which had been prepared), which I was to arrange to be published in a variety of places.

Similar letters of demand were received by the person who had made the original tweet (Ken McAlpine); by Ketan Joshi, who while watching the committee hearing online had tweeted about Xenophon's question; and by the *Sydney Morning Herald* journalist Peter Hannam, who had been in the Senate committee room to report on the proceedings and simply retweeted Joshi's tweet.

As I had said under oath in the committee hearing, I regretted my retweet because I knew Laurie was unregistered, not deregistered. I genuinely did not recall clicking the retweet button, something I have done thousands of times since joining Twitter in 2009. I have always been fastidious in describing Laurie as an unregistered doctor. So when Xenophon produced the text of the retweet in the Senate committee, I was embarrassed and without hesitation said that I would apologise to Laurie.

I later checked all of my publications, including tweets, in which I had ever mentioned Laurie, which confirmed I had never referred to her as being 'deregistered' in the past.

On receiving the letter of demand I was immediately curious about how many people would have seen my retweet. This would have been relevant to the claims being made of damage to Laurie's reputation. I located it in my Twitter archive and took a screenshot. The tweet had only received six 'impressions' and four 'engagements'. Impressions count those who see a tweet, while 'engagements' count those who retweet (in this case, three) or 'like' (one) a tweet.

I searched for the four who had engaged with tweet. One was obviously me. The others were Ray Walker @funkygibbing (unknown to me and not someone who follows me on Twitter), and two anonymous parties who had set their security settings so as to keep their identities secret.

Ray Walker retweeted the McAlpine tweet on 29 June 2015, the day Senator Xenophon publicised the tweet in the Senate. That coincidence points to the strong likelihood that Ray Walker may have been watching the committee broadcast, searched for the original tweet and retweeted it. There was no evidence that anyone else had further retweeted (or had even seen) my retweet.

My lawyers may have conveyed that we had this evidence and soon afterwards, the demand for $50,000 in damages dropped to less than a tenth of that amount. I had no problem at all apologising, as I had been careless in retweeting the original tweet and the imputation that Laurie had been deregistered was both wrong and potentially harmful to her reputation, despite it being already subject to correction in the Hansard record. My lawyers recommended closing down the case by settling for the reduced amount and issuing the apology, which I was happy to do.

I was more than astonished that Xenophon had not declared, when asking his question about my retweet under parliamentary privilege, that his legal firm had a professional relationship with Laurie. The letter I received from his company indicated that they would be demanding that I also pay Laurie's 'legal costs to date', thus benefitting his private legal practice. It also referred to evidence that I had given under parliamentary privilege.

Xenophon's firm has also worked pro bono representing the Waubra Foundation in their appeal to the Administrative Review Tribunal over their problems with the Australian Charities and Not-for-profits Commission over the revocation of the foundation's charitable status.[31]

Laurie published my apology on the Waubra Foundation website, noting that 'the wind industry and its supporters have stooped to new lows, including wrongly publicly describing the CEO as a "deregistered" doctor despite knowing full well that was untrue. This is grossly and deliberately defamatory.' Anti-windfarm websites were cock-a-hoop at my apology and Graham Lloyd in the *Australian* dutifully wrote it up.[32]

Laurie was fully aware that I had never before 'stooped' to calling her deregistered (because I knew it was untrue). Indeed, on her own website in September 2014, she published a lengthy article by anti-

31 Cook 2016.
32 Cook, Lewandowsky and Ecker 2017.

windfarm activist Jackie Rovensky, who wrote about Laurie's medical registration status:

> Indeed anyone with any awareness of this issue would be well aware of her current unregistered status because of the wide and frequent publicity this issue was given by the wind industry and its vocal supporters, particularly Professor Simon Chapman, the ABC and Fairfax media.[33]

I started writing this book in the months following the publication of the 2015 Senate report on wind turbines, which we have discussed many times throughout the book. In the nearly two years that have passed, other than the continued anonymous never-say-die flailings of Stop These Things, anti-windfarm activists in Australia have been extraordinarly muted and all but absent from news media. The Wind Farm Commissioner has not exactly been inundated with work. State governments of both political complexions have taken enlightened attitudes to windfarm developments. Three of the most virulent critics of windfarms (Madigan, Day and Back) are no longer in parliament. And globally, wind energy developments are moving like a brakeless train, making those agitating against them look like relics of a time that is fast disappearing, as nations embrace renewable energy.

In the final chapter of the book, we consider principles and best practices in efforts to reduce pockets of community anxiety about windfarms.

33 Banas 2010.

8

Strategies for reducing anxiety and complaints

We have emphasised throughout the book that claims about noise and health problems said to be caused by wind turbines are not distributed in any way that is compatible with a 'direct causation' hypothesis. As we have summarised, the overwhelming majority of windfarms around the world do not experience hostility and complaints from their neighbours. Complaints instead tend to concentrate around particular windfarms, in particular states or regions of a small minority of generally Anglophone nations.

Those that do attract complaints often have a history of being targeted by organised anti-windfarm lobby groups who set about trying to spread concern and anxiety among local residents. The central argument of this book has been that for some, concern and anxiety can be contagious, 'infecting' others who are exposed to it. Some of those develop symptoms of anxiety and can express these somatically in ways that can be objectively measured and which can be experienced as highly unpleasant. They really *are* ill.

Many people who worry themselves sick are highly resistant to accepting that this is what is happening to them. They feel it is some sort of character defect to be susceptible in this way and are embarrassed by the idea. They rationalise that the agents concerned (here, wind turbines) must be directly noxious. They become preoccupied with confirming this belief. They link up with others and share evidence, often regardless of its abject quality, that confirms their conviction that the agent really *is* harmful.

Since first showing an interest in this phenomenon, we have both heard people working in the windfarm industry talk about examples of companies that have brought trouble on themselves. Comments like '[X company] took a really arrogant and cavalier attitude toward neighbours of their turbine hosts. It's no wonder it blew up in their face', and 'They broke just about every rule about community engagement there was to break' are typical. However, these comments referred to a very small number of Australian windfarms. By far the more common remarks were those of utter frustration about the intractability of a small, determined group of objectors.

When presenting our research to international audiences we have often found a level of incredulity, particularly among Europeans, that windfarms have become contentious on health grounds in Australia. At a renewable energy conference in Sydney, an executive from a German wind-energy company asked 'What is it about Australia that it gets these complaints? We very rarely see anything like this in Germany.' We have noted the virtual absence of complaints from most nations that have windfarms, and from most windfarms within the few countries that have seen complaints.

So in this, our final chapter, we consider the implications of findings that 'wind turbine syndrome' is a disease spread by communication. We outline practical steps that can be taken by the developers of windfarm projects to minimise the potential for health anxiety to take hold in nearby communities and thereby reduce the likelihood of later nocebo responses. To this end, we set out important components of early community engagement and consultation processes that should improve community satisfaction with developer interactions, increase community acceptance of windfarms, and enhance resistance to the effects of misleading anti-windfarm messages. We specifically look at effective ways to address windfarm health concerns incorporating techniques designed to avoid the backfire effect, a phenomenon commonly seen when refutational information reinforces, rather than corrects, misperceptions.

We also consider procedural justice issues – the fairness of decision-making procedures – which have been shown to influence views about windfarms. Finally, we look at principles of distributive justice and argue that a key strategy to minimise local opposition to windfarms and reduce all concerns, including health anxiety, involves some form of benefit sharing. This involves communities having some significant financial stake in the project, or other benefits of value that accrue to the community as a whole.

Going forward

One of the most compelling reasons to garner an understanding of factors contributing to health concern and symptom reports attributed to windfarms is that this knowledge can be used to inform appropriate strategies to reduce anxiety and health complaints. We have argued that media facilitated and socially transmitted negative expectations provide a pathway for symptom reporting in windfarm communities. While it is difficult in the age of the internet to prevent exposure to negative health messages and misinformation about windfarms, there are ways to reduce the scope for such exposure to trigger anxiety and nocebo responses.[1]

As we discussed in Chapter 5, not everyone accessing negative health messages will experience health anxiety and attribute their symptoms to wind turbines. Whether exposure to health misinformation leads to nocebo responses will depend on whether residents are likely to be concerned by and believe the narrative that turbines cause health effects. Evidence suggests people are less likely to be vulnerable to the effects of negative health information about wind turbines if they have already formed positive views of windfarms.[2] It is therefore important that strategies are undertaken very early in the windfarm development process that are conducive to creating positive attitudes to the proposed windfarm and which lead to social acceptance of the wind energy project.[3] This generally requires that the windfarm developer cultivates a relationship of trust with the community and is seen as adopting fair and consultative processes.[4]

In particular, public engagement and community consultation undertaken in the planning process have been shown to improve community views about windfarms and increase acceptance and support for proposed windfarm development.[5] The emphasis must be

1 Langford and Wessely 2015.
2 Crichton and Petrie 2015.
3 D'Souza and Yiridoe 2014.
4 Khorsanda, Kormos, MacDonald and Crawford 2015.
5 Walker, Baxter and Ouellette 2015.

on 'meaningful' engagement, where there is a two way information flow – such as an opportunity for the developer to share the proposal with the community, and a chance for the public to provide the developer with their vision for the community in which they live.[6]

A recent study analysed the effect of government-mandated minimum community-engagement requirements, such as the requirement for windfarm developers to hold two public meetings, as a pre-requisite to planning approval.[7] It was found that setting minimum engagement requirements could lead to perfunctory, 'tick the box' community engagement, where the minimum requirements might be, in effect, treated by the developer as the maximum requirement rather than the starting point, and which did not enable meaningful public participation based on the particular needs and concerns of the community. Such cursory engagement has the potential to lead to lower levels of community support for the windfarm project and more divided communities.[8]

Meaningful engagement should extend beyond public meetings and also incorporate initiatives involving the early provision of information and education opportunities for community members to be exposed to a more comprehensive understanding of the impacts of windfarms, and allow for questions and concerns to be raised and addressed.[9] In the 2016 report by the Office of the National Wind Farm Commissioner there are a number of recommended initiatives for windfarm developers to facilitate this aim, including the following:

- Establish a 'shop front' in the community town centre that provides project and permit information, a map and model of the project and information about windfarms, and that can address questions or concerns raised by community members
- Provide an informal channel for community members to ask questions and provide feedback about the project, and be able to do so anonymously if required
- Provide opportunities for community members to visit operating windfarms
- Provide a windfarm noise simulator event to explain windfarm noise and experience simulated windfarm noise conditions

6 Fast et al. 2016.
7 Fast et al. 2016.
8 Office of the National Wind Commissioner 2017.
9 Office of the National Wind Commissioner 2017.

- Provide and maintain an up-to-date project website with full transparency on project and permit information
- Provide information sessions about the project and windfarms more generally, at convenient locations within the community, including presentations from key stakeholders, along with regular project newsletters and updates.

Addressing health concerns and correcting misinformation

Given that anticipatory fear of windfarm health effects is apparent in some communities faced with the prospect of windfarm development, effective processes to address and reduce health concerns may be necessary during community consultation and engagement.[10] Addressing health concerns is likely to be more effective early in the consultation process, before concerns have time to develop and strengthen over time.[11] Recent research also indicates that resistance to wind energy developments on health grounds has been prompted by perceptions of unfair treatment in relation to those raising health concerns, particularly when concerns were seen to be ignored or pejoratively dismissed as NIMBYism.[12] Therefore consultation and engagement processes which answer health concerns respectfully, rather than ignoring them or dismissing them out of hand, is likely to be important to minimise threat perceptions and stress at the community level.[13]

However, where residents are raising concerns about windfarm health issues based on information accessed via the media, or disseminated by anti-windfarm campaigners, it is important to be aware that reversing beliefs created by misinformation tends to be difficult. According to Stephan Lewandowsky, a cognitive psychologist with expertise in correcting misinformation, this is because misinformation is 'sticky', and often continues to influence people's thinking even when they are made aware it is wrong, and despite the fact they may accept the information is false.[14] Further, attempts to

---

10 Baxter, Morzaria and Hirsch 2013; Mroczek, Banas, Machowska-Sewczyk and Kurpas 2015.

11 D'Souza and Yiridoe 2014.

12 Songsore and Buzzelli 2014.

13 Walker, Baxter and Oullette 2015.

correct misinformation can backfire or create a 'boomerang effect' where such corrections create or further entrench erroneous beliefs.[15]

We often see the backfire phenomenon in studies designed to address misinformation about the side effects and risks of vaccination that proliferate on the internet, such as the discredited and untrue claim that the measles, mumps and rubella (MMR) vaccine causes autism.[16] In one such study, which assessed effective messages in vaccine promotion using a nationally representative sample of parents in the United States, pro-MMR vaccine messages reduced misperceptions about the vaccine–autism link, but backfired by decreasing the intent to vaccinate in some parents, while some pro-vaccine messages increased beliefs in serious vaccine side-effects.[17]

In addition, research has shown a backfire effect connected to handouts designed to refute common misperceptions about vaccinations.[18] These handouts, often distributed to patient populations, outline misperceptions, such as that the side effects of the influenza vaccine 'are worse than the flu', and counter them with opposing information, such as evidence that the side effects of the influenza vaccine are 'rare and mild'. While individuals given such a flyer were able to correctly identify myths and facts about vaccinations immediately after reading the flyer, within 30 minutes they confused more myths with facts, and reported a lower intention to vaccinate than individuals who had read a flyer that simply presented the facts about vaccination without mentioning the myths.

Therefore, when addressing misinformation about the health effects of windfarms, strategies should be designed to limit the potential for the backfire effect.[19] A number of techniques have been identified which may be useful during public engagement and community consultation processes.[20]

---

14 Lewandowsky, Ecker, Seifert, Schwarz and Cook 2012.
15 Hart and Nisbet 2011; Sanna, Schwarz and Stocker 2002.
16 Betsch and Sachse 2013.
17 Nyhan, Reifler, Richey and Freed 2014.
18 Schwarz, Sanna, Skurnik and Yoon 2007.
19 Langford and Wessely 2015.
20 Cook 2016.

Corrections should be presented simply and concretely, and repeated

One technique shown to be effective in countering misinformation is to use simple, concrete messages that address misperceptions by reiterating the facts, rather than focusing on misleading information.[21] Corrections to misinformation should also be repeated to strengthen their effect and be framed to command attention and stick in the memory.[22] In the case of correcting misinformation about infrasound, messages could emphasise the fact that infrasound is a normal component of environmental sound and a natural phenomenon occurring throughout nature, and that levels of windfarm infrasound are the same as those found when walking by a beach.[23]

Corrections should be accompanied by coherent alternative explanations for events

It is also important to note that field evidence suggests that answering health concerns with the simple assertion that scientific evidence does not indicate windfarms cause health effects may be regarded with suspicion, is unlikely to allay fears, and may even *reinforce* misperceptions.[24] Applying work by Lewandowsky, this may be explained by the fact that people build mental models to make sense of events that occur in the world.[25]

In a hypothetical windfarm case, where an individual has been exposed to media misinformation about the health effects of windfarms, such a cognitive model could be depicted in the following way: *I have come across accounts that, in 2013, a windfarm became operational in X community. Windfarms emit infrasound, which Dr Pierpont says is dangerous to health. Since 2013 previously healthy residents in X community have reported a number of new health issues, such as headaches, tinnitus, and sleep disturbance. Therefore exposure to windfarm infrasound is responsible for health complaints.*

21 Lewandowsky, Ecker, Seifert, Schwarz and Cook 2012.
22 Cook, Ecker and Lewandowsky 2015.
23 Crichton and Petrie 2015a.
24 Fast et al. 2016; Walker, Baxter and Ouellette 2015.
25 Lewandowsky, Ecker, Seifert, Schwarz and Cook 2012.

A simple disclaimer that health risks are not posed by exposure to windfarm-generated infrasound (or windfarms in general) leaves an explanatory gap in the 'event representation', so that the mental model now lacks logical coherence – it no longer makes sense: *Residents were healthy before the windfarm started operating and when the windfarm started operating they became ill. But the windfarm is not responsible? That seems most unlikely.*

To make sense of events, people are then apt to revert to the repudiated information, thereby reinforcing the misperception: *Infrasound must be responsible for the reported health effects*. This can be avoided if corrections to misinformation are accompanied by coherent alternative explanations to prevent the appearance of causal gaps in the representation of events.[26]

Experimental evidence discussed in Chapter 5 indicates that an effective method to address the continued influence of misinformation is to provide a cogent alternative explanation for symptom reporting attributed to windfarms; an explanation of the nocebo effect that normalises the nocebo response and eliminates blame.[27] In keeping with experimental findings, directly answering residents' health concerns by explaining that reported symptom complaints are the likely effects of anxiety, negative expectations, and symptom misattribution may be one way to address this explanatory void.

If residents are not convinced by this explanation it may be useful to have a psychologist or medical professional with expertise in the nocebo effect address a community meeting, or for particularly worried individuals to have the opportunity for a one-on-one meeting with such an expert. The persuasiveness and plausibility of a message is enhanced when the communicator is seen as independent and credible, with an expertise in the subject at issue.[28] Reinforcing this message with information from the National Wind Commissioner showing that health complaints are very rare and the vast majority of windfarms have no complaints at all should helpfully illustrate that the problem does not lie with exposure to windfarms.[29]

We have noticed that in online debate, windfarm opponents invariably avoid any engagement with the very obvious fact that most

---

26 Cook, Ecker and Lewandowsky 2015.

27 Crichton and Petrie 2015b.

28 Lewandowsky, Ecker, Seifert, Schwarz and Cook 2012.

29 Office of the National Wind Commissioner 2017.

windfarms have been complaint-free, often for many years. It is as if this information is too subversive to acknowledge. It may be an example of what some have called a 'killer fact'.[30]

Pre-emptive inoculation messages ('prebunking')

Another approach is to provide people with advanced warning that they may be exposed to misleading information in the future and to debunk that information before it is accessed, a technique known colloquially as 'prebunking'.[31] In essence, the intent is to 'inoculate' against anticipated forthcoming misinformation through prior exposure to a rebutted version of the future message.[32] Evidence indicates that individuals exposed to inoculation messages are more likely to resist misinformation than individuals exposed to messaging that conveys accurate information, but which does not allude to the misinformation.[33] Inoculating messages have been shown to be effective to reduce the influence of science misinformation about issues such as climate change[34] and genetically modified food, as well as increasing resistance to conspiracy theory propaganda.[35]

In the case of windfarms, it may certainly be useful during initial community consultation meetings to explain to community members that they may come across misinformation. However, the utility of specifically refuting health misinformation about windfarms to inoculate against the possible negative effects of future misinformation about windfarm health risks has yet to be researched. There may be a risk of backfire effects, particularly in areas where windfarm opponents are not particularly active and there is no specific campaign to disseminate negative health information. Still, given promising indications that this technique is one of the most useful ways to reduce the influence of misinformation,[36] pre-emptive 'inoculation' may be a particularly effective way to counter the effects of exposure to misinformation in communities where windfarms are proposed,

---

30 Bowen, Zwi, Sainsbury and Whitehead 2009.
31 Cook 2016.
32 Cook, Lewandowsky and Ecker 2017.
33 Banas 2010.
34 van der Linden, Leiserowitz, Feinberg and Maibach 2015.
35 Banas 2013.
36 Cook et al. 2017.

particularly in cases where it is obvious from the outset that anti-windfarm activists are likely to target the project.

Fair process

Procedural justice issues, such as fairness of process in relation to negotiations with landowners and consultation with neighbours, are integral to achieving acceptance and support for any proposed windfarm development.[37] If residents view processes unfavourably and consider interactions with the developer to be unsatisfactory, this can create resentment and hostility, and a susceptibility to negative rhetoric disseminated by anti-windfarm campaigners. A number of steps can be taken to minimise discord and improve perceptions of procedural fairness. In this section we draw on the exemplary 2016 report of the Australian Wind Farm Commissioner[38] and also include discussion about noise regulation.

Fairness of negotiations with potential host landowners

In his 2016 report, the Australian Wind Farm Commissioner identified a number of factors important for developers to consider during negotiations with landowners to improve the overall experience for the landowner.[39] Managing landowners' expectations was highlighted as a key component of the negotiation process.

As we discussed in Chapter 6, sometimes a landowner initially agrees to host wind turbines on an understanding that they will received compensation for a specific number of turbines, and in the latter stages of the process that number is significantly reduced or even eliminated. This eventuality can lead to disappointment, resentment, or a feeling of being cheated. Such a landowner is likely to be further aggrieved if neighbouring properties are receiving an income stream from wind turbines, particularly if these turbines can be seen and/or heard from the disappointed landowner's property.

37 Khorsanda et al. 2015
38 Office of the National Wind Commissioner 2017.
39 Office of the National Wind Commissioner 2017.

It is important to mitigate the potential for landowner disenchantment with the negotiation process and dissatisfaction with the final development by ensuring that they are aware from the outset that they may end up hosting fewer turbines than discussed during preliminary negotiation, and that changes may be made to the proposed windfarm layout. One practical recommendation is for developers to consider offering some level of compensation to all potential host landowners, irrespective of the final allocation of turbines on individual properties.

Fairness to neighbours

The residents of neighbouring properties are often impacted by the development, construction, and eventual operation of wind turbines. However, they are not always included by developers in the consultation process. A failure to properly consult with neighbours can create feelings of hostility, mistrust and anxiety, making these residents more likely to seek out and believe negative information about windfarms, and more prone to vehemently oppose windfarm development.

A fair consultation processes would provide neighbours with information about the layout and design of the proposed windfarm, and about noise exposure and testing processes. The developer would appoint a contact person, through whom concerned residents could raise questions and concerns and have them answered directly in a timely fashion. As part of the consultation process, agreements may be negotiated to provide compensation for the possible impact of the windfarm, such as changes to visual amenity, or reimbursement for expenses such as visual screening. While these agreements are likely to be confidential, they should not include clauses that could be interpreted as restricting the neighbours' right to make a complaint.

Complaint-handling procedures

Windfarm developers and operators should also have the facility to receive, investigate, and resolve complaints. Residents should be made aware of how to make a complaint. Community resentment can quickly arise and escalate where complaints are left unanswered or are not dealt with expeditiously.

Noise should be measured in decibels, not metres

In his 2016 report, the Wind Farm Commissioner noted a need for consistent windfarm noise regulations across Australia.[40] When standards vary from state to state there is the potential for perceptions of injustice to arise in residents who live in jurisdictions with less stringent requirements, which may also create suspicion that these noise regulations are not sufficiently rigorous to protect health. This raises the question of how standardised noise regulations should be formulated, and about the usefulness of minimum setback provisions (regulations governing how close turbines can be to other buildings) in setting noise guidelines.

While there is some variability around the world, windfarm noise guidelines are, on average, set at a daytime limit of 40 to 45 dBA and a night-time outdoor limit of 40 dBA.[41] This night-time sound limit is based on the World Health Organization's recommended noise limit of 30 dBA inside bedrooms to prevent sleep disturbance, which, given attenuation of sound as it travels through walls and windows, equates to an outdoor level of 40 dBA.[42] Recent analysis has confirmed that the development and enforcement of health-based A-weighted audible noise limits is an effective method of assessing and monitoring noise and protecting the public in relation to exposure to all the components of windfarm sound, including low frequency noise and infrasound exposure.[43] The evidence also indicates that regulatory guidelines setting a daytime outdoor limit of 45 dBA, and a night-time limit of 40 dBA, are effective in protecting the health and safety of residents.[44]

We would argue that decisions about where to locate windfarms should not be based on prescribed minimum setback distances, but should instead be guided by noise standards set out above. We also suggest adopting recommendations set by the New Zealand standard NZS 6808:2010,[45] which in special circumstances, for particularly quiet locations, recommend a lower limit during the evening and night-time

40 Office of the National Wind Commissioner 2017.
41 McCunney et al. 2014.
42 World Health Organisation 2009.
43 Berger et al. 2015.
44 Berger et al. 2015.
45 Chiles 2010.

of 35 dBA or 5 dBA more than the background sound level, whichever is the greater.

Wind-energy companies are always required to include noise studies in their development applications. These model the noise of the entire proposed windfarm and provide a noise contour map showing the projected maximum noise impact at every point in the vicinity of the farm. If the project is ultimately approved, the approval comes with a large set of conditions, one of which is that the project produces a post-construction noise study to determine whether or not the farm is compliant. As with any development, there is a suite of regulatory measures to enforce compliance.

If, at post-construction testing, noise levels are excessive, there are noise-mitigation options. These include reducing turbine power and turning off particular turbines. Such options can seriously negatively affect the economics of the project. It is therefore in the developers' interests to be conservative during the development phase. It is far preferable to change a prospective turbine location before it is constructed than to be forced to operate a non-compliant turbine in reduced-power mode for its entire life.

The problem inherent in incorporating prescribed minimum setback distances as part of noise regulation is that they are arbitrary, and may be greater or smaller than necessary.[46] Therefore, minimum setback distances can needlessly impede or even stymie suitable windfarm development, or fail to properly protect residents. Further, fixed minimum setback requirements may convey the erroneous impression that there is something inherently dangerous or bad about living near wind turbines, creating unnecessary anxiety or hostility. As one expert told us, 'Noise should be measured in decibels, not metres.'

Distributive justice

In this section we discuss broader social justice issues and explore some of the most important contextual considerations influencing community acceptance of windfarms. An article by David Roberts, a staff writer for *Vox*, sets the tone.[47] Roberts' insightful and poignant piece was written in answer to a story about a town meeting held in

46 Godden and Kallies 2011.
47 Roberts 2015.

Woodland, a small town in North Carolina, at which a number of residents voiced their opposition to a proposed solar farm being built in their neighbourhood (there were already three solar farms around the town).

The story, originally published by the local newspaper, had bounced around the internet, reaching 220 sites and attaining viral status, mostly because of reports that a retired science teacher's stated concern was that solar panels, as well as posing a cancer risk, would prevent photosynthesis in the area, which would harm local vegetation, and because another resident had expressed worries that solar panels would suck up all the energy from the sun. The residents were widely derided online, prompting some social commentators to admonish the ridiculers for their elitism. The story then died down.

In his *Vox* piece, Roberts looks at the lessons in the story. He paints a picture of a struggling small town of 800 residents, with unemployment well above national and state averages, most residents having only a high-school education or less, and with a disproportionately large population of middle-aged adults, the young adults having left the town. Residents were worried that their town was becoming a ghost town. The promise of the American dream had eluded them and they were faced with grim economic realities, which, for some, led to a conviction that corrupt powers were shaping the country, motivated by secret agendas.

Roberts makes the compelling point that lack of trust breeds conspiracy theories (solar panels will suck all the energy from the sun and new businesses will stay away). Importantly, even for residents who do not buy the conspiracy theories, the appearance of solar panels around their town is a visible and ever-present reminder of social and economic changes that benefit others but not them. Roberts sums it up eloquently:

> The land around the town, once its future, is being industrialized by a company from Somewhere Else, for the profits and benefits of people Somewhere Else, as Woodland continues to struggle.

In answer to residents' concerns, the town council blocked the proposed solar farm and issued a moratorium on future farms. As Roberts concludes, this decision was not really propelled by cancer fears or by barmy beliefs about photosynthesis – it was an entirely rational response to a request for something valuable that offered nothing of substance in return. The solar farm was an unappealing deal for a community suspicious of modernity and for whom the local economic forecast offered little in the way of hope for improvement.

This story is a familiar one. We can find similar issues arising in the case of windfarms. Distributive justice can be broadly conceptualised as the equitable distribution of outcomes. In the context of renewable energy projects, this generally relates to how benefits are introduced and shared within communities in which renewable energy developments are sited.[48] It has been noted that distributive justice issues are of particular relevance in the United Kingdom, where many of the rural and coastal areas in which wind energy developments are located are comparatively disadvantaged, characterised by aging populations, youth outmigration, higher than average levels of poverty, dependence on low-paid seasonal employment, and geographical isolation.[49]

One argument put forward is that the distribution of benefits by windfarm developers should not merely be seen as a means to cultivate acceptance of the project, but should also be viewed as a way to redress uneven social and economic consequences that can arise from wind-energy development, particularly when the project is located in areas already suffering from social, environmental, and economic disadvantage.[50]

Beyond payments to host landowners, wider economic benefits to the community can be slight.[51] Further, in the UK, windfarm-related construction and manufacturing jobs have rarely materialised in the rural areas in which windfarms are sited.[52] While support for local windfarm development has been found to be predicted by a belief that windfarms will provide economic benefits, this has not been found to reflect individual self-interest, but rather a broader concern about the community as a whole.[53] It is the fair distribution of local benefits that appears to matter most (although the overall amount no doubt matters as well).[54]

There are a number of mechanisms for benefit-sharing:[55]

---

48 Walker and Baxter 2017.
49 Cowell, Bristow and Munday 2012.
50 Cowell, Bristow and Munday 2012.
51 Cowell, Bristow and Munday 2012.
52 Munday, Bristow and Cowell 2011.
53 Bidwell 2013.
54 Walker and Baxter 2017.

1. Local ownership or co-ownership, whereby shares in the windfarm project are granted or offered to the community
2. Community funds, whereby the developer provides funds for community projects
3. Compensation packages
4. Benefits in kind, whereby the developer creates improvements to the community
5. Local employment opportunities
6. Energy-price reduction packages
7. Indirect social benefits, such as eco-tourism.

Overall, local support for wind energy development is improved if benefits offered are viewed as having substantive value and as being appropriate for the community in which they are to be shared.[56] On the flip side, perceptions that the benefits proposed are token in nature or generally unfair can stimulate community mistrust in the developer and opposition to the project.[57]

The extent to which perceptions of distributive justice are affected by different approaches to community benefit strategies has been recently assessed in an important study comparing the views of stakeholders in the Canadian provinces of Ontario and Nova Scotia.[58] In Ontario, windfarm profits are, in the main, distributed to developers, with the only other benefits allotted to the relatively small number of large-parcel land holders hosting wind turbines under lease agreements (an arrangement known as the technocratic model). By contrast, in Nova Scotia, legislative policy has supported community-owned wind-energy development, ensuring that more benefits stay within the community (the community model).

Results of the study showed that local support for and approval of windfarm planning and construction was three times higher in Nova Scotia. One of the messages from developers was that, in their experience, where landowners holding turbine leases were the only community beneficiaries, this created feelings of envy and resentment in other residents and therefore community discord. Interestingly, residents from Ontario, when introduced to the possibility that

55 van Erk 2011.

56 Bronfman, Jiménez, Arévalo and Cifuentes 2012; Cohen, Reichl and Schmidthaler 2014.

57 Aitken 2010.

58 Walker and Baxter 2017.

windfarms could bring additional financial benefits to the community, viewed these potential benefits with aversion; receiving benefits without addressing the perceived health issues felt 'toxic' to people already concerned about health risks. In the same vein, one windfarm supporter recognised that, in Ontario, introducing community benefits could be seen by residents as a bribe or being 'bought off'. However, as the researchers pointed out, this does not mean that financial benefits should not be channelled to local communities, as the technocratic model adopted in Ontario had increased dissatisfaction with windfarms.

Considering the experience of residents of Nova Scotia, it might have been the case that, if community-based models had been adopted at the initial planning stages, mistrust of developers could have been allayed, envy of host landowners avoided, and the overall perception of windfarms improved. As we have discussed in previous chapters, health concerns about windfarms have proliferated in Ontario. It is relevant that anticipation of economic benefits has been found to influence beliefs about the effects of windfarms, a finding consistent with risk-perception research indicating that when people view something as providing economic benefit, they consider it to be less risky.[59]

Community-based models, by improving the anticipated economic benefit to the community and enhancing distributive justice outcomes, should reduce perceptions of risk, and so make resident less susceptible to the kind of negative rhetoric about windfarms seen in Ontario. Overall, a key strategy to minimise local opposition to windfarms and reduce anxiety is likely to involve some form of benefit sharing whereby the community has a significant financial stake in the project, or where some other benefits accrue to the community as a whole.

As an interesting aside, more than 75 percent of all survey respondents supported the concept of a program that would lower household electricity bills for residents living close to wind turbines.[60] Support for reduced electricity costs was even more resounding in those who opposed their local wind-energy project, with 83.1 percent of this subset of respondents in favour of lower power bills. The study suggests another avenue to improve distributive justice outcomes likely to appeal even to those resistant to the idea of windfarms.

---

59 Bidwell 2013.

60 Walker and Baxter 2017.

In the Australian context, the National Wind Farm Commissioner has recognised the importance of distributive justice considerations by making the following observations and recommendations:

> The developer should establish and maintain a community engagement fund and ensure there is appropriate community involvement in the governance and management of the fund. This should include appropriate opportunities for community originated submissions to obtain funding for project proposals. Prioritisation of funded projects that may be of benefit to those community members more directly affected by the presence of the wind farm should be encouraged.
>
> The developer should seek out opportunities to help facilitate improvements to other related infrastructure, such as mobile phone coverage, which would benefit both the wind farm and the community.
>
> There may also be innovative opportunities for landowners and other community members to have an ownership stake in the project, which could be in the form of a community-owned wind farm through to equity or debt participation in the commercial ownership structure.[61]

The natural history of complaints

We have often been asked by journalists and wind-industry employees about our predictions for the future of windfarm complaints. Our advice usually follows the suggestions we have just described, although these are not guaranteed antidotes to future complaints.

However, there is a final important consideration. As we discussed in the Introduction, the phenomenon of complaints about windfarms is by no means the first time we have seen communities expressing anxiety about new technology, and a minority of those who are anxious somaticising that anxiety in symptoms.

Perhaps the most recent and pertinent comparison here is with mobile phone towers and the phones themselves. The heyday of anxiety about these was in the mid-1990s, when cell phone use began to

61 Office of the National Wind Commissioner 2017.

accelerate rapidly. Within a few years, a large and soon a very large proportion of the population was using cell phones. The resulting service demands required that transmission towers mushroom across all countries.

Mobile phones and towers rapidly moved from being exotic technologies to being near-ubiquitous in every nation on earth. While outbreaks of health concerns were quite common in the early years of phone use,[62] today they have long been a phenomenon of the past. It is now around 20 years since reports of protests about mobile phone towers regularly featured in news media.

While there are still die-hard enclaves of passionate crusaders against mobile phones and wi-fi, these are tiny. Their dire warnings in the face of no evidence of any increase in the diseases they have constantly warned us all about[63] have rendered them as marginal and eccentric as the occasional person we have all encountered who tells us they would never have a microwave oven, a computer or a television in their home because 'those things are deadly'. Here, there is probably no rival for heroic predictions gone badly wrong than that made in 2006 by two 'researchers' who predicted that by 2017, half of all the world's population would have developed electrosensitivity.[64]

We believe it is quite likely that the few complaint hotspots around the world today where we still see a dribble of complaints about wind turbines and health will continue to reduce. The very small number of complaints received by Australia's Wind Farm Commissioner in the first year of its establishment is plainly a sign that this process is well underway.

That is a very good thing. The world is in desperate need of a rapid transition to renewable energy. Wind is a critical part of that.

We hope our book will be helpful in accelerating that process.

---

62 Chapman and Wutzke 1997.
63 Chapman et al. 2016.
64 Chapman 2017.

Appendix: 247 symptoms, diseases and aberrant behaviours attributed to wind turbine exposure

In January 2012, I commenced building the list shown below of ever-growing claims made about problems in humans and animals that windfarm opponents attribute to exposure to wind turbines. All the claims below can be found in online sources, mostly websites of opponents of windfarms and submissions they have made to governments.

The list is now permanently located on the University of Sydney's scholarship repository (http://hdl.handle.net/2123/10501), where links to sources for each claim can also be found.

Teresa Simonetti (2012) and Vince Cakic (2013) both assisted with locating many complaints during vacation placements at the Sydney Medical School.

'arcing' teeth

ADHD, aggravated

alcohol abuse

allergy-like sensations

anger

angina pectoris

appetite loss

accelerated ageing

arthritis, aggravated

asthma, aggravated

autism, aggravated

aversive learning

back pain

balance disturbance

bats, death of

bats, exploding lungs in

bees, threatened extinction of

benzodiazepine abuse

bleeding ears

blood in the urine

blurred vision
bowl cancer
bowels, 'loss of'
brain pathology
brain tumours
brain-derived neurotrophic factor, reduced
breast pain
breathing difficulties
bronchitis
bruxism
burst blood vessels in the eyes
cardiac arrhythmias
cataracts
cats, social problems in
cattle, aggression in
cattle, birth defects in
cattle, dancing in
cattle, death of
cattle, decreased weight gain in
cattle, electric shocks of
cattle, haemorrhaging of adrenal glands in
cattle, infertility in
cattle, reduced calving rates in
cattle, social problems in
cattle, spontaneous abortions in
chest pain
chicken, birth defects in
chicken, egg abnormalities in
chicken, infertility in
cognitive dysfunction
cold sores (herpes)
collagen, destruction of
collagen, excess
colon cancer
concentration problems
confidence loss
confusion
conjunctival haemorrhages
conjunctivitis
crabs, delayed metamorphosis in
crickets, increased mortality in
crying
deaths from 'unusual' cancers
decrease in visual acuity
delayed brain development
delayed healing of wounds
dental infections
dental injuries
depression
diabetes, adult-onset
diabetes, aggravated
diarrhoea

difficulty praying
dogs, bad behaviour in
dogs, ear problems in
dogs, inappropriate urination in
dogs, stunted growth in
dolphins, beaching of
dry eyes
duodenal ulcers
ear pain
eardrum perforation
electromagnetic spasms
emotionality
epilepsy
excessive sleep
eye discharge
fatigue
fibromyalgia, aggravated
foot sores
formication
fungal skin infections
groundwater contamination
hair greying
hallucinations
headache
hearing, unprecedented ability
heart palpitations
heartburn
hippocampal atrophy

gastrointestinal haemorrhages
dogs, behavioural changes in
dogs, epilepsy in
dogs, itchy skin in
dogs, reduced litters in
dream disturbances
dry retching
dysmenorrhoea
ear popping
echidnas, disorientation in
elevated salivary cortisol levels
emus, death of
excessive urination
exhaustion
family discord
fever
fluttering heartbeat
forgetfulness
frustration
goats, death of
haemorrhoids
hair loss
hares, internal haemorrhaging in
hearing loss
heart attack
heart valve problems
hip pain
horses, behavioural problems in

hyperacusis
hypertensive crisis
hyperthyroidism
immunodeficiency
increased climatic temperature
increased violent crime
indigestion
infertility
inflammatory bowel disease
intellectual delay
internal pulsations
irritability
ischaemic heart disease
joint pain
kidney damage
lethargy
leukaemia
lip vibrations
loose stools
loss of libido
lower respiratory tract infections
lung cancer
lung ciliary factor disturbance
lupus, aggravated
lymphoma
mania
memory loss, long-term
memory loss, short-term
Meniere's disease, aggravated
migraine
minks, birth defects in
minks, premature births in
mood swings
motor paralysis
mouth ulcers
multiple sclerosis
muscle hypotonia
muscle pain
muscle twitches
nausea
nerve pain
nerve twitching
nervousness
neurological disturbances
night sweats
night terrors
nocturia (excessive night-time urination)
noise pollution
non-convulsive mental defects
non-Hodgkin's lymphoma
nosebleeds
pacemaker interference
painful urination
panic attacks

parasitic skin infection
peacocks, behavioural problems in
pericardial thickening
pigs, increased mortality in
pituitary gland destruction
pruritis
psychiatric disturbance
PTSD, aggravated
reduced visual acuity
retching
scleroderma, aggravated
shaking head
sheep, behavioural problems in
sheep, birth defects in
sheep, blurred vision in
sheep, gastric ulcers in
sheep, infertility in
sheep, reduced wool quality in
shoulder pain
sick building syndrome
sinus tightening
sinusitis
skin cancer
skin rashes
sleep disturbance
sore eyeballs
sore legs
sound hypersensitivity
spastic colitis
speech delay
speech problems
staring blankly
stomach inflammation
stress
stroke
stunted growth of internal organs
suicidal ideation
suicide
sunken eyes
swollen glands
tachycardia
throat infections
thyroid problems
tinnitus
transient ischaemic attack
triglyceride elevation
unusual noises
uterine haemorrhaging
varicose veins
vertigo
vestibular illusions
vibrations in the body
vibroacoustic disease
viral skin infections

visceral vibratory vestibular disturbance

visual sensitivity

vomiting blood

water pollution

watery eyes

weight gain

weight loss

whales, disorientation in

worms, behavioural issues in

worms, death of

yawning

Works cited

Abbasi, M., M.R. Monazzam, A. Akbarzadeh, S. A. Zakerian and M. H. Ebrahimi (2015). 'Impact of wind turbine sound on general health, sleep disturbance and annoyance of workers: a pilot-study in Manjil wind farm, Iran.' *Journal of Environmental Health Science and Engineering* 13(71) doi:10.1186/s40201-015-0225-8

Aberdeenshire Council (2016). 'Sunnyside Royal Hospital, Montrise.' http://bit.ly/2zQKWvU

Abrams, L. (2013). 'Wind turbines are either making people sick or driving them crazy.' *Salon*, 16 September. http://bit.ly/2lhj7tr

Adler, I. (1912). *Primary malignant growths of the lungs and bronchi*. London, Longmans.

Aitken, M. (2010). 'Wind power and community benefits: challenges and opportunities.' *Energy Policy* 38(10) doi:10.1016/j.enpol.2010.05.062

Akerman, P. (2010). 'Baillieu policy bodes ill for Victorian wind farmers.' *Australian*, 3 December. http://bit.ly/2zPPZMY

Alberta Utilities Commission (2014). 'Errata to Decision 2014-040. Bull Creek Wind Project.' 10 March. http://bit.ly/2zEYrxC

Allsop, J. (2013). 'Practice note CM 7: expert witnesses in proceedings in the Federal Court of Australia.' Federal Court of Australia, 4 June. http://bit.ly/2gKm04v

Alves-Pereira M and N.A.A. Castelo Branco (2007). 'Public health and noise exposure: the importance of low frequency noise.' *Inter-Noise*, 28 August. http://bit.ly/2yOBetU

Alves-Pereira M. and N.A.A. Castelo Branco (2011). 'Low frequency noise and health effects.' Presentation to Wind Farms and Human Health Scientific Forum, Canberra, 7 June. http://bit.ly/2z7XaD9

Alves-Pereira, M. and N.A.A. Castelo Branco (2014). 'Letter to the editor re: "how the factoid of wind turbines causing "vibroacoustic disease" came to be "irrefutably demonstrated"'. *Australian and New Zealand Journal of Public Health*, 38(2) doi:10.1111/1753-6405.12229

Ambrose, S., R. Rand and C. Krogh (2012). 'Wind turbine acoustic investigation: infrasound and low-frequency noise – a case study.' *Bulletin of Science, Technology and Society* 32(2) doi:10.1177/0270467612455734

American Wind Energy Association (2017). 'US wind generation reached 5.5 percent of the grid in 2016.' http://bit.ly/2y8rdKZ

American Wind Energy Association, n.d. 'Wind power facts.' American Wind Energy Association. http://bit.ly/2zS47Fz

Anon. (1889). 'The telephone as a cause of ear troubles.' *British Medical Journal* 2(1499): 671–72.

Anon. (2005). 'Turbine a health risk, warns Foster doctor.' *The Star* (Gippsland), 1 March: 3.

Anon. (2009). 'Wind farm "kills Taiwanese goats"'. *BBC News UK*, 21 May. http://bbc.in/2gMML8y

Anon. (2013). *Hamilton Spectator*, 13 April.

Anon. (2014). 'King Island anti-wind campaign funded by "Rich List" absentee landowners.' *Renew Economy*, 1 October.

Anon. (2016). 'Global wind power capacity tops nuclear energy for first time.' *Japan Times*, 20 February.

Association for Research of Renewable Energy in Australia (2015). Submission 372 to the Senate Select Committee on Wind Turbines, March. http://bit.ly/2gMfeLG

Association of Australian Acoustical Consultants (2015). Submission 194 to the Senate Select Committee on Wind Turbines, 1 June. http://bit.ly/2zHZE7B

Aston, H. (2013). 'Huff and puff as Alan Jones leads wind farm protest.' *Sydney Morning Herald*, 18 June. http://bit.ly/11lIsmY

Atav, R. (2013). 'The use of new technologies in dyeing of proteinous fibers, eco-friendly textile dyeing and finishing'. *InTech*, doi:10.5772/53912.

Australian Associated Press (2013). 'Alan Jones lacks wind at protest,' *Australian*, 18 June. http://bit.ly/2xrEQ3z

Australian Broadcasting Corporation (2017). 'Mining report finds 60,000 abandoned sites, lack of rehabilitation and unreliable data.' *Lateline*. 16 February. http://ab.co/2y7udHs

Australian Broadcasting Corporation (2015). 'Turbine torture: do wind farms make you sick?' *Media Watch*, 16 February. http://ab.co/1zi29Go

Australian Broadcasting Corporation. (2013). '"Wind turbine syndrome" blamed for mysterious symptoms in Cape Cod town'. *ABC News,* 21 October, http://abcn.ws/2yOkncN

Australian Broadcasting Corporation. (2011). 'Law group questions wind gag clauses.' 8 March http://ab.co/2yUPy6c

Australian Broadcasting Corporation. (2011). 'Wind turbines and the flock.' *The 7.30 Report,* 12 October. http://ab.co/2hcYSZg

Australian Broadcasting Corporation (2010). Tony Abbott interviewed by Kerry O'Brien. *The 7.30 Report*, 2 February. http://ab.co/2yQupYP

Australian Bureau of Statistics (2016). *4631.0 – Employment in renewable energy activities, Australia, 2014–15.* http://bit.ly/2yNaJqX

Australian Charities and Not-for-profits Commission (2016). 'The Waubra Foundation'. http://bit.ly/2gFa1Bi

Australian Greens (2015). 'Richard Di Natale questions the NHMRC on wind farms and health.' Video published 25 February, http://bit.ly/2hcTXrr

Back, C. (2012). 'Wind turbines the untold story'. Blog post, 9 July. http://bit.ly/2xqHrL3

Bacon, F. ([1597] 2005). 'Of envy', in *The essays or counsels civil and moral of Francis Bacon.* Digital edition at http://bit.ly/2yOMpm4

Bakker, R.H., E. Pedersen, G.P. van den Berg, R.E. Stewart, W. Lok, and J. Bouma (2012). 'Impact of wind turbine sound on annoyance, self-reported sleep disturbance and psychological distress.' *Science of the Total Environment* 425 doi:10.1016/j.scitotenv.2012.03.005.

Banas, J.A. and G. Miller (2013). 'Inducing resistance to conspiracy theory propaganda: Testing inoculation and metainoculation strategies.' *Human Communication Research* 39(2) doi:10.1111/hcre.12000

Banas, J.A. and S.A. Rains (2010). 'A meta-analysis of research on inoculation theory.' *Communication Monographs.* 77(3) doi:10.1080/03637751003758193

Barnard, M. (2015). 'Do wind turbines reduce the value of nearby properties?' *Quora*, 24 May. http://bit.ly/2hc6Ce6

Barnard, M. (2014). 'Wind health impacts dismissed in court.' Energy and Policy Institute, August. http://bit.ly/2gH4xGn

Barnard, M. (2013). 'Issues of wind turbine noise.' *Noise Health* 15(63) doi:10.4103/1463-1741.110305

Barnard, M. (2012). 'Bad day in court for anti-wind campaigner Sarah Laurie.' *Renew Economy*, 27 November. http://bit.ly/2i7LdT0

Bastasch, M. (2014). 'Wind turbine "infrasound" may be making thousands sick in UK, US.' *Daily Caller*, 11 August. http://bit.ly/1Ba2U7N

Bauer, M. Sander-Thömmes, A. Ihlenfeld, S. Kühn, R. Kühler and C. Koch. (2015). 'Investigation of perception at infrasound frequencies by functional magnetic resonance imaging (FMRI) and magnetoencephalography (MEG).' Paper presented to the 22nd International Congress on Sound and Vibration, Florence, 12–16 July. http://bit.ly/2gMgjDe

Baxter, J., R. Morzaria and R. Hirsch (2013). 'A case-control study of support/opposition to wind turbines: perceptions of health risk, economic benefits, and community conflict.' *Energy Policy* 63 doi:10.1016/j.enpol.2013.06.050

Benedetti, F., J. Durando and S. Vighetti (2014). 'Nocebo and placebo modulation of hypobaric hypoxia headache involves the cyclooxygenase-prostaglandins pathway.' *Pain* 155(5) doi:10.1016/j.pain.2014.01.016

Benedetti, F., M. Lanotte, L. Lopiano and L. Colloca (2007). 'When words are painful: unraveling the mechanisms of the nocebo effect.' *Neuroscience* 147(2) doi:10.1016/j.neuroscience.2007.02.020

Berger, R.G., P.Ashtiani, C.A. Ollson, M.W. Aslund, L.C. McCallum, G. Leventhall and L.D. Knopper (2015). 'Health-based audible noise guidelines account for infrasound and low-frequency noise produced by wind turbines.' *Frontiers in Public Health* 3 doi:10.3389/fpubh.2015.00031

Berglund, B., P. Hassmen and R.F. Job (1996). 'Sources and effects of low-frequency noise.' *Journal of the Acoustical Society of America* 99(5) doi:10.1121/1.414863

Betsch, C. and K. Sachse (2013). 'Debunking vaccination myths: strong risk negations can increase perceived vaccination risks.' *Health Psychology* 32(2) doi:10.1037/a0027387

Bidwell, D. (2013). 'The role of values in public beliefs and attitudes towards commercial wind energy.' *Energy Policy* 58 doi:10.1016/j.enpol.2013.03.010

Boland-Rudder, H. (2013). 'Collector wind farm opponents angry about government approval.' *Canberra Times*, 5 December. http://bit.ly/2yOOi4Q

Bolin, K., G. Bluhm, G. Eriksson and M.E. Nilsson (2011). 'Infrasound and low frequency noise from wind turbines: exposure and health effects.' *Environmental Research Letters* 6(3) doi:10.1088/1748-9326/6/3/035103

Booth, M (2017). 'AFL boss Gillon McLachlan withdraws from wind farm case.' *Australian*, 8 March. http://bit.ly/2gMtunv

Bourke, L. (2014). 'Joe Hockey says wind turbines "utterly offensive," flags budget cuts to clean energy schemes.' *ABC News*, 2 May. http://ab.co/SfMlFS

Bourke, L. and L. Cox (2014). 'Phillip Morris donated to Liberal Democrat senator David Leyonhjelm.' *Sydney Morning Herald*, 1 October. http://bit.ly/1v5f3Gh

Bowen, S., A. Zwi, P. Sainsbury and M. Whitehead (2009). 'Killer facts, politics and other influences: what evidence triggered early childhood intervention policies in Australia?' *Evidence and Policy: A Journal of Research, Debate and Practice* 5(1) doi:10.1332/174426409X395394

Boykoff, M.T. and J.M. Boykoff (2004). 'Balance as bias: global warming and the US prestige press.' *Global Environmental Change* 14(2) doi:10.1016/j.gloenvcha.2003.10.001

Branco, N. and M. Alvez-Pereira (2004). 'Vibroacoustic disease.' *Noise Health* 6(23): 3–20.

Broderick, J.E., E. Kaplan-Liss and E. Bass (2011). 'Experimental induction of psychogenic illness in the context of a medical event and media exposure.' *American Journal of Disaster Medicine* 6(3): 163–172.

Bronfman, N.C., R.B. Jiménez, P.C. Arévalo and L.A. Cifuentes (2012). 'Understanding social acceptance of electricity generation sources.' *Energy Policy* 46 doi:10.1016/j.enpol.2012.03.057

Burgess, K. (2016). '90,000 Canberra homes to be powered by two new wind farms.' *Sydney Morning Herald*, 12 December. http://bit.ly/2ljYbC5 .

Calvert, A.M., C.A. Bishop, R.D. Elliot, E.A. Krebs, T.M. Kydd, C.S. Machtans and G.J. Robertson (2013). 'A synthesis of human-related avian mortality in Canada.' *Avian Conservation and Ecology* 8(2) doi:10.5751/ACE-00581-080211

Canadian Broadcasting Corporation News (2013). 'Expert doubts Digby wind turbines killed emus.' CBC News, 18 November. http://bit.ly/2i80jYJ

Canadian Broadcasting Corporation News (2015). 'Timeline: a history of wind power.' CBC, http://bit.ly/1S57v48

Caneva, L. (2016). 'Noise impact charity challenges regulator over revocation.' Pro Bono Australia, 29 September. http://bit.ly/2dAExdm

Carey, V., S. Chapman and D. Gaffney (1994). 'Children's lives or garden aesthetics? A case study in public health advocacy.' *Australian Journal of Public Health* 18(1) doi:10.1111/j.1753-6405.1994.tb00190.x

Carpenter, D.O. (2012). 'Radiation from your washing machine? Hair dryer?' *Bottom Line Health*, 1 January. http://bit.ly/2dJKRSe

Chapman, S. (2017). 'Apocalypse now: wifi and radiation sickness sweeping the world.' *Conversation*, 21 March. http://bit.ly/2hcUlpR

Chapman, S. (2015a). 'Infrasound phobia spreads … to solar energy cells! What's next?' *Conversation*, 12 August. http://bit.ly/2yPW4LQ

Chapman, S. (2015b). Submission 369 to the Senate Select Committee on Wind Turbines. http://bit.ly/2Acjx74

Chapman, S. (2015c). 'Answers to questions taken on notice during 29 June public hearing, received from Simon Chapman 27 July 2015.' Submitted to the Senate Select Committee on Wind Turbines, 23 June. http://bit.ly/2llBI7G

Chapman, S. (2015d). 'A $2.5m investment in wind farms and health won't solve anything.' *Conversation*, 6 March. http://bit.ly/2zbUCE9

Chapman, S. (2015e). 'Copernicus, tobacco, UFOs: the wild logic of Leyonhjelm's wind inquisition.' *Australian*, 12 June. http://bit.ly/2y785gh

Chapman, S. (2015f). 'Mobile phone goes into charge mode near wind turbines!' Video published 1 July. http://bit.ly/2yPTKC2

Chapman, S. (2014a). 'Symptoms, diseases and aberrant behaviours attributed to wind turbine exposure.' Sydney eScholarship Repository, http://hdl.handle.net/2123/10501.

Chapman, S. (2014b). 'Factoid forensics: have "more than 40" Australian families abandoned their homes because of wind farm noise?' *Noise Health* 16(71) doi:10.4103/1463-1741.137043

Chapman, S. (2014c). 'Author response.' *Australian and New Zealand Journal of Public Health* 38(2) doi:10.1111/1753-6405.12230

Chapman, S. (2014d). 'Persuant to Resolution 5(7)(b) to the Senate of 25 Feb 1988: Reply to speech by Senator John Madigan.' 14 June. http://bit.ly/2iCQGVK

Chapman, S. (2013a). *Over our dead bodies: Port Arthur and Australia's fight for gun control.* Sydney, Sydney University Press.

Chapman, S. (2013b). 'Questions a prominent wind farm critic needs to answer.' *Australian*, 7 November. http://bit.ly/2zaBM0f

Chapman, S. (2013c). 'Sydney mobile phone tower panic in 1995'. Video published 16 April. http://bit.ly/2zahGTC

Chapman, S. (2011). 'Wind farms and health: who is fomenting community anxieties?' *Medical Journal of Australia* 195(9) doi:10.5694/mja11.11253

Chapman, S (2010). 'Can wind farms make people sick?' *Crikey*, 23 February. http://bit.ly/2xrnYK1

Chapman, S. (1997). 'It's the government's call over phone tower debate.' *Sydney Morning Herald*, 6 March.

Chapman, S. (1980). 'A David and Goliath story: tobacco advertising and self-regulation in Australia.' *British Medical Journal* 281(6249): 1187– 90.

Chapman, S., L. Azizi, Q. Luo and F. Sitas (2016). 'Has the incidence of brain cancer risen in Australia since the introduction of mobile phones 29 years ago?' *Cancer Epidemiology* 42 doi:10.1016/j.canep.2016.04.010.

Chapman, S., K. Joshi and L. Fry (2014). 'Fomenting sickness: nocebo priming of residents about expected wind turbine health harms.' *Frontiers in Public Health* 2 doi:10.3389/fpubh.2014.00279

Chapman, S., B. Morrell, R. Forsyth, I. Kerridge and C. Stewart (2012). 'Policies and practices on competing interests of academic staff in Australian universities.' *Medical Journal of Australia* 196(7) doi:10.5694/mja11.11224

Chapman, S. and T. Simonetti (2015). 'Summary of main conclusions reached in 25 reviews of the research literature on wind farms and health.' Sydney eScholarship Repository. http://bit.ly/2zQs9k9

Chapman, S. and A. St George (2013). 'How the factoid of wind turbines causing "vibroacoustic disease" came to be "irrefutably demonstrated".' *Australian and New Zealand Journal of Public Health* 37(3) doi:10.1111/1753-6405.12066
Chapman, S., A. St George, K. Waller and V. Cakic (2013). 'The pattern of complaints about Australian wind farms does not match the establishment and distribution of turbines: support for the psychogenic, "communicated disease" hypothesis.' *Public Library of Science One* 8(10) doi:10.1371/journal.pone.0076584.
Chapman, S. and S. Wutzke (1997). 'Not in our backyard: media coverage of community opposition to mobile phone towers: an application of Sandman's outrage model of risk perception.' *Australian and New Zealand Journal of Public Health* 21(6) doi:10.1111/j.1467-842X.1997.tb01765.x
Charlier, R. and J. Justus (1993). *Ocean energies: Environmental, economic and technological aspects of alternative power sources*. Amsterdam, Elsevier Science.
Chiles, S. (2010). 'NZS 6808: 2010 Acoustics – wind farm noise.' *New Zealand Acoustics* 23(2): 20–22.
Clarke, D. (2017). 'Wind turbine fires.' *Ramblings*, 20 January. http://bit.ly/2yOn8Lb
Clarke, D. (2016). 'Dr Roger Sexton: How wrong can one man be?' *Ramblings*, 20 May. http://bit.ly/2gHjHve
Claude Moore Health Sciences Library. (2007). 'Cures for women. Cures for men.' University of Virginia. https://at.virginia.edu/2i7F1dT
Clean Energy Council (2013). 'Wind industry statement on confidentiality clauses in landowner contracts.' http://bit.ly/2i827Rv
Clean Energy Regulator (n.d.). 'The renewable energy target explained.' Australian Government. http://bit.ly/2y7Otsm
Cohen, J.J., J. Reichl and M. Schmidthaler (2014). 'Re-focussing research efforts on the public acceptance of energy infrastructure: a critical review.' *Energy* 76 doi:10.1016/j.energy.2013.12.056
Commonwealth of Australia (2015a). *Official Committee Hansard: Senate Select Committee on Wind Turbines*, 29 June. parlinfo.aph.gov.au.
Commonwealth of Australia (2015b). *Select Committee on Wind Turbines: Final Report*. Senate Printing Unit, Canberra.
Commonwealth of Australia (2015c). *Official Committee Hansard: Senate Select Committee on Wind Turbines*, 19 June. parlinfo.aph.gov.au.
Commonwealth of Australia (2015d). *Official Committee Hansard: Senate Select Committee on Wind Turbines*, 19 May. parlinfo.aph.gov.au.
Commonwealth of Australia (2015e). *Australian Labor Party Senators' Dissenting Report*. http://bit.ly/2gH70AD

Commonwealth of Australia (2011). *Official Committee Hansard: Senate Community Affairs References Committee*, 28 March. http://bit.ly/2xzndPf.

Conroy, J. (2014). 'Waubra loses "health promotion" charity status.' *Australian*, 19 December. http://bit.ly/2xrGhyA

Cook, J. (2016). *Countering climate science denial and communicating scientific consensus*. London, Oxford University Press.

Cook, J., S. Lewandowsky and U.K.H. Ecker (2017). 'Neutralizing misinformation through inoculation: exposing misleading argumentation techniques reduces their influence.' *Public Library of Science One* 12(5) doi:10.1371/journal.pone.0175799

Cook, J., U. Ecker and S. Lewandowsky (2015). 'Misinformation and how to correct it.' *Emerging Trends in the Social and Behavioral Sciences: An Interdisciplinary, Searchable, and Linkable Resource,* 1–17 doi:10.1002/9781118900772

Cooper, S. (2015a). 'The results of an acoustic testing program – Cape Bridgewater wind farm.' Pacific Hydro, 21 January. http://bit.ly/2zH74rB

Cooper, S. (2015b). 'Answers to questions taken on notice during 30 March public hearing, received from Steven Cooper.' Submitted to the Senate Select Committee on Wind Turbines, 20 April. http://bit.ly/2iENNDT

Cooper, S. (2013). 'Curriculum vita (sic) Steven E. Cooper.' Acoustic Group, September. http://bit.ly/2i7d7yt

Coote, G. (2017). 'More divisions within small rural NSW community surface as Rye Park wind farm goes under microscope.' *ABC News,* 31 March. http://ab.co/2nQpof0

Covello, V. and P.M. Sandman (2001). *Risk communication: evolution and revolution. Solutions to an environment in peril.* Baltimore, John Hopkins University: 164–78

Cowell, R., G. Bristow and M. Munday. (2012). 'Wind energy and justice for disadvantaged communities.' Research Gate, 19 May. http://bit.ly/2y7SnBy

Cox, L. and T. Arup (2015). 'The one wind turbine Tony Abbott has ever seen up close was funded by the Howard government.' *Sydney Morning Herald*, 13 June. http://bit.ly/2yOLGnE

Crichton, F. and K.J. Petrie (2015a). 'Accentuate the positive: counteracting psychogenic responses to media health messages in the age of the internet.' *Journal of Psychosomatic Research* 79(3) doi:10.1016/j.jpsychores.2015.04.014

Crichton, F. and K.J. Petrie (2015b). 'Health complaints and wind turbines: the efficacy of explaining the nocebo response to reduce symptom reporting.' *Environmental Research* 140 doi:10.1016/j.envres.2015.04.016

Crichton, F., G. Dodd, G. Schmid and K.J. Petrie (2015). 'Framing sound: using expectations to reduce environmental noise annoyance.' *Environmental Research* 142 doi:10.1016/j.envres.2015.08.016.

Crichton, F., G. Dodd, G. Schmid, G. Gamble and K.J. Petrie (2014). 'Can expectations produce symptoms from infrasound associated with wind turbines?' *Health Psychology* 33(4) doi:10.1037/a0031760.

Crichton, F., G. Dodd, G. Schmid, G. Gamble, T. Cundy and K.J. Petrie (2014). 'The power of positive and negative expectations to influence reported symptoms and mood during exposure to wind farm sound.' *Health Psychology* 33(12) doi:10.1037/hea0000037.

Crichton, F., S. Chapman, T. Cundy and K.J. Petrie (2014). 'The link between health complaints and wind turbines: support for the nocebo expectations hypothesis.' *Frontiers in Public Health* 2 doi:10.3389/fpubh.2014.00220

Cubby, B. (2012). 'Climate change a hoax, Jones tells tax protestors.' *Sydney Morning Herald*, 2 July. http://bit.ly/2gFgtIJ

D'Angelo C. (2016). 'Warren Buffett wants to build the nation's largest wind farm.' *Huffington Post*, 14 April. http://bit.ly/1qt7EEd

D'Souza, C. and E.K. Yiridoe (2014). 'Social acceptance of wind energy development and planning in rural communities of Australia: a consumer analysis.' *Energy Policy* 74 doi:10.1016/j.enpol.2014.08.035.

Danker-Hopfe, H., H. Dorn, C. Bornkessel and C. Sauter (2010). 'Do mobile phone base stations affect sleep of residents? Results from an experimental double-blind sham-controlled field study.' *American Journal of Human Biology* 22(5) doi:10.1002/ajhb.21053.

David, A.S. and S.C. Wessely (1995). 'The legend of Camelford: medical consequences of a water pollution accident.' *Journal of Psychosomatic Research*, 39(1) doi:10.1016/0022-3999(94)00085-J

Day, B. (2015). 'Opinion – wind turbines' inconvenient truth.' Senator Bob Day, 30 April. http://bit.ly/2xqq2Sp

Dean, N. (2011a). Submission 647 to the Senate Committee on the Social and Economic Impact of Rural Wind Farms. http://bit.ly/2xqaazm

Dean, N. (2011b). Senate Committee on the Social and Economic Impact of Rural Wind Farms. http://bit.ly/2xqaazm

Dechene, A., C. Stahl, J. Hansen and M. Wanke (2009). 'The truth about the truth: a meta-analytic review of the truth effect.' *Personality and Social Psychology Review* 14(2) doi:10.1177/1088868309352251

Deignan, B. and L. Hoffman-Goetz (2015). 'Emotional tone of Ontario newspaper articles on the health effects of industrial wind turbines before and after policy change.' *Journal of Health Communication* 20(5) doi:10.1080/10810730.2014.999894

Deignan, B., E. Harvey and L. Hoffman-Goetz (2013). 'Fright factors about wind turbines and health in Ontario newspapers before and after the Green Energy Act.' *Health, Risk & Society* 15(3) doi:10.1080/13698575.2013.776015
Delgermaa, V., K. Takahashi, E.-K. Park, V.L. Giang, T. Hara and T. Sorahan (2011). 'Global mesothelioma deaths reported to the World Health Organization between 1994 and 2008.' *Bulletin of the World Health Organisation* 89(10) doi:10.2471/BLT.11.086678.
Delingpole, J. (2012). 'Wind farm scam a huge cover-up.' *Australian*, 3 May. http://bit.ly/2zJUl7v
Department of Energy, February. http://bit.ly/2gG9FdK
Department of Infrastructure and Regional Development (n.d.). 'National Airports Safeguarding Framework. Managing the risk to aviation safety of wind turbine installations (wind farms)/wind monitoring towers.' http://bit.ly/2yTpSGY
Desai, A. (2014). 'Freak collision with a wind turbine brings down a plane killing four in South Dakota.' *Inquisitr*, 29 April. http://bit.ly/2gHPDzQ
Devlin, C. (2014). 'Is big wind the new big tobacco?' Wind Turbine Syndrome, 17 February. http://bit.ly/2yPcBzL
Dieudonne, M. (2016). 'Does electromagnetic hypersensitivity originate from nocebo responses? Indications from a qualitative study.' *Bioelectromagnetics* 37(1) doi:10.1002/bem.21937.
Dingle, S. (2013). 'An ill wind.' *ABC RN*, 26 May. http://ab.co/2liW6pT
Doll, R. and A. B. Hill (1950). 'Smoking and carcinoma of the lung; preliminary report.' *British Medical Journal*, 2(4682): 739–48.
Donaldson, B. (2013). 'Comment posted: Where are Australia's wind farm refugees?' Renew Economy, 4 October. http://bit.ly/2zI9qGA
Dutton, D. (1995). 'Speaker's other interests.' Skeptics, 1 May. http://bit.ly/2i7PTIp
Eknoyan, D., R. A. Hurley and K. H. Taber (2013). 'The neurobiology of placebo and nocebo: how expectations influence treatment outcomes.' *Journal of Neuropsychiatry and Clinical Neurosciences* 25(4) doi:10.1176/appi.neuropsych.13090207
Eldridge-Thomas, B. and G. J. Rubin (2013). 'Idiopathic environmental intolerance attributed to electromagnetic fields: a content analysis of British newspaper reports.' *Public Library of Science One* 8(6) doi:10.1371/journal.pone.0065713.
Ellermeier, W., M. Eigenstetter and K. Zimmer (2001). 'Psychoacoustic correlates of individual noise sensitivity.' *Journal of the Acoustical Society of America* 109(4) doi:10.1121/1.1350402
EM Watch, n.d.a 'TV radiation.' EM Watch. http://bit.ly/2hd38Ie
EM Watch, n.d.b 'Is computer radiation damaging your health?' EM Watch. http://bit.ly/2xqKL8Z

EMR Australia (2015). 'Devra Davis: the truth about mobile phones and wireless radiation', EMR Australia, 8 December. http://bit.ly/2iBy4Wi

EMR Australia, (n.d.) 'Smart meters', EMR Australia. http://bit.ly/2lkecYC

Enck, P., U. Bingel, M. Schedlowski and W. Rief (2013). 'The placebo response in medicine: minimize, maximize or personalize?' *Natural Review Drug Discovery* 12(3) doi:10.1038/nrd3923

Environment, Resources and Development Court of South Australia (2014). *TRU Energy Renewable Developments Pty Ltd v Regional Council of Goyder & Ors.* http://ab.co/2gMN5UE

Environment, Resources and Development Court of South Australia (2011). *Paltridge & Ors v. District Council of Grant & Anor [2011]*, SAERDC 23. http://bit.ly/2yVGmyg

Environmental Review Tribunal of Ontario (2013). *Bovaird v Director, Ministry of the Environment*, case nos 13-070–13-075. http://bit.ly/2zS0krK

Environmental Review Tribunal of Ontario (2012). *Middlesex-Lambton Wind Action Group Inc v Director, Ministry of the Environment*, case no. 11-208. http://bit.ly/2cUYwnD

European Platform Against Wind Farms (n.d.) 'Professionals voice concern.' EPAW. http://bit.ly/2lkbX7I

Evans T., J. Cooper and V. Lenchine (2013). 'Infrasound levels near windfarms and in other environments.' EPA South Australia and Resonate Acoustics, January. http://bit.ly/2hcSt0m

Ewbank, L. (2014). 'Pollie Watch: Angus Taylor, Liberal against renewable energy.' *Renew Economy*, 13 May. http://bit.ly/2hdL8NO

Faasse, K., A. Grey, R. Jordan, S. Garland and K.J. Petrie (2015). 'Seeing is believing: impact of social modeling on placebo and nocebo responding.' *Health Psychology* 34(8) doi:10.1037/hea0000199

Fair Dinkum Radio (2014). Interview with Annie Gardner, 18 May. http://bit.ly/2lhe5wZ (at 8 minutes, 12 seconds).

Farber, T. (2012). 'Rewind re wind.' Miller Thomson, April. http://bit.ly/2ljcsyJ

Fast, S., W. Mabee, J. Baxter, T. Christidis, L. Driver, S. Hill, J.J. McMurtry and M. Tomkow (2016). 'Lessons learned from Ontario wind energy disputes.' *Nature Energy* 1(2) doi:10.1038/nenergy.2015.28

Fazeli Farsani, S., M.P. van der Aa, M.M. van der Vorst, C.A. Knibbe and A. de Boer (2013). 'Global trends in the incidence and prevalence of type 2 diabetes in children and adolescents: a systematic review and evaluation of methodological approaches.' *Diabetologia* 56(7) doi:10.1007/s00125-013-2915-z.

Fedak, K.M., A. Bernal, Z.A. Capshaw and S. Gross (2015). 'Applying the Bradford Hill criteria in the 21st century: how data integration has changed causal inference in molecular epidemiology.' *Emerging Themes in Epidemiology* 12 doi:10.1186/s12982-015-0037-4.

Ferrer, M., M. de Lucas, G.F.E. Janss, E. Casado, A.R. Muñoz, M.J. Bechard, and C.P. Calabuig (2012). 'Weak relationship between risk assessment studies and recorded mortality in wind farms.' *Journal of Applied Ecology* 49 doi:10.1111/j.1365-2664.2011.02054.x

Ferrucci, L.M., B. Cartmel, Y.E. Turkman, M.E. Murphy, T. Smith, K.D. Stein and R. McCorkle (2011). 'Causal attribution among cancer survivors of the 10 most common cancers.' *Journal of Psychosocial Oncology* 29(2) doi:10.1080/07347332.2010.548445.

First Dog on the Moon (2015a). 'Dr Onthemoon's self diagnosis windfarm syndrome check list!' *Guardian*, 12 June. http://bit.ly/1FcCrom

First Dog on the Moon (2015b). 'Symptoms of wind turbine syndrome.' *ABC Radio National*, 21 June http://ab.co/2yTPQds

Fowler, A. (2011). Against the wind. *ABC Four Corners*, 25 July. http://ab.co/2gGzvhW

Fowles, S. (2016). '$275 million wind farm to be built at Winchelsea's Mt Gellibrand.' *Geelong Advertiser*, 6 July. http://bit.ly/2lldUAz

Francis, A. (2013). 'Wind farm court action blowing in the wind.' *ABC News*, 30 October. http://ab.co/2zII5V0

Frew, W. (2006). 'It's an ill wind.' *Sydney Morning Herald*, 19 May. http://bit.ly/2gMtwMb

Froese, M. (2016). 'How tall are wind turbines? Nordex installs the world's tallest turbine.' Windpower Engineering and Development, 28 June. http://bit.ly/29psuxF

Fyfe, M. (2002). 'Turbines spark coastal controversy.' *Age*, 8 July. http://bit.ly/2hd1Ugl

Fyfe, M. (2004). 'Just tilting at windmills.' *Age*, 28 August. http://bit.ly/2yQptTA

Gallandy-Jakobson, G. (2015). 'Submission 380.' Submission to the Select Committee on Wind Turbines, Denmark, 2 April. http://bit.ly/2yPYU0S

Gardner, A. (2015a). 'Response to adverse comment made by Professor Simon Chapman to the Senate Select Committee on Wind Tubines.' Submitted to the Senate Select Committee on Wind Turbines, 19 April. http://bit.ly/2za7NW4

Gardner, A. (2015b). 'Study is world first research' (letter to the editor), *Hamilton Spectator*, 7 February.

Gardner, A. (2013). 'Rally – Annie Gardner.' Stop These Things, 6 July. http://bit.ly/2ljS54I

Garnett, S. (2013). 'Australian endangered species: orange-bellied parrot.' *Conversation*, 28 November. http://bit.ly/2qN7vQk

Gartrell, A. (2017). 'Liberal Party–linked fundraising body Cormack Foundation bankrolling two Senate crossbench parties.' *Age*, 4 February. http://bit.ly/2l5MDhJ

Giulivo, M., M. Lopez de Alda, E. Capri and D. Barcelo (2016). 'Human exposure to endocrine disrupting compounds: their role in reproductive systems, metabolic syndrome and breast cancer. A review.' *Environmental Research* 151 doi:10.1016/j.envres.2016.07.011

Glenday, J. (2015). 'Tony Abbott launches another attack on "ugly", "noisy" wind turbines.' *ABC News*, 18 June. http://ab.co/2zaJVSa

Global Wind Energy Council. (2017). 'Global Wind Report 2016: annual market update.' Global Wind Energy Council, http://bit.ly/2oXrSp9

Global Wind Energy Council. (2016). 'Wind in numbers.' Global Wind Energy Council, n.d. http://bit.ly/1keW2e5

Godden, L. and A. Kallies. (2011). 'Regulating wind farms out of Victoria.' *Conversation,* 7 September. http://bit.ly/2lkdURA

Goldberg, L.R., J.A. Johnson, H.W. Eber, R. Hogan, M.C. Ashton, C.R. Cloninger and H.G. Gough. (2006). 'The international personality item pool and the future of public domain personality measures.' *Journal of Research in Personality* 40(1) doi:10.1016/j.jrp.2005.08.007

Green, L-A. (2015). 'Submission 467: key findings.' Evidence Submitted to Select Committee on Wind Turbines.' 21 June. http://bit.ly/2gHTGMe

Group, E. (2015). '10 shocking facts about the health dangers of wi-fi'. Global Healing Center, 2 October. http://bit.ly/VMSbPU

Gullifer, B. (2010). 'A win for the little bloke.' Wind Watch, 15 November. http://bit.ly/2lk7Mc7

Haapala, K.R. and P. Prempreeda (2014). 'Comparative life cycle assessment of 2.0 MW wind turbines.' *International Journal of Sustainable Manufacturing* 3(2): 170–85.

Hahn, R.A. (1997). 'The nocebo phenomenon: concept, evidence, and implications for public health.' *Preventive Medicine* 26: 607–11.

Hall, N., P. Ashworth and H. Shaw. (2012). 'Exploring community acceptance of rural wind farms in Australia: a snapshot.' CSIRO Science into Society Group http://bit.ly/2gGu5n4

Hamilton, M. (2014). 'A re-evaluation of the wind concerns Ontario Health Survey: a comparison to the general population.' Barnard on Wind, 28 July. http://bit.ly/2gQlKkl

Hannam, P. (2015). 'NSW, Victorian health officials objected to federal wind farm study conclusion.' *Sydney Morning Herald,* 14 February. http://bit.ly/2i8ua3g

Harding, G.W., B.A. Bohne, S.C. Lee and A.N. Salt (2007). 'Effect of infrasound on cochlear damage from exposure to a 4 kHz octave band of noise.' *Hearing Research* 225(1–2) doi:10.1016/j.heares.2007.01.016

Harrington, N. (2005). 'The frustration discomfort scale: development and psychometric properties.' *Clinical Psychology and Psychotherapy* 12(5) doi:10.1002/cpp.465.

Harry, A. (2007). 'Wind turbines, noise and health.' Wind Watch, 15 April. http://bit.ly/2zS3vj6

Hart, P. S. and E.C. Nisbet (2011). 'Boomerang effects in science communication: How motivated reasoning and identity cues amplify opinion polarization about climate mitigation policies.' *Communication Research* 39(6) doi:10.1177/0093650211416646.

Health Canada (2014). 'Wind Turbine Noise and Health study: summary of results.' Government of Canada, 30 October. http://bit.ly/1wn3Joc

Health Protection Agency (2010). 'Health effects of exposure to ultrasound and infrasound. Report of the Independent Advisory Group on non-ionising radiation.' Report presented to the UK government, February. http://bit.ly/2xrKjr6

Henderson, G. (2015). 'Defending David Hicks and bagging Tony Abbott.' *Australian,* 20 February. http://bit.ly/2heIlnC

Hoepner, J. and W. Grant. (2015). 'Wind turbine studies: how to sort the good, the bad, and the ugly.' *Conversation,* 22 January. http://bit.ly/2iCObTB

Hogan, J. (2006). 'Fury over wind farm decision.' *Age,* 5 April. http://bit.ly/2gI7mHp

Holmes à Court, S. 'How much "subsidy" has wind energy received in Australia?' *Quora,* 13 June. http://bit.ly/2hcbUpY

Hotelling, B.A. (2013). 'The nocebo effect in childbirth classes.' *Journal of Perinatal Education* 22(2) doi:10.1891/1058-1243.22.2.120

Houtveen, J.H. and N.Y. Oei (2007). 'Recall bias in reporting medically unexplained symptoms comes from semantic memory.' *Journal of Psychosomatic Research* 62(3) doi:10.1016/j.jpsychores.2006.11.006

Hubbert, M. (1956). 'Nuclear energy and the fossil fuel.' One Petro, http://bit.ly/2zQuQ5f

Huson, L.W. (2015b). 'Stationary wind turbine infrasound emissions and propagation loss measurements.' Presented at the 6th International Conference on Wind Turbine Noise, Glasgow, 20–23 April. http://bit.ly/2gMPRcn

Huson, W.L. (2015a). 'Stationary wind turbine infrasound emissions and propagation.' Waubra Foundation, 20–23 April. http://bit.ly/2yOQ3fK

Inagaki, T., Y. Li and Y. Nishi (2015). 'Analysis of aerodynamic sound noise generated by a large-scaled wind turbine and its physiological evaluation.' *International Journal of Environmental Science and Technology* 12(6) doi:10.1007/s13762-014-0581-4

Ingielewicz, R. and A. Zagubien (2014). 'Infrasound noise of natural sources in the environment and infrasound of wind turbines.' *Polish Journal of Environmental Science* 23(4) doi:10.1007/s13762-014-0581-4.

Iser, D. (2004). 'Report to Council.' Waubra Foundation, 19 May. http://bit.ly/2yOye2Y

Jakobsen, J. (2005). 'Infrasound emission from wind turbines.' *Journal of Low Frequency Noise, Vibration and Active Control* 24: 145–55.

Jalali, L., P. Bigelow, M.R. Nezhad-Ahmadi, M. Gohari, D. Williams and S. McColl (2016). 'Before-after field study of effects of wind turbine noise on polysomnographic sleep parameters.' *Noise Health* 18(83) doi:10.4103/1463-1741.189242

Janda, M., S. Frazer and A. Caldwell. (2014). 'Michael Wooldridge fined, banned as company director over collapse of retirement village company.' *ABC News,* 3 December. http://ab.co/2gF7CGS

Jansson-Frojmark, M. and K. Lindblom (2008). 'A bidirectional relationship between anxiety and depression, and insomnia? A prospective study in the general population.' *Journal of Psychosomatic Research* 64(4) doi:10.1016/j.jpsychores.2007.10.016.

Jauchem, J.R. (1992). 'Epidemiologic studies of electric and magnetic fields and cancer: a case study of distortions by the media.' *Journal of Clinical Epidemiology* 45(10): 1137–42.

Jeffery, R., C. Krogh and B. Horner (2014). 'Industrial wind turbines and adverse health effects.' *Canadian Journal of Rural Medicine* 19(1): 21–26.

Johansson, M. (2015). Submission No. 385 to the Select Senate Committee on Wind Turbines. Canberra, 2 May. http://bit.ly/2hcZyOr

Johnson, J. n.d. 'EHS Symptoms'. EMF Analysis. http://bit.ly/2vITmWT

Johnston, I. (2009) 'Wind turbines cause heart problems, headaches and nausea, claims doctor.' *Telegraph* (*UK*), 3 August. http://bit.ly/2zaGSJN

Jones, A. (2016). Interview with Dr Mariana Alves Periera. 2GB Radio, 27 October. http://bit.ly/2zHfHT8

Joshi, K. (2015a). 'Creating a spurious correlation: how the most recent "wind syndrome" study ditches the scientific method.' *Etwas Luft*, 27 January. http://bit.ly/2xrJSNv

Joshi, K. (2015b). 'A follow up – are German doctors trying to ban wind turbines?' *Etwas Luft*, 27 May. http://bit.ly/2gGHBas

Joshi, K. (2015c). 'Why aren't Australian wind farm workers suffering a plague of "wind syndrome"?' *Etwas Luft*, 28 May. http://bit.ly/2y7xIgU

Joshi, K. (2012a). 'The range of wind turbine syndrome – update.' *Etwas Luft*, 28 October, http://bit.ly/2hd3ZbP

Joshi, K. (2012b). 'The European platform against horses, rice and maybe some windfarms.' *Etwas Luft*, 5 November. http://bit.ly/2zTTVwb

Jung, S., W.-S. Cheung, C. Cheung and S.-H. Shin. (2008). 'Experimental identification of acoustic emission characteristics of large wind turbines with emphasis on infra-sound and low-frequency noise.' *Journal of the Korean Physical Society* 53(4): 1897–905.

Karp, P. (2016). 'Scott Morrison faces pressure to cut $7.7bn fossil fuel subsidies.' *Guardian,* 26 April. http://bit.ly/1VUjy7o

Keane, S. (2011). 'The ugly landscape of the guardians.' *Independent Australia,* 24 July. http://bit.ly/1KLxQlL

Kelley N.D., H.E. McKenna, E. W. Jacobs, R.R. Hemphill and N.J. Birkenhauer. (1988). 'The MOD-2 turbine: aeroacoustical noise sources, emissions, and potential impact.' Report presented to the US Department of Energy, January. http://bit.ly/2lhAOsG

Kelley N.D., H.E. McKenna, R.R. Hemphill, C.I. Etter, R.I. Garrelts and N.C. Linn. (1985). 'Acoustic noise associated with the MOD. 1 wind turbine: its source, impact, and control.' Report presented to the US Department of Energy, February. http://bit.ly/2hL2dCi

Kelley, M. (2014). 'Kooragang wind turbine sold to Tasmanian poultry farm.' *Herald,* 15 August. http://bit.ly/2zIJRp8

Kellner, T. (2014). 'How loud is a wind turbine?' *GE Reports*, 2 August. http://invent.ge/2y8dAv2

Kermond, B.F. (2015). Submission 204 to the Senate Select Committee on Wind Turbines. http://bit.ly/2gH9gYD

Khorsand, I., C. Kormos, E.G. MacDonald and C. Crawford (2015). 'Wind energy in the city: an interurban comparison of social acceptance of wind energy projects.' *Energy Research & Social Science* 8 doi:10.1016/j.erss.2015.04.008.

King, S. 'Legal move threatened over Media Watch report.' *Australian*, 23 February. http://bit.ly/2yQ0z6q

Knapton, K. (2015). 'Wind turbines may trigger danger response in brain.' *Telegraph,* 13 July. http://bit.ly/2pulLxG

Knopper L.D. and C.A. Ollson (2011). 'Health effects of wind turbines: a review of the evidence.' *Environmental Health* 10(78) doi:10.1186/1476-1069X-1110–178.

Kroesen, M., E.J. Molin and B. van Wee (2008). 'Testing a theory of aircraft noise annoyance: a structural equation analysis.' *Journal of the Acoustical Society of America* 123(6) doi:10.1121/1.2916589.

Krogh, C. (2011). 'Industrial wind turbine development and loss of social justice.' *Bulletin of Science, Technology and Society* 31(4) doi:10.1177/0270467611412550

Krogh, C.M.E., L. Gillis, N. Kouwen and J. Aramini (2011). 'WindVoice, a self-reporting survey: adverse health effects, industrial wind turbines, and the need for vigilance monitoring.' *Bulletin of Science, Technology and Society* 31(4) doi:10.1177/0270467611412551

Lafarge (2012). 'Lafarge cement used in giant commercial wind energy project.' Lafarge, 12 December. http://bit.ly/2iBBMzc

Lambie, J. (2015). 'Government's pledge to be tougher on wind farm noise wins Lambie's support.' 17 June. http://bit.ly/2zTV4DZ

Land and Environment Court of NSW (2007). *Taralga Landscape Guardians Inc v Minister for Planning and RES Southern Cross Pty Ltd [2007] NSWLEC 59 (12 February 2007).* http://bit.ly/2yVe2Mo

Landgrebe, M., W. Barta, K. Rosengarth, U. Frick, S. Hauser, B. Langguth, R. Rutschmann, M.W. Greenlee, G. Hajak and P. Eichhammer (2008). 'Neuronal correlates of symptom formation in functional somatic syndromes: A fMRI study.' *Neuroimage* 41(4) doi:10.1016/j.neuroimage.2008.04.171

Langford, A. and S. Wessely (2015). 'Breaking news: can the media make you sick?' *Journal of Psychosomatic Research* 79(3) doi:10.1016/j.jpsychores.2015.06.007

Laurie S. (2012a). 'To all responsible individuals, including the Planning Minister and the Director General of the NSW Planning Department.' Letter submitted to NSW Department of Planning, 24 September. http://bit.ly/2yQOGgS

Laurie S. (2012b). 'Couple who sued Big Wind, are gagged, home is sold (UK)'. Wind Turbine Syndrome, 16 March. http://bit.ly/2gI94Zl

Laurie, S. (2011a). 'And what about people who work under those turbines, collecting bird & bat carcasses?' Wind Turbine Syndrome, 25 January. http://bit.ly/2yPvDFO

Laurie S. (2011b). Submission to the Joint Senate Committee on Australia's Clean Energy Future Legislation. http://bit.ly/2zHVcWp

Laurie S. n.d. 'Is it the turbines?' Waubra Foundation. http://bit.ly/2d4Fezz

Leask, J. and S. Chapman (1998). 'An attempt to swindle nature: press anti-immunisation reportage 1993–1997.' *Australian and New Zealand Journal of Public Health* 22(1) doi:10.1111/j.1467-842X.1998.tb01140.x

Lee J. (2013). *No. 1 Position in Google Gets 33% of Search Traffic [Study]. Search Engine Watch*. http://searchenginewatch.com/article/2276184/No.-1-Position-in-Google-Gets-33-of-Search-Traffic-Study

Leslie, G.B. (2000). 'Health risks from indoor air pollutants: public alarm and toxicological reality.' *Indoor and Built Environment*. 9(1): 5–16.

Leventhall, G. (2017). 'Why do some people believe that they are "made ill" by wind turbine noise?' Paper presented to the 7th International Conference on Wind Turbine Noise, Rotterdam, 2–5 May.

Leventhall, G. (2013). 'Concerns about infrasound from wind turbines.' *Acoustics Today* 9: 30–38.

Leventhall G. (2011). 'Wind farms and human health.' Presentation to Wind Farms and Human Health Scientific Forum, 7 June. http://bit.ly/2zHp456

Leventhall, G. (2009a). 'Low frequency noise: what we know, what we do not know, and what we would like to know.' *Journal of Low Frequency Noise, Vibration and Active Control* 28(2): 79–104.

Leventhall, G. (2009b). 'Vibroacoustic disease (VAD) and wind turbines. Critique by Geoff Leventhall. Exhibit 20. Public Service Commission of Wisconsin PSC, ref. 121879 20.

Leventhall, G. (2007). 'What is infrasound?' *Progress in Biophysics and Molecular Biology* 93(1–3) doi:10.1016/j.pbiomolbio.2006.07.006

Leventhall, G. (2006). 'Infrasound from wind turbines – fact, fiction or deception.' *Canadian Acoustics* 34(2): 29–36.

Lewandowsky, S., U.K. Ecker, C.M. Seifert, N. Schwarz and J. Cook (2012). 'Misinformation and Its correction: continued influence and successful debiasing.' *Psychological Science in the Public Interest* 13(3) doi:10.1177/1529100612451018

Leyonhjelm, D. (2015). 'End the smug untouchability of the wind industry.' *Australian*, 10 June. http://bit.ly/2gQpSkl

Liberal Democrats (Australia) (2015). 'Lindt cafe siege and self defence'. Video published 8 February. http://bit.ly/2hdiFrJ

Liden, E., E. Bjork-Bramberg and S. Svensson (2015). 'The meaning of learning to live with medically unexplained symptoms as narrated by patients in primary care: a phenomenological-hermeneutic study.' *International Journal of Qualitative Studies in Health and Well-being* 10 doi:10.3402/qhw.v10.27191.

Lloyd, G. (2015a). 'Turbines may well blow an ill wind over locals, "first" study shows.' *Australian*, 21 January. http://bit.ly/2z9YNAa.

Lloyd, G. (2015b). 'Wind-farm workers suffer poor sleep, international studies find'. *Australian*, 28 May.

Lloyd, G. (2015c). 'Brains "excited" by wind turbines study.' *Australian*, 16 July.

Lloyd, G. (2015d). 'Wind farm advocate Simon Chapman sorry for false allegations.' *Australian,* 19 August.

Lloyd, G. (2013). 'Wind turbine dangers known since '87.' *Australian*, 9 July.

Lorber, W., G. Mazzoni and I. Kirsch (2007). 'Illness by suggestion: expectancy, modeling, and gender in the production of psychosomatic symptoms.' *Annals of Behavioral Medicine* 33(1) doi:10.1207/s15324796abm3301_13

Loss, S., T. Will and P. Marra (2013). 'Estimates of bird collision mortality at wind facilities in the contiguous United States.' *Biological Conservation* 168 doi:10.1016/j.biocon.2013.10.007.

Lowell Capital Ltd (2011). 'Lowell resources fund product disclosure statement.' Lowell Capital, 17 June. http://bit.ly/2yQ2GqS

Ludlow, M. (2015). 'Dick Warburton slams RET deal.' *Australian Financial Review,* 11 May. http://bit.ly/2yU4v8i

Lynch, J. and E. Himmelreich. (2009). 'Minister still keen to talk after hurt by wind farm protesters.' *Standard,* 28 August. http://bit.ly/2zSKRHX

MacGregor, D.G. and R. Fleming (1996). 'Risk perception and symptom reporting.' *Risk Analysis* 16(6): 773–83.

Madigan, J. (2015). 'It's the great wind farm scam'. Video published 17 June. http://bit.ly/2cT2nko

Magari, S.R., C.E. Smith, M. Schiff and A.C. Rohr (2014). 'Evaluation of community response to wind turbine-related noise in western New York state.' *Noise Health* 16(71) doi:10.4103/1463-1741.137060.

Marciniak, A. (2012a). 'This man abandoned his home to live in a shed.' Wind Turbine Syndrome, 13 March. http://bit.ly/2yNtZET

Marciniak, A. (2012b). Submission 35 to the Senate Standing Committee on Environment and Communications, inquiry into the Renewable Energy (Electricity) Amendment (Excessive Noise from Wind Farms) Bill 2012. http://bit.ly/2gFVyFl

Marks, K. (2012). 'Australian developers see red as rare bird foils plans.' *National,* 30 March. http://bit.ly/2y8DTS5

Martin, C.L. (2013). 'U.S. government has known about wind turbine syndrome since 1987 (U.S. Dept. of Energy).' Wind Turbine Syndrome, 6 July. http://bit.ly/2lkXfx0

Martin, C.L. (2011). 'WTS.com's "Journalist of the Year" award.' Wind Turbine Syndrome, 1 January. http://bit.ly/2lhwJog

Martin, C.L. (2009). 'How to fight the big wind onslaught.' American Wind Energy Association, January. http://bit.ly/2gGD5bS

Martin, L.L. (2015). Submission 356 to the Senate Select Committee on Wind Turbines. http://bit.ly/2gH9gYD

Maugh, T.H. (1982). 'The dump that wasn't there.' *Science* 215(4533) doi:10.1126/science.215.4533.645.

Maughan, B., R. Rowe, J. Messer, R. Goodman and H. Meltzer (2004). 'Conduct disorder and oppositional defiant disorder in a national sample: developmental epidemiology.' *Journal of Child Psychology and Psychiatry* 45(3): 609–21.

Mauney, M. (2017). 'Mesothelioma in Australia.' Asbestos.com, 1 May. http://bit.ly/2yT0jG4

Mazzoni, G., L. Foan, M.E. Hyland and I. Kirsch (2010). 'The effects of observation and gender on psychogenic symptoms.' *Health Psychology* 29(2) doi:10.1037/a0017860.

McAteer, A., A.M. Elliott and P.C. Hannaford (2011). 'Ascertaining the size of the symptom iceberg in a UK-wide community-based survey.' *The British Journal of General Practice* 61(582) doi:10.3399/bjgp11X548910.

McCluskey, J.J., N. Kalaitzandonakes and Swinnen (2016). 'Media coverage, public perceptions, and consumer behavior: Insights from new food technologies.' *Annual Review of Resource Economics* 8: 467–86.

McCunney, R.J., K.A. Mundt, W.D. Colby, R. Dobie, K. Kaliski and M. Blais (2014). 'Wind turbines and health: a critical review of the scientific literature.' *Journal of Occupational & Environmental Medicine* 56(11) doi:10.1097/JOM.0000000000000313.

McCunney, R.J., P. Morfeld, W.D. Colby and K.A. Mundt (2015). 'Wind turbines and health: an examination of a proposed case definition.' *Noise Health* 17(77) doi:10.4103/1463-1741.160678.

McGrath, G. (2013). 'Waubra wind farm: locals petition to save town's name.' *Courier*, 5 November. http://bit.ly/2gNPbUp

McMurtry, R. (2011). 'Toward a case definition of adverse health effects in the environs of industrial wind turbines: facilitating a clinical diagnosis.' *Bulletin of Science, Technology and Society* 31(4): 0.1177/0270467611415075.

McMurtry, R.Y. and C.M. Krogh (2014). 'Diagnostic criteria for adverse health effects in the environs of wind turbines.' *Journal of the Royal Society of Medicine* 5(10) doi:10.1177/2054270414554048.

McVeigh, J., D. Burtraw, J. Darmstadter and K. Palmer. (1999). 'Winner, loser, or innocent victim? Has renewable energy performed as expected?' Discussion Paper, Washington, 28 June. http://bit.ly/2yUGJt8

Mechanic, D. and E.H. Volkart (1961). 'Stress, illness behavior and the sick role.' *American Sociological Review* 261(1): 51–58.

Mercola, J. (2009). 'Is your electric blanket safe?' Mercola, 24 February. http://bit.ly/2gGwqhQ

Mercola, J. (2016). 'How LED lighting may compromise your health.' Mercola, 23 October. http://bit.ly/2fZ1FqX

Meridian Energy Limited (2015). Submission to the Hearings Commissioners, Palmerston North City Council, on the proposed Plan Change 15 under the Resource Management Act 1991. http://bit.ly/2z9Xa5z

Merlin, T., S. Newton, B. Ellery, J. Milverton and C. Farah. (2015). 'Systematic review of the human health effects of wind farms.' Commissioned report from the National Health and Medical Research Council. http://bit.ly/2hdSEZ7

Michaels, D. and C. Monforton (2005). 'Manufacturing uncertainty: contested science and the protection of the public's health and environment.' *American Journal of Public Health* 95(S1) doi:10.2105/AJPH.2004.043059.

Michaud, D. (2015). 'Health and well-being related to wind turbine noise exposure: summary of results.' *Journal of the Acoustical Society of America* 137(4) doi:10.1121/1.4920604.

Michaud, D.S., S. Fidell, K. Pearsons, K.C. Campbell and S.E. Keith (2007). 'Review of field studies of aircraft noise-induced sleep disturbance.' *Journal of the Acoustical Society of America* 121(1) doi:10.1121/1.2400613.

Michaud, D., K. Feder, S.E. Keith, and S.A. Voicescu (2016a) 'Self-reported and measured stress related responses associated with exposure to wind turbine noise.' *Journal of the Acoustical Society of America* 139(3) doi:10.1121/1.4942402

Michaud, D., K. Feder, S.E. Keith, and S.A. Voicescu (2016b). 'Exposure to wind turbine noise: perceptual responses and reported health effects.' *Journal of the Acoustical Society of America* 139(3) doi:10.1121/1.4942391

Michaud, D., K. Feder, S. Keith, S. Voicescu, L. Marro, J. Than, M. Guay, A. Denning, B.J. Murray, S.K. Weiss, P.J. Villeneuve, F. van den Berg, and T. Bower. (2016). 'Effects of wind turbine noise on self-reported and objective measures of sleep.' *Sleep* 39(1) doi:10.5665/sleep.5326.

Michaud, D., S.E. Keith, K. Feder, and S.A. Voicescu (2016c). 'Personal and situational variables associated with wind turbine noise annoyance.' *Journal of the Acoustical Society of America* 139(3) doi:10.1121/1.4942390.

Millar, R. and A. Morton. (2012). 'Against the wind.' *Age*, 31 March.

Mitchell, D. (2011). Submission 274 to the Senate Committee on the Social and Economic Impact of Rural Wind Farms. http://bit.ly/2xqaazm

Mitric-Andjic, A. (2012). Submission 141 to the Senate Standing Committee on Environment and Communications, inquiry into the Renewable Energy (Electricity) Amendment (Excessive Noise from Wind Farms) Bill 2012. http://bit.ly/2gFVyFl

Moore, A. (2013). 'Too late for pre-turbine study: residents.' Niagara This Week, 13 April. http://bit.ly/2yQyqfK

Moorhouse, A., M. Hayes, S. von Hünerbein, B. Piper and M. Adams. (2007). 'Research into aerodynamic modulation of wind turbine noise: final report.' Department for Business, Enterprise and Regulatory Reform, UK.' http://bit.ly/2heebRo

Morris, C. (2010). 'Waubra wind farm: critics' property bought.' *Courier,* 11 February. http://bit.ly/2zHkC6y

Moss-Morris, R. and K.J. Petrie (1999). 'Link between psychiatric dysfunction and dizziness.' *Lancet* 353(9152) doi:10.1016/S0140-6736(98)00348-1

Mroczek, B., J. Banas, M. Machowska-Szewczyk and D. Kurpas (2015). 'Evaluation of quality of life of those living near a wind farm.' *International Journal of Environmental Research and Public Health* 12(6) doi:10.3390/ijerph120606066

Munday, M., G. Bristow and R. Cowell (2011). 'Wind farms in rural areas: how far do community benefits from wind farms represent a local economic development opportunity?' *Journal of Rural Studies* 27 doi:10.1016/j.jrurstud.2010.08.003

Munk, A.K. (2014). 'Mapping wind energy controversies online: introduction to methods and datasets.' *Social Science Research Network:* doi:10.2139/ssrn.2595287.

Murray, P. (2014). An ill wind blows as the surge of turbines stirs fears of silent danger to our health. *Sunday Express*, 10 August. http://bit.ly/1tslOT3

Muse, C.J. (2013). 'Town of Falmouth vs. Town of Falmouth Zoming Board of Appeals & others.' Superior Court Civil Action, Commonwealth of Massachusetts, 13 November. http://bit.ly/2yVmNGv

NASA (2013). 'Scientific consensus: earth's climate is warming.' Climate NASA, 31 May. https://go.nasa.gov/1zmXghN

National Health and Medical Research Council (2015a). 'National statement on ethical conduct in human research.' Australian Government, May. http://bit.ly/2gLl8fR

National Health and Medical Research Council (2015b). 'Wind turbines and health: a rapid review of the evidence.' National Health and Medical Research Council, 2 November. http://bit.ly/2gMTtvc

National Health and Medical Research Council (2015c). 'NHMRC statement and information paper: Evidence on wind farms and human health.' National Health and Medical Research Council, 17 July. http://bit.ly/1gC2yRy

Newman, M. (2012). 'Against the wind.' *Spectator,* 21 January. http://bit.ly/2yPSQFz

Newton, D. (2015). Wind energy: a reference handbook. Santa Barbara, Ca.: ABC-CLIO Greenwood.

Nissenbaum, M.A., J.J. Aramini and C.D. Hanning (2012). 'Effects of industrial wind turbine noise on sleep and health.' *Noise Health* 14(60) doi:10.4103/1463-1741.102961.

Novello, A.C. (1990). 'The surgeon general's 1990 report on the health benefits of smoking cessation executive summary – preface.' Centres for Disease Control and Prevention, 5 October. http://bit.ly/2i8knKj

Nyhan, B., J. Reifler, S. Richey and G.L. Freed (2014). 'Effective messages in vaccine promotion: a randomized trial.' *American Academy of Pediatrics* 133(4) doi:10.1542/peds.2013-2365.

O'Donoghue, G.M., N. Fox, C. Heneghan and D.A. Hurley (2009). 'Objective and subjective assessment of sleep in chronic low back pain patients compared with healthy age and gender matched controls: a pilot study.' *BMC Musculoskeletal Disorders* 10 doi:10.1186/1471-2474-10-122

Office of the National Wind Commissioner (2017). 'Annual Report to the Parliament of Australia.' Report presented to the Parliament of Australia, Canberra, 31 March. http://bit.ly/2y7dzrn

Oiamo, T.H., J. Baxter, A. Grgicak-Mannion, X. Xu and I.L. Luginaah (2015). 'Place effects on noise annoyance: cumulative exposures, odour annoyance and noise sensitivity as mediators of environmental context.' *Atmospheric Environment* 116 doi:10.1016/j.atmosenv.2015.06.024.

Olesen, K.B. (2015). Submission 416 to the Senate Select Committee on Wind Turbines. http://bit.ly/2xs8Dc6

Ollson, C.A., L.D. Knopper, L.C. McCallum and M.L. Whitfield-Aslund (2013). 'Are the findings of "effects of industrial wind turbine noise on sleep and health" supported?' *Noise Health* 15(63) doi:10.4103/1463-1741.110302.

Omachi, T.A. (2011). 'Measures of sleep in rheumatologic diseases: Epworth Sleepiness Scale (ESS), Functional Outcome of Sleep Questionnaire (FOSQ), Insomnia Severity Index (ISI), and Pittsburgh Sleep Quality Index (PSQI).' *Arthritis Care Research (Hoboken)* 63(11) doi:10.1002/acr.20544.

Ontario Highlands Friends of Wind Power (2012). 'When tears are not enough.' Ontario Highlands Friends of Wind Power, 2 March. http://bit.ly/2yTzT6Z

Osborne, R.B., J.W. Hatcher and A.J. Richtsmeier (1989). 'The role of social modeling in unexplained pediatric pain.' *Journal of Pediatric Psychology* 14(1): 43–61.

Pacific Hydro and the Acoustic Group (2015). 'Joint statement – Pacific Hydro & the Acoustic Group.' Pacific Hydro, 16 February. http://bit.ly/2lkhQBM

Page, L.A., K.J. Petrie and S.C. Wessely (2006). 'Psychosocial responses to environmental incidents: a review and a proposed typology.' *Journal of Psychosomatic Research* 60(4) doi:10.1016/j.jpsychores.2005.11.008

Paine, S.J., P.H. Gander, R.B. Harris and P. Reid (2005). 'Prevalence and consequences of insomnia in New Zealand: disparities between Maori and non-Maori.' *Australian and New Zealand Journal of Public Health* 29(1): 22–28.

Papadopoulos, G. (2013). 'Comment on Waubra locals set record straight on wind farms.' Yes2Renewables, 22 September. http://bit.ly/2y8gHmY

Papadopoulos, G. (2012a). 'Comment on a wind up of the 2km setback.' *Climate Spectator*, 1 March.

Papadopoulos, G. (2012b). 'Wind turbines and low frequency noise: implications for human health.' Wind Watch, 24 September. http://bit.ly/2ciZ7lk

Papadopoulos, G. (2011). 'Public health: Don Quixote vs the wind turbines.' Redland Bay Homeopathy, 24 May. http://bit.ly/2yOsZk0

Parker, J. (2017). 'Elon Musk's offer to halve Tesla's battery price for SA a game changer, says Mike Cannon-Brookes.' *ABC News*, 15 March. http://ab.co/2nihU51

Parkinson, G. (2016). 'Wind energy hits 100% of South Australia demand on Sunday.' *Renew Economy*, 24 May. http://bit.ly/2zaZJEj

Parkinson, S. (2015). 'Video of the day: The Bald Hills wind farm.' *Renew Economy*, 27 August. http://bit.ly/2yOwJle

Parkinson, G. (2014). 'Anti-wind, climate denying crusader behind Leyonhjelm RET campaign.' *Renew Economy*, 27 November. http://bit.ly/2iCCFYm

Parliament of Australia (n.d). 'Matters constituting contempts.' Parliament of Australia. http://bit.ly/2xWNsir.

Parliament of South Australia, Legislative Council (2012). Select Committee on Wind Farm Developments in South Australia. http://bit.ly/2lkcsyH

Parnell, S. and P. Akerman (2014). 'Health check on wind power farms.' *Australian*, 8 January.

Pearen, G. (2010). 'Dunlite wind turbines.' Pearen Ventures, 4 July. http://bit.ly/2hdmiOn

Pedersen, E. and H.I. Halmstad (2003). 'Noise annoyance from wind turbines – a review.' Swedish Environmental Protection Agency, Stockholm, August. http://bit.ly/2gMxmVB

Pedersen, E. and K.P. Waye (2004). 'Perception and annoyance due to wind turbine noise – a dose-response relationship.' *Journal of the Acoustical Society of America* 116(6): 3460–70.

Pedersen, E., F. van den Berg, R. Bakker and J. Bouma (2009). 'Response to noise from wind farms in the Netherlands.' *Journal of the Acoustical Society of America* 126(2) doi:10.1121/1.3160293.

Pennebaker, J.W. (1994). 'Psychological bases of symptom reporting: perceptual and emotional aspects of chemical sensitivity.' *Toxicology Industrial Health* 10(4–5): 497–511.

Pennebaker, J.W. and J.A. Skelton (1981). 'Selective monitoring of physical sensations.' *Journal of Personality and Social Psychology* 41(2): 213–23.

Petrie, K.J. and Wessely, S. (2002). 'Modern worries, technological change and medicine: New technologies mean new health complaints.' *BMJ* 324(7339) doi:10.1136/bmj.324.7339.690.

Petrie, K.J., E.A. Broadbent, N. Kley, R. Moss-Morris, R. Horne and W. Rief (2005). 'Worries about modernity predict symptom complaints after environmental pesticide spraying.' *Psychosomatic Medicine* 67(5) doi:10.1097/01.psy.0000181277.48575.a4.

Petrie, K.J., K. Faasse, F. Crichton and A. Grey (2014). 'How common are symptoms? Evidence from a New Zealand national telephone survey.' *BMJ Open* 4(6): e005374.

Petrie, K.J., R. Moss-Morris, C. Grey and M. Shaw (2004). 'The relationship of negative affect and perceived sensitivity to symptom reporting following vaccination.' *British Journal of Health Psychology* 9(Pt 1) doi:10.1348/135910704322778759.

Phillips, C. (2011). 'Properly interpreting the epidemiologic evidence about the health effects of industrial wind turbines on nearby residents.' *Bulletin of Science, Technology and Society* 31(4) doi:10.1177/0270467611412554.

Pierpont, N. (2009a). *Wind turbine syndrome: a report on a natural experiment.* Santa Fe, K-Selected Books.

Pierpont, N. (2009b). 'Reviews by other scientists and clinicians.' Wind Turbine Syndrome. http://bit.ly/2zHlWq2

Pierpont N. (2006). 'Clinical study of "wind turbine syndrome".' We Oppose Wind Farms, 4 March. http://bit.ly/2xq5SIn

Potter, B. and M. Ludlow. (2017). 'Budget 2017: Turnbull's $5b Snowy Hydro plunge.' *Australian Financial Review*, 9 May, http://bit.ly/2xrJXRe

PR Resources Inc. (2011) *Pandora's Pinwheels: the reality of life with wind turbines – Australia and New Zealand.* Film. http://bit.ly/2hd8q6t

Price, S. (2013). Interview with David Mortimer and Sarah Laurie. *Nights with Steve Price*, 2GB Radio, 28 March. http://bit.ly/2gMlhQ3

Put, C., O. Van den Bergh, E. Van Ongeval, S. De Peuter, M. Demedts and G. Verleden (2004). 'Negative affectivity and the influence of suggestion on asthma symptoms.' *Journal of Psychosomatic Research* 57(3): 249–55.

Pyper, J. (2017). 'Global clean energy investment fell 18% in 2016 with slowdown in China.' Green Tech Media, 12 January. http://bit.ly/2jIfA5x

Quinn, W. (2015). Submission 118 to Senate Select Committee on Wind Turbines.

Raferty, M. (2012). 'Wind spin: blowing holes in industry's denial of health impacts.' *East County Magazine*, 22 April. http://bit.ly/2iClg1W

Raymo, D. (2005). 'Wind-power firm, critics spar over claims.' *Press-Republican*, 23 April.

Rehn, A. (2011). 'Wind farms set up farmers.' *Daily Telegraph*, 26 July. http://bit.ly/2gGxF0u

Rheese M. (2011). 'The windmills in our minds.' *Online Opinion*, 25 November. http://bit.ly/2i7UPxc

Rief, W., J. Avorn and A.J. Barsky (2006). 'Medication-attributed adverse effects in placebo groups: implications for assessment of adverse effects.' *Archives of Internal Medicine* 166(2): 155–60.

Roberts, D. (2015). 'The North Carolina town that's scared of solar panels, revisited.' *Vox*, 18 December. http://bit.ly/2yRNgTn

Rodriguez-Monforte, M., E. Sanchez, F. Barrio, B. Costa and G. Flores-Mateo (2016). 'Metabolic syndrome and dietary patterns: a systematic review and meta-analysis of observational studies.' *European Journal of Nutrition* 56(3) doi:10.1007/s00394-016-1305-y.

Roper, R. (2015). 'No more studies needed to debunks wind farm kills (letter).' 13 May.

Rosenzweig, P., S. Brohier and A. Zipfel (1993). 'The placebo effect in healthy volunteers: influence of experimental conditions on the adverse events profile during phase I studies.' *Clinical Pharmacology and Therapeutics* 54(5): 578–83.

Rovensky, J. (2014). 'Open letter, Mike Barnard's disreputable wind industry propagandist role revealed.' Waubra Foundation, 11 September. http://bit.ly/2zSpbM8

Royal Society for the Protection of Birds (n.d.). 'Why has the RSPB built a wind turbine?' Royal Society for the Protection of Birds. http://bit.ly/2hd4pzb

Rubin, G.J., A.J. Cleare and S. Wessely (2008). 'Psychological factors associated with self-reported sensitivity to mobile phones.' *The Journal of Psychosomatic Research* 64(1) doi:10.1016/j.jpsychores.2007.08.016.

Rubin, G.J., M. Burns and S. Wessely (2014). 'Possible psychological mechanisms for "wind turbine syndrome". On the windmills of your mind.' *Noise Health* 16(69) doi:10.4103/1463-1741.132099.

Rubin, G.J., R. Nieto-Hernandez and S. Wessely (2010). 'Idiopathic environmental intolerance attributed to electromagnetic fields (formerly "electromagnetic hypersensitivity"): an updated systematic review of provocation studies.' *Bioelectromagnetics* 31(1) doi:10.1002/bem.20536.

Russell, K. (2010). 'The great renewable energy rort.' *Quadrant*, http://bit.ly/2gMnrQ3

Rydell, J., L. Bach, M.-J. Douourg-Savage, M. Green, L. Rodrigues and A. Hedenstrom (2010). 'Bat mortality at wind turbines in Northwestern Europe.' *Acta Chiropterologica* 12(2) doi:10.3161/150811010X537846.

Safespace (n.d.). 'EMF pollution from living near power lines.' Safespace. http://bit.ly/2y93REY

Sakula, B. (2016). 'Pyroluria is a real disease or just a myth?' Dr Bill Sakula, 12 December. http://bit.ly/2gHWM38

Salt, A.N. (2016). 'Wind turbines can be hazardous to human health.' Web Archive, 21 October. http://bit.ly/2ljKR0v

Salt, A.N. and J.E. DeMott (1999). 'Longitudinal endolymph movements and endocochlear potential changes induced by stimulation at infrasonic frequencies.' *Journal of the Acoustical Society of America* 106(2) doi:10.1121/1.427101.

Salt, A.N. and T.E. Hullar (2010). 'Responses of the ear to low frequency sounds, infrasound and wind turbines.' *Hearing Research* 268(1–2) doi:10.1016/j.heares.2010.06.007.

Sandman, P. (1989). 'Hazard versus outrage in the public perception of risk.' In V.T. Covello, D.B. McCallum and M.T. Pavlova, eds, *Effective risk communication*. New York: Plenum Press.

Sandman, P. (1991). 'Twelve principal outrage components.' P. Sandman. http://bit.ly/2hcfUXl

Sanna, L.J., N. Schwarz and S.L. Stocker (2002). 'When debiasing backfires: accessible content and accessibility experiences in debiasing hindsight.' *Journal of Experimental Psychology: Learning, Memory, and Cognition* 28(3) doi:10.1037/0278-7393.28.3.497.

Save the Eagles International (2012). 'Spanish wind farms kill 6–18 million birds & bats a year.' Save the Eagles International, 12 January. http://bit.ly/2xrObs9

Sawa, M. (2015). 'Australian households chase sun to lead world on solar adoption.' 16 May. http://bit.ly/2hdmDk7

Schaefer, C. (2015). Submission 165 to the Senate Select Committee on Wind Turbines. http://bit.ly/2yQifiw

Schmid, J., N. Theysohn, F. Gass, S. Benson, C. Gramsch, M. Forsting, E.R. Gizewski and S. Elsenbruch (2013). 'Neural mechanisms mediating positive and negative treatment expectations in visceral pain: a functional magnetic resonance imaging study on placebo and nocebo effects in healthy volunteers.' *Pain* 154(11) doi:10.1016/j.pain.2013.07.013.

Schutte, M., A. Marks, E. Wenning and B. Griefahn (2007). 'The development of the noise sensitivity questionnaire.' *Noise Health* 9(34): 15–24.

Schwarz, N., L. Sanna, I. Skurnik and C. Yoon (2007). 'Metacognitive experiences and the intricacies of setting people straight: implications for debiasing and public information campaigns.' *Advances in Experimental Social Psychology*, 39 doi:10.1016/S0065-2601(06)39003-X.

Scollo, M.M. and M.H. Winstanley (2017). 'The pricing and taxation of tobacco products in Australia' in *Tobacco in Australia: Facts and Issues*. Melbourne: Cancer Council Victoria. http://bit.ly/2i7MUA1

Seven Network Pty Ltd (2015). 'Cape Bridgewater report.' *Today Tonight*, 16 March. http://bit.ly/1O3K88N

Seven Network Pty Ltd (2012a). '*Today Tonight* report on wind farms'. *Today Tonight*, 5 June. http://bit.ly/2cIupB8

Seven Network Pty Ltd (2012b). '*Today Tonight* follow up to wind farm report.' *Today Tonight*, 6 June. http://bit.ly/2gMVW8Q

Shepherd, D. (2017). 'Comment on Mroczek et al. "Evaluation of quality of life of those living near a wind farm" *International Journal of Environmental Research and Public Health*, 2015, 12, 6066-83.' *International Journal of Environmental Research and Public Health* 14(2) doi:10.3390/ijerph14020141.

Shepherd, D. and R. Billington (2011). 'Mitigating the acoustic impacts of modern technologies: acoustic, health and psychosocial factors informing wind farm placement.' *Bulletin of Science, Technology, and Society*. 31(5) doi:10.1177/0270467611417841.

Shepherd, D., D. McBride, D. Welch, K.N. Dirks and E.M. Hill (2011). 'Evaluating the impact of wind turbine noise on health-related quality of life.' *Noise Health* 13(54) doi:10.4103/1463-1741.85502

Simon, L. (2005). *Dark light: electricity and anxiety from the telegraph to the X-ray*. Orlando, Harcourt.

Singer, S. (2012). 'Bad vibrations: health hazards of geothermal and wind turbine noise.' *Killer Culture*, 26 November. http://bit.ly/2zTaFUu

Sky News (2015). Interview with Anne Gardner. *Richo + Jones*, 15 August. http://bit.ly/2heaWK3

Smith, R. (2002). 'In search of "non-disease".' *British Medical Journal* 324(7342) doi:10.1136/bmj.324.7342.883.

Society for Wind Vigilance (n.d.). 'Advisory Group.' Wind Vigilance. http://bit.ly/2gMSNFQ

Songsore, E. and M. Buzzelli (2014). 'Social responses to wind energy development in Ontario: the influence of health risk perceptions and associated concerns.' *Energy Policy* 69 doi:10.1016/j.enpol.2014.01.048.

SourceWatch (n.d.). 'Australian Landscape Guardians Association Inc.' Source Watch. http://bit.ly/2xr0lBm

Sovaccol, B.K. (2009). 'Contextualizing avian mortality: a preliminary appraisal of bird and bat fatalities from wind, fossil-fuel, and nuclear electricity.' *Energy Policy* 37(6) doi:10.1016/j.enpol.2009.02.011.

Spurgeon, A. (2002). 'Models of unexplained symptoms associated with occupational and environmental exposures.' *Environmental Health Perspectives* 110(S4): 601–05.

Stead M., J. Cooper and T. Evans (2014). 'Comparison of infrasound measured at people's ears when walking to that measured near wind farms.' *Acoustics Australia* 42(3): 197–203.

Stewart, M. (2013). 'Wind-farm "illnesses" blamed on bad publicity.' Stuff, 22 March. http://bit.ly/2yNxVW1

Stop These Things (2016). 'Transcript of radio interview Nov 1 2016.' Stop These Things, November. http://bit.ly/2yNygrL

Stop These Things (2015a). 'Alan Jones: Victims – like turbine host David Mortimer – vindicated by Steven Cooper's groundbreaking wind farm study.' Stop These Things, 25 January. http://bit.ly/2i89IiZ

Stop These Things (2015b). 'STT's Australian of the Year awards.' Stop These Things, 26 January. http://bit.ly/2heXBRH

Stop These Things (2015c). 'Three magnificent women take on Australia's monstrous wind power outfits & their pathetic political backers.' Stop These Things, 12 August. http://bit.ly/2xrRob9

Stop These Things (2014). 'Andy's rant: how much CO2 gets emitted to build a wind turbine?' Stop These Things, 16 August. http://bit.ly/2gwbHyC

Stop These Things (2013a). 'Victims: Carl and Sam Stepnell.' Stop These Things, 31 May. http://bit.ly/2y70Chr

Stop These Things (2013b). 'Victims: Noel and Janine Dean.' Stop These Things, 1 June. http://bit.ly/2hda87T

Stop These Things (2013c). 'Victims: Brian and Joanne Kermond.' Video published 13 April. http://bit.ly/2iET9Pv

Stop These Things (2013d). 'Victim: Melissa Ware and Rikki Nicholson.' Stop These Things, 4 April. http://bit.ly/2zGJQ4X

Stop These Things (2013e). 'The national wind power fraud rally; June 18 2013; Australia.' Video published on 7 July. http://bit.ly/2zbERNe

Stop These Things (2013f). 'Cape Bridgewater: Sonia.' Video published on 24 March. http://bit.ly/2xqtUTD

Stop These Things (2013g). 'The rally in pictures: we will prevail.' Video published on 20 June. http://bit.ly/2zSYvLl

Stop These Things (2013h). 'What "community" wind farms are really like.' Stop These Things, 3 September. http://bit.ly/2zTYsyH

Stop These Things (n.d.). 'These people get it.' Stop These Things. http://bit.ly/2dbRjBE

Stovner, L.J., G. Oftedal, A. Straume and A. Johnsson (2008). 'Nocebo as headache trigger: evidence from a sham-controlled provocation study with RF fields.' *Acta Neurologica Scandinavica* 188 doi:10.1111/j.1600-0404.2008.01035.x.

Sturmer, J. (2014). 'Waubra Foundation, prominent anti-wind farm lobby, stripped of health promotion charity status.' *ABC News*, 19 December. http://ab.co/13htoXT

Sugimoto T., K. Koyama, Y. Kurihara and K. Watanabe (2008). 'Measurement of infra-sound generated by wind turbine generator.' Paper presented to the SICE Annual Conference, Tokyo, 20–22 August. http://bit.ly/2gMEmSl

Sweet, M.A., S. Chapman, R. N. Moynihan and J. H. Green (2009). 'CHAMP: a novel collaboration between public health and the media.' *Medical Journal of Australia* 190(4): 206–207.

Swinbanks, M. (2015). 'Direct experience of low frequency noise and infrasound within a windfarm community.' Presented at the 6th International Meeting on Wind Turbine Noise, Glasgow, 20–23 April. http://bit.ly/2yOh2dV

Szemerszky, R., F. Koteles, R. Lihi and G. Bardos (2010). 'Polluted places or polluted minds? An experimental sham-exposure study on background psychological factors of symptom formation in "idiophatic environmental intolerance attributed to electromagnetic fields".' *International Journal of Hygiene and Environmental Health* 213(5) doi:10.1016/j.ijheh.2010.05.001.

Szemerszky, R., Z. Domotor, T. Berkes and F. Koteles (2016). 'Attribution-based nocebo effects: perceived effects of a placebo pill and a sham magnetic field on cognitive performance and somatic symptoms.' *International Journal of Behavioral Medicine* 23(2) doi:10.1007/s12529-015-9511-1.

Taylor, J., C. Eastwick, C. Lawrence and R. Wilson (2013). 'Noise levels and noise perception from small and micro wind turbines.' *Renewable Energy* 55 doi:10.1016/j.renene.2012.11.031

Taylor, L. (2013). 'Top Abbott business adviser wants renewables target scrapped.' *Guardian*, 13 June. http://bit.ly/2gN5ukg

ten Veen, P. M., M. Morren and C.J. Yzermans (2009). 'The influence of news events on health after disaster: a longitudinal study in general practice.' *Journal of Traumatic Stress* 22(6) doi:10.1002/jts.20462.

Tharpaland International Retreat Centre (2012). 'Three windfarm studies and an assessment of infrasound.' *National Wind Watch*, 24 May. http://bit.ly/2i7GC34

Thorne, R. (2011). 'The problems with "noise numbers" for wind farm noise assessment.' *Bulletin of Science, Technology & Society* 31 doi:10.1177/0270467611412557.

Tobacco Tactics (2013). 'Carl V Phillips.' University of Bath, 26 September. http://www.tobaccotactics.org/index.php/Carl_V_Phillips.

Tobacco Tactics (n.d.). 'Alliance of Australian retailers.' Tobacco Tactics. http://bit.ly/2y7PctJ

Topsfield, J. (2006). 'Minister's backflip on wind farm.' *Age*, 22 December. http://bit.ly/2gFd3FM

Trist, C. (2015). Submission 251 to the Senate Select Committee on Wind Turbines. http://bit.ly/2y8uSIM

Turvey, C. and D. Sparling (2002). 'The great emu bubble: A retrospective look at a new industry failure.' *Current Agriculture, Food & Resource Issues* (3): 49–61.

Tyrer, P., S. Thompson, U. Schmidt, et al. (2003). 'Randomized controlled trial of brief cognitive behaviour therapy versus treatment as usual in recurrent deliberate self-harm: The POPMACT study.' *Psychological Medicine* 33(6): 969–76.

Umwelt, F., and M. Landesanstalt (2016). 'Low-frequency noise incl. infrasound from wind turbines and other sources.' Report presented to Ministry for the Environment, Climate and Energy of the Federal State of Baden-Wuerttemberg. http://bit.ly/2iy3pcn

van der Linden, S.L., A.A. Leiserowitz, G.D. Feinberg and E.W. Maibach (2015). 'The scientific consensus on climate change as a gateway belief: experimental evidence.' *PLoS One* 10(2): e0118489.

van Erk, R. (2011). 'Benefit sharing mechanisms in renewable energy.' Report presented for the European Commission, Brussels. http://bit.ly/2gJrZXm

van Renterghem, T., A. Bockstael, V. De Weirt and D. Botteldooren (2013). 'Annoyance, detection and recognition of wind turbine noise.' *Science of the Total Environment* 456–7 doi:10.1016/j.scitotenv.2013.03.095.

von Gierke, H. (2002). 'Vibroacoustic disease.' *Aviation Space Environmental Medicine* 73: 828.

Vorrath, S. and G. Parkinson. (2017). 'Origin stuns industry with record low price for 530MW wind farm.' *Renew Economy*, 8 May. http://bit.ly/2ptfihC

Walentynowicz, M., K. Bogaerts, I. Van Diest, F. Raes and O. Van den Bergh (2015). '"Was it so bad? The role of retrospective memory in symptom reporting": correction to Walentynowicz et al. (2015).' *Health Psychology* 34(12) doi:10.1037/hea0000266

Walker, C. (2011). 'Yes to renewable energy: disclosure needed on anti-windfarm group's motives.' Yes2Renewables, 12 September. http://bit.ly/2gIkH25

Walker, C. and J. Baxter. (2017). '"It's easy to throw rocks at a corporation": wind energy development and distributive justice in Canada.' *Journal of Environmental Policy & Planning* doi:10.1080/1523908X.2016.1267614

Walker, C., J. Baxter and D. Ouellette (2015). 'Adding insult to injury: the development of psychosocial stress in Ontario wind turbine communities.' *Social Science & Medicine Journal* 133 doi:10.1016/j.socscimed.2014.07.067.

Ware, M. (2015). 'Submission 206: Melissa Ware.' Submitted to the Select Committee on Wind Turbines, Canberra, 25 March. http://bit.ly/2z8QhBq

Warren, C.R., C. Lumsden, S. O'Dowd and R.V. Birnie (2005). 'Green on green: public perceptions of wind power in Scotland and Ireland.' *Journal of Experimental Planning and Management* 48(6) doi:10.1080/09640560500294376.

Watson, D. and J.W. Pennebaker (1989). 'Health complaints, stress, and distress: exploring the central role of negative affectivity.' *Psychological Review* 96(2): 234–54.

Waubra Foundation (2011a). 'Wind turbines and public health'. Video published 8 December. http://bit.ly/2y9FwP8

Waubra Foundation (2011b). 'Explicit cautionary notice to those responsible for wind turbine siting decisions.' Waubra Foundation, 29 June. http://bit.ly/2yRi9as

Wayne, A. and L. Newell (n.d.). 'The hidden hazards of microwave cooking,' Health Science. http://bit.ly/2mnImKl

Wells, R.E. and T.J. Kaptchuk (2012). 'To tell the truth, the whole truth, may do patients harm: the problem of the nocebo effect for informed consent.' *American Journal of Bioethics* 12(3) doi:10.1080/15265161.2011.652798.

Weston, S. (2013). 'Dereel residents outraged over NBN tower.' Dereel, 22 January.

Whisson, M. (2011). 'Wind power and ecology.' Wind Watch, 4 November. http://bit.ly/2zRH8dN

Whiteford, H.A., L. Degenhardt, J. Rehm, A.J. Baxter, A.J. Ferrari, H.E. Erskine, F.J. Charlson, R.E. Norman, A.D. Flaxman, N. Johns, R. Burstein, C.J. Murray and T. Vos (2013). 'Global burden of disease attributable to mental and substance use disorders: findings from the Global Burden of Disease Study 2010.' *Lancet* 382(9904) doi:10.1016/S0140-6736(13)61611-6.

Whitmore, J. (2016). 'Public support for climate action on the up after dark days: Climate Institute survey.' *Conversation,* 26 September. http://bit.ly/2dkHmmR

Whyte, S. 'The rich list absentee landowners behind Tassie anti-windfarm campaign'. *Crikey,* 1 October.

Wilsmore, B.R., R.R. Grunstein, M. Fransen, M. Woodward, R. Norton and S. Ameratunga (2013). 'Sleep habits, insomnia, and daytime sleepiness in a large and healthy community-based sample of New Zealanders.' *Journal of Clinical Sleep Medicine* 9(6) doi:10.5664/jcsm.2750.

Wilson, C. (2013). 'Blowing in the wind.' *ABC News Bush Telegraph,* 7 October. http://ab.co/2cB1rCl

Wilson, G.A. and S.L. Dyke (2009). 'Pre-and post-installation community perception of wind farm projects: the case of Roskrow Barton (Cornwall, UK).' *Land Use Policy* 52 doi:10.1016/j.landusepol.2015.12.008.

Wind Europe (2017). 'Daily wind power numbers – archive.' Wind Europe. http://bit.ly/2mT79ot

Winters, W., S. Devriese, I. Van Diest, B. Nemery, H. Veulemans, P. Eelen, K. Van de Woestijne and O. Van den Bergh (2003). 'Media warnings about environmental pollution facilitate the acquisition of symptoms in response to chemical substances.' *Psychosomatic Medicine* 65(3) doi:10.1097/01.PSY.0000041468.75064.BE

Wittert, G. (2011). 'Analysis of personal journal recordings, as provided by Dr Sarah Laurie, of morning blood pressure in relation to wind turbine output, of three individuals living within 5km of Waubra wind farm.' Evidence submitted to the Environment Resources and Development Court in *Richard Paltridge, Thomas Paltridge and Louise Paltridge vs District Council of Grant vs Acciona Energy Oceania Ptd Ltd.* http://bit.ly/2i5syr7

Witthoft, M. and G.J. Rubin (2013). 'Are media warnings about the adverse health effects of modern life self-fulfilling? An experimental study on idiopathic environmental intolerance attributed to electromagnetic fields (IEI-EMF).' *Journal of Psychosomatic Research* 74(3) doi:10.1016/j.jpsychores.2012.12.002.

Wolff, N., A.S. Darlington, J. Hunfeld, F. Verhulst, V. Jaddoe, A. Hofman, J. Passchier and H. Tiemeier (2010). 'Determinants of somatic complaints in 18-month-old children: the generation R study.' *Journal of Pediatric Psychology* 35(3) doi:10.1093/jpepsy/jsp058.

Wong, M. (2011). 'Coming second: Victoria's first wind farm.' *Waking Up in Geelong*, 24 October. http://bit.ly/2yRvE9Z

Wood, M. L. (2007). 'Rethinking the inoculation analogy: effects on subjects with differing preexisting attitudes.' *Human Communication Research* 33(3) doi:10.1111/j.1468-2958.2007.00303.x.

World Health Organization. (2009). 'WHO Night noise guidelines for Europe.' World Health Organization Europe. http://bit.ly/1tV3wN1

Wynder, E.L. and E.A. Graham (1950). 'Tobacco smoking as a possible etiologic factor in bronchiogenic carcinoma; a study of 684 proved cases.' *Journal of American Medical Association* 143(4): 329–36.

Further reading

In addition to the sources directly cited in the footnotes, this book draws on some of our previous research papers, opinion pieces and other public writing on the subject, including those listed below.

Research papers

Chapman, S. (2014). 'Vibroacoustic disease' is recognised only by the heavily self-citing research group promoting it: a reply to Alves-Pereira and Castelo Branco.' *Australia New Zealand Journal of Public* 38: 192–3 doi:10.1111/1753-6405.12230.

Chapman, S. (2014). 'Major problems with recent systematic review on wind farms and distress.' *Cureus*, 19 June.

Chapman, S. (2014). 'Factoid forensics: have "more than 40" Australian families abandoned their homes because of wind farm noise?' *Noise and Health* 16: 208–12.

Chapman, S. (2012). 'Editorial ignored 17 reviews on wind turbines and health.' *BMJ* 344 doi:10.1136/bmj.e3366.

Chapman, S., K. Joshi and L. Fry (2014). 'Fomenting sickness: nocebo priming of residents about wind farm health harms' *Frontiers in Public Health*, 28 November doi:10.3389/fpubh.2014.00279.

Chapman, S. and A. St George (2013). 'How the factoid of wind turbines causing "vibroacoustic disease" came to be "irrefutably demonstrated".' *Australia New Zealand Journal of Public Health* 33: 244–49.

Chapman, S., A. St George, and K.V. Waller (2013). 'The pattern of complaints about Australian wind farms does not match the establishment and

distribution of turbines: support for the psychogenic, "communicated disease" hypothesis.' *PLoS One* 8(10) doi:10.1371/journal.pone.0076584.
Crichton, F., S. Chapman, T. Cundy and K.J. Petrie (2014). 'The link between health complaints and wind turbines: support for the nocebo expectations hypothesis.' *Frontiers in Public Health*, 11 November:doi:10.3389/fpubh.2014.00220.
Crichton, F., G. Dodd, G. Schmid, G. Gamble and K.J. Petrie (2014). 'Can expectations produce symptoms from infrasound associated with wind turbines? *Health Psychology* 33: 360–4 doi:10.1037/a0031760.
Crichton, F., G. Dodd, G. Schmid and K.J. Petrie (2015). 'Framing sound: using expectations to reduce environmental noise annoyance.' *Environmental Research* 142: 609–14 doi:10.1016/j.envres.2015.08.016.
Crichton, F., G. Dodd, G. Schmid, G. Gamble, T. Cundy and K.J. Petrie (2014). 'The power of positive and negative expectations to influence reported symptoms and mood during exposure to wind farm sound.' *Health Psychology* 33: 1588–92 doi:10.1037/hea0000037.
Crichton, F. and K.J. Petrie (2015). 'Accentuate the positive: counteracting psychogenic responses to media health messages in the age of the internet.' *Journal of Psychosomatic Research* 79:185–9 doi:10.1016/j.jpsychores.2015.04.014.
Crichton F. and K.J. Petrie (2015).'Health complaints and wind turbines: the efficacy of explaining the nocebo response to reduce symptom reporting.' *Environmental Research* 140: 449–55 doi:10.1016/j.envres.2015.04.016.

Opinion pieces and blog posts

Chapman, S. (2017). 'The wind farm complaints stampede that never happened.' *Conversation*, 7 April.
Chapman, S. (2017). 'Wind farms are hardly the bird slayers they're made out to be. Here's why.' *Conversation*, 16 June.
Chapman, S. (2016). 'Alan Jones goes after wind farms again, citing dubious evidence.' *Conversation*, 4 November.
Chapman, S. (2016). 'World's largest wind farm study finds sleep disturbances aren't related to turbine noise.' *Conversation*, 30 May.
Chapman, S. (2015). 'A $2.5m investment in wind farms and health won't solve anything.' *Conversation*, 6 March.
Chapman, S. (2015). 'Infrasound phobia spreads to solar energy cells. What's next?' *Conversation*, 12 August.

Chapman, S. (2015). 'Let's appoint a judge to investigate bizarre wind farm health claims.' *Conversation*, 14 May.

Chapman, S. (2015). 'The Australian's campaign against wind farms continues but the research doesn't stack up.' *Conversation*, 15 July.

Chapman S. (2015). 'Copernicus, tobacco, UFOs: the wild logic of Leyonhjelm's wind inquisition.' *Climate Spectator,* 12 June.

Chapman, S. (2015). 'What's next? A senate inquiry into infrasound from trees, waves or air conditioners?' *Conversation*, 18 November.

Chapman, S. (2015). 'Why a dedicated research fund for wind farms and health?' *Conversation*, 11 February.

Chapman S. (2014). 'Chilean earthquakes in Australia and other wacky myths from wind farm opponents.' *Crikey*, 17 November.

Chapman, S. (2014). 'Abandoning homes due to wind farms: the deep fragrance of factoid.' *Renew Economy*, 25 July.

Chapman, S. (2014). 'New study: wind turbine syndrome is spread by scaremongers.' *Conversation*, 18 March.

Chapman, S. (2014). 'Study finds no evidence wind turbines make you sick – again.' *Conversation*, 25 February.

Chapman, S. (2014). 'Who exactly are these wind farm refugees?'*Drum*, 10 February.

Chapman, S. (2014). 'Wind farm noise complainants and anti-wind groups: how many, how large?' *Renew Economy*, 13 January.

Chapman, S. (2013). 'Questions a prominent wind farm critic needs to answer.' *Climate Spectator*, 8 November.

Chapman, S. (2013). 'Relax – wind farms are not stressing out your emus.' *Drum*, 27 November.

Chapman, S. (2013). 'Wind farm factoids: the VAD non-disease.' *Drum*, 2 June.

Chapman, S. (2013). 'Wind turbine hosts tell a very different story.' *Conversation*, 24 September.

Chapman, S. (2012). 'Fanning fear: the wind farm nocebo effect.' *Drum*, 28 November.

Chapman, S. (2012). 'The sickening truth about wind turbine syndrome.' *New Scientist*, 6 October.

Chapman, S. (2012). 'There's still no evidence that wind farms harm your health.' *Conversation*, 2 November.

Chapman, S. (2012). 'Where are Australia's wind farm refugees?' *Renew Economy*, 3 October.

Chapman, S. (2012). 'Wind turbine syndrome: a classic "communicated" disease.' *Conversation*, 20 July.

Chapman, S. (2012). 'Wind turbine syndrome: mass hysteria in the 21st century?' *Climate Spectator*, 6 June.
Chapman, S. (2012). 'Wind turbines power mass hysteria.' *Drum*, 23 May.
Chapman, S. (2012). 'Wind farms, the Waubra Foundation and a post-office box.' *Crikey*, 2 February.
Chapman, S. (2011). 'Is "wind turbine syndrome" mass hysteria?' *ABC Unleashed*, 2 September.
Chapman S. (2011). 'The quality of medical evidence promoted by the anti-windfarm lobby.' *Crikey*, 16 July.
Chapman, S. (2011). 'Much angst over wind farms is just hot air.' *Sydney Morning Herald*, 21 December.
Chapman, S. (2011). 'The web of vested interests behind the anti-wind farm lobby.' *Crikey*, 13 October.
Chapman, S. (2011). 'Wind turbine sickness prevented by money drug.' *ABC Unleashed*, 29 March.
Chapman, S. (2010). 'Can wind farms make people sick?' *Croakey*, 23 February.
Crichton, F. (2014). 'How the power of suggestion generates wind farm symptoms.' *Conversation*, 15 March.
Crichton, F. (2013). 'A matter of spin.' *Conversation*, 29 November.

Index

abandoned homes 90–99, 119, 182, 190, 210
Abbott, Tony xviii, xxii, 12, 15, 132, 193, 221, 223, 223
Acoustic Research Centre (New Zealand) 160
Adler, Isaac 101
aesthetic objections to windfarms 18, 136, 159, 223
aggregate wind energy 17
AGL (energy company) 63, 83, 113, 212
AHE/IWT (syndrome) 48
aircraft safety 29
Alves-Pereira, Mariana 47, 226
Anderson, Warwick 132
Andjic, Andja Mitric 201
animals 60, 61, 71, 220; *see also* bats, birds, cattle, dogs, livestock, poultry, sheep
anti-vaccination movement 221, 225, 264
anxiety 109, 130, 148, 152, 157, 166, 172
Aramini, Jeffery 106, 230
Arnott, Charlie 187, 193
asbestos industry 99–102
Association for Research of Renewable Energy in Australia Limited (ARREA) 194
Association of Australian Acoustical Consultants 121
Auckland University of Technology 108
Australian and New Zealand Journal of Public Health 47
Australian Charities and Not-for-profits Commission (ACNC) 188
Australian Environment Foundation 10, 168, 208
Australian Greens 188
Australian Landscape Guardians 10, 192
Australian (newspaper) 111, 113, 117, 183, 223, 232–235
Australian Securities and Investment Commission (ASIC) 188
Australian Wind Alliance 100
Australian Wind Energy Forecasting System (AWEFS) 17

Back, Chris 92, 98, 188, 219, 221, 230, 257
backfire effect 264, 267
background noise 50, 52, 56

Bacon, Francis 150
Baillieu, Ted 8, 195
Bald Hills windfarm (Vic.) 28, 194, 198
Ballarat Courier 184, 190, 223
Barnard, Mike 24, 130
Batchelor, Peter 228
bats 25–29
battery storage 18
Beard, George Miller xvii
behavioural problems 128
benefit-sharing 137, 199, 260, 273, 274; *see also* distributive justice
birds 8, 25, 60, 61, 172
blood pressure 135
Blue Creek windfarm (USA) 21
Bluegrass (consulting firm) 194
Blyth, James 1
Boco Rock (NSW) 198
Boorowa District Landscape Guardians 193
Boswell, Ron 221
bovine spongiform encephalopathy (BSE) 38
Bray, Andrew 100
Breamlea windfarm (Vic.) 7
Brush, Charles 2
Bucknell, Douglas 194
Buffett, Warren 13
Bulletin of Science, Technology and Society 108, 125–127
Business Advisory Council 12, 193

Cameron, Doug 91
Campbell, Ian 28
Campbell, Steve 168
Canada 60, 69, 72, 79, 81, 107, 126, 130, 133–137, 140, 146, 203–207, 274
Canavan, Matt 221
Cancer Council Victoria 217
Cape Bridgewater windfarm (Vic.) 94, 117–125, 232, 253
Capital windfarm (NSW) 82
case reports 45, 64, 77–79, 129
Cathedral Rocks windfarm (NSW) 31
cattle 37, 38, 71
Cherry Tree windfarm (Vic.) 168, 181, 237
China xxiv, 5, 12
Clarke, David 21
class divisions 195–197, 272, 273
Clean Energy Council 88, 104
climate change denial 10, 190, 192, 208, 226
climate change xxvii, 4, 182, 192, 267
clinical studies 113, 155, 160–167
Codrington windfarm (Vic.) 70
Collector (NSW) 194–197
Commonwealth Scientific and Industrial Research Organisation (CSIRO) 177, 182
community engagement 261–276
complaint-handling procedures 269
confidentiality clauses 82, 88, 199, 269
confirmation bias 175
conspiracy theories 272
Conversation, The (media outlet) 120, 124, 253
Coonooer Bridge windfarm (Vic.) 177
Cooper, Steven 117–125, 201, 213, 232, 253
Crawford, Michael 187
Crikey (media outlet) xxiii
Croakey (blog) 226
Crookwell and District Landscape Guardians 193
Crookwell (NSW) 198
Crouch, Michael 195
Crystal Brook Energy Park (SA) 198, 202

Dale, Helen 249–252
Davis, June 230
Day, Bob xxii, 22, 132, 221, 230, 257
Daylesford and Districts Landscape Guardians 34, 208
Daylesford (Vic.) 208, 240
Dean, Noel 168, 175, 210–212
decibels 51–57, 270–271
decommissioned wind turbines 19
defamation 246, 253–257
Delingpole, James 96
Democratic Labour Party (Australia) 221
Denmark 5, 76, 114, 130
depression 35, 61
Di Natale, Richard 133, 188
Dingle, Sarah 132
distributive justice 271–276
dogs 60, 71
Doolan, Con 201
drug trials 149
Duchamp, Mark 27, 76
Dunlite Electrical Company 6
Dunn, Lloyd 6
Dyer, Andrew xxii, 180

economic objections to windfarms 11, 14, 23, 199, 212, 272, 273
eco-tourism 274
Edney, Tony 187
electricity, early anxieties about xv
electrosensitivity 58, 116, 151, 155, 277
emus 60
energy crisis (1970s) 5
energy storage 18
English-speaking countries 72–77, 130
Environment, Resources and Development Court of South Australia 204
environmental objections to windfarms 20–23
Environmental Protection Authority (South Australia) 56
Epworth sleepiness scale 112
European Platform Against Windfarms 76, 201, 218
Excessive Noise from Wind Farms Bill 2012 222

factoids 47
Fair Dinkum Radio 223
Fielding, Steve 221
fires 29
First Dog on the Moon (cartoonist) 57
Flyers Creek windfarm 191
fossil fuel industries 16, 185, 192
France xxi, 1, 77
Friends of Collector 191, 193
Fry, Luke 168
functional magnetic resonance imaging (fMRI) 115, 150

Gardner, Andrew 'Gus' 212
Gardner, Ann 212, 214
Gare family 83
Geovital Academy 216
Germany 13, 53, 110, 115–117, 116, 130, 147, 260
GetUp! 222
Global Wind Energy Council 5
goats 60
Godfrey family 93
Goodman, Steve 50
Green, Lilli-Anne 62, 75, 230
Grimwade family 6
Gullifer, Brendan 190, 223

Hannam, Peter 255
Hanning, Christopher 106

Hansen, Colin 201
Harry, Amanda 34–36
Hartwich, Lyn 212
Hartwich, Noel 212
Health Canada 81, 133–137, 160
health complaints about windfarms
  correction of 263–268
  history of 33–65
  psychogenics of 139–177
  scientific reviews of 130–137
Health Protection Agency (UK) 48
hearing loss 35, 43
hearing thresholds 52
Henderson, Gerard 232
Hepburn Community Wind Project 11, 21, 181, 240
hertz 51
Hetherington, Jan 64
Hockey, Joe 13, 221
Hodgson, Tony 187, 193
Hogan, Paul 225
Holcroft, Michael 88
Holmes à Court, Simon 21, 181, 240–244
Howard, John 194
Hulls, Rob 28
human ethics reviews 43, 126, 248
Hungary 116
Huson, Les 201, 214
hydroelectricity 15
hyperbolic language 62

Infigen Energy 84, 168, 174
infrasound 46, 49–57, 119, 265
  clinical studies of 114–117, 161–168, 214
  in nature 165
insomnia *see* sleep disturbance
Institute of Public Affairs 10
International Classification of Diseases 45
Iran 111–113
Iser, David 34, 36, 201

James, Bill 195
James, Rick 107
Japan 113
job creation 7, 199
Jones, Alan 20, 47, 63, 84, 183, 224, 229
Joshi, Ketan 76, 112, 114, 120, 168, 255
Journal of the Acoustical Society of America 134

Keane, Sandi 185, 192
Kelley, Neil 103
Kelly, Craig 221, 242
Kermond, Brian 118
Kermond, Joanne 118
King Island (Tas.) 84, 86, 195
King, Simon 232
Knopper, Loren 140
Korea 133
Krogh, Carmen 48, 125, 230
Kruszelnicki, Karl 101

La Cour, Poul 5
Lake Bonney windfarm 31, 84
Lambie, Jacquie 221
Landscape Guardians Association 184–186, 192
Laurie, Sarah 19, 69, 91, 97, 132, 187, 189, 202–210
legal actions 130, 185, 195, 203, 209, 237, 253–257, 253
Leonards Hill (Vic.) 34, 94, 174, 208, 240
Leventhall, Geoff 114, 141, 226
Lewandowsky, Stephan 263

Leyonhjelm, David xxii, 10, 75, 100–102, 132, 221, 230, 249
Liberal Democratic Party (Australia) 100, 221
Liberal Party of Australia 221
livestock 61, 72
Lloyd, Graham 111, 113, 117, 120, 223, 234, 256
low frequency noise 38, 46, 53, 104, 145, 146, 270

Macarthur windfarm (Vic.) 7, 63, 94, 212
Madigan, John xxii, 84, 92, 98, 117, 132, 168, 221–222, 230, 234, 246, 252, 257
Makara Valley sleep study 108–111
Marsh, Russell 104
Martin, Calvin Luther 37, 44, 190
Martin, Murray 81
Massey University (New Zealand) 218
May, Robert 43
McAlpine, Ken 255
McHarg Ranges 195
McLachlan, Gillon 195
measuring sound 51–57, 270–271
media reporting 117, 120, 141–147, 152, 155, 169–171, 175, 197, 208–209, 223–224
Media Watch (TV program) 120, 232, 253
mental illness 43, 47
micro turbines 81
migraine 35, 43, 135, 172
mining industry 16, 89, 185, 186, 192
Miskelly, Andrew 185
Mitchell, Peter 7, 34, 186, 187, 192, 201, 227
mobile telephones xviii, xxvi, 110, 116, 147, 151, 225, 276
money as an antidote to windfarm complaints 81, 137, 159, 199, 269, 275
Morris, Mary 85, 191
Mortimer, David 84–88, 222
Mortlake (Vic.) 69
Mount Gambier (SA) 84
Mount Lofty Landscape Guardians 195
Mount Pollock windfarm (Vic.) 186, 198
Musk, Elon 18

National Health and Medical Research Council 102, 131, 200, 226, 234
National Party of Australia 221
National Wind Farm Commissioner xxii, 167, 180–182, 257, 262, 268, 276
negative expectations 109–111, 116, 131, 136, 139–177, 261
negative personality types 157–159
Netherlands, the 130, 155
neuroimaging techniques 150
neuroticism 157
New South Wales 7
New Zealand 60, 108–111, 130, 148, 161, 218, 270
New Zealand Skeptics Society 220
Newman, Maurice 12, 193
News Corporation 117
Nicholson, Rikki 118
Nicol, Alexandra 188
Nine Mile Beach windfarm (WA) 7
Nissenbaum, Michael 106
Nixon, Richard 4
nocebo effect 37, 116, 149–152, 156, 163, 167, 219–220, 266
noise complaints 24, 33, 70, 103
noise reduction 271
noise regulations 270

noise sensitivity 165
Noise Watch (website) 191
North Brown Hill windfarm (SA) 83
nuclear energy industry 185

Oaklands Hill windfarm (Vic.) 94
Ollson, Christopher 140
online anti-windfarm communities 42, 47, 144
Ontario Environmental Review Tribunal 203–208
orange-bellied parrot 28
Origin Energy (energy company) 186
outrage factors 140–148

Pacific Hydro (energy company) 117, 120, 253
Pahl, Rodd 193
Pandora's pinwheels (film) 62, 69, 211, 218, 227
Papadopoulos, George 93, 201, 215–218, 230
Pedersen, Eja 230
peer review 43, 75, 124, 125–127, 126, 131, 133
personality types 157
Petrie, Keith 148
Phillips, Carl 107, 127, 230
Phipps, Robyn 230
Pierpont, Nina 37–45, 78, 154, 190
Pittard, Leon 223
placebo effect 116, 149, 156
planning laws 195, 262, 270
Poland 55
Portugal 46
poultry 71
Price, Steve 84
property values 23, 89, 96, 158
psychogenic illnesses 156
psychogenics of windfarm complaints 139–177
public meetings 147, 168, 175, 197, 208, 211, 221, 262
public opinion polls 182
PubMed 125
pumped hydro energy storage (PHES) 18
pyroluria 58

Quadrant 186
Queensland 34, 37, 180

Rapley, Bruce 74, 218, 230
rare earths 22
Rauch, Steven 78
recall bias 153
Renewable Energy Certificate (REC) Registry 15
renewable energy xxi, 4, 13, 182, 192
Renewable Energy Target Scheme 15
research funding 102, 133
research methods 35, 36, 38, 47, 49, 108, 114, 117, 126
Resonate Acoustics 56
Rheese, Max 10, 168
risk communication xxvii
risk perception xxvi, 140–148, 275
Roberts, David 271
Robertstown windfarm (SA) 83
Rogers, Gail 230
Roper, Roly 49
Rovensky, Jackie 246, 257
Russell, Kathy 168, 185, 187

Salmon Beach windfarm (WA) 6
Salt, Alec 105
Sandman, Peter 141
Save the Eagles International 27
Schmidt, Norma 230

Schneider, Patina 191
Schultz, Alby 187, 221, 234
self-citation 46
Senate inquiries into windfarms (Australia) xxii, 73
of 2012 91, 211
of 2015 82, 105, 119, 121–123, 132, 137, 180, 203, 214, 218, 228, 252
Sexton, Roger 21
Seymour (Vic.) 168
sheep xxv, 60, 71, 212
Shepherd, Daniel 108–111
Simon, Linda xv
sleep disturbance 35, 36, 47, 61, 106–113, 135, 152, 172
Sleep (journal) 135
Snowy Hydro scheme 18
social media 30, 144, 249–252, 254–256
social scientists xxxi–xxxi, 228
social transmission of symptoms 154–159
Society for Wind Vigilance 105, 107, 108, 125, 128
socio-economics of windfarm opposition 195–197
solar energy 4, 15, 16, 272
Solar Energy Resarch Institute (USA) 4, 103
South Australia 56, 132, 205, 209
Southey, Lady Marigold 195
Spain xxiii, 26, 73
Spectator, The (magazine) 193
Spring, Wayne 201
Starfish Hill windfarm (SA) 31
Stockyard Hill windfarm (Vic.) 7, 186, 193, 198
Stop These Things (website) 23, 71, 84, 92, 183, 190–191, 221, 239
stress 135
subject selection bias 39
subsidies 14–17
susceptibility to health complaints 70–79
Swinbanks, Malcolm 68
Sydney Morning Herald 185
symptoms attributed to windfarms 57, 152–159

Tadgell, Robert 188
Taiwan 60
Taralga Landscape Guardians 185
Tarwin Valley Coastal Guardians 28
Tasmania 71, 84, 180, 195
Taylor, Angus 221, 222
Taylor, Scott 201
Tehran University 112
Ten Mile Lagoon windfarm (WA) 70
thalidomide 99
Tharpaland International Retreat Centre 58
Thomas, Donald 168, 227
Thorne, Bob 201
tinnitus 35, 43, 135, 152, 172
tobacco industry 99, 225
Today Tonight (television program) 125
Tooborac (Vic.) 195
Toora (Vic.) 34, 36, 93, 97
transmission lines 17
Trawool Valley Landscape Guardians 168
Trawool (Vic.) 168
Trist, Sonia 118
Turnbull, Malcolm 18

unemployment 96, 272, 273
United Kingdom 34, 35, 130, 182, 273
United States of America 4, 5, 13, 104, 130
New York 38
North Carolina 272

Wisconsin 38
Ohio 2, 21
University of Auckland 160, 235
University of Sydney 57, 228, 233, 238, 247–249
Urquhart, Anne xxii, 75, 121, 137, 194

vibroacoustic disease 45, 59
Vic Wind 176
victim testimonies 175
Victoria 7, 10, 28, 130, 168, 180
Victorian Civil and Administrative Tribunal (VCAT) 168, 176, 181
visceral vibratory vestibular disturbance 45

Warburton, Dick 12
Ware, Melissa 118
Waterloo Concerned Citizens Group 191
Waterloo windfarm (SA) 29, 94, 95, 191
Watts, Alan 201
Watts, Colleen 201
Waubra 95
Waubra Foundation xxiv, 24, 34, 36, 69, 168, 172, 174, 186–190, 190, 194, 202
Waubra (Vic.) xxiii, 93, 188, 210, 227
Wessely, Simon 220
Western Australia 71, 180, 223
Western Plains Landscape Guardians 147, 186
Wheatley, Libby 230
Whitehead's Creek (Vic.) 168
wi-fi 58, 116, 155, 225, 277
Winchelsea (Vic.) 198
wind energy, history of 1–6
wind turbine syndrome, origins of 37–43
wind turbines, manufacture of 21
windfarm developers 197, 260, 261, 268–269, 271
windfarm employees 82, 111–113, 208, 228
windfarm hosts 197–201, 268, 274
windfarm 'refugees' 90–99
Windy Hill (Qld) 34, 37
Wittert, Gary 204
Woakine windfarm (SA) 84
Wonthaggi (Vic.) 37
Wooldridge, Michael 28, 187, 194
World Health Organization 101, 270

Xenophon, Nick xxii, 84, 92, 99, 132, 221, 222, 230, 254

Yass (NSW) 111, 215

www.ingramcontent.com/pod-product-compliance
Lightning Source LLC
Chambersburg PA
CBHW050331270326
41926CB00016B/3413
* 9 7 8 1 7 4 3 3 2 4 9 6 7 *